Multiple Sclerosis

Recovery of Function and Neurorehabilitation

Multiple Sclerosis

Recovery of Function and Neurorehabilitation

Edited by

Jürg Kesselring
Department of Neurology and Neurorehabilitation, Rehabilitation Centre, Valens, Switzerland

Giancarlo Comi
Institute of Experimental Neurology and Department of Neurology, University Vita-Salute and Scientific Institute S. Raffaele, Milan, Italy

Alan J. Thompson
University College London, Institute of Neurology, London, UK

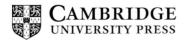

CAMBRIDGE UNIVERSITY PRESS
Cambridge, New York, Melbourne, Madrid, Cape Town, Singapore,
São Paulo, Delhi, Dubai, Tokyo, Mexico City

Cambridge University Press
The Edinburgh Building, Cambridge CB2 8RU, UK

Published in the United States of America by
Cambridge University Press, New York

www.cambridge.org
Information on this title: www.cambridge.org/9780521888325

© Cambridge University Press 2010

First published 2010

Printed in the United Kingdom at the University Press, Cambridge

A catalogue record for this publication is available from the British Library

Library of Congress Cataloging-in-Publication Data

Multiple sclerosis : recovery of function and neurorehabilitation / editors,
Jürg Kesselring, Giancarlo Comi, Alan J. Thompson.
    p. ; cm.
  Includes bibliographical references and index.
  ISBN 978-0-521-88832-5 (Hardback)
  1. Multiple sclerosis.   2. Multiple sclerosis–Patients–Rehabilitation.
I. Kesselring, Jürg.   II. Comi, G. (Giancarlo), 1947–   III. Thompson,
Alan J., M. D.   IV. Title.
  [DNLM: 1. Multiple Sclerosis.   2. Multiple Sclerosis–rehabilitation.
WL 360 M9577 2010]
  RC377.M8635 2010
  616.8′34–dc22

                                                                    2010022872

ISBN 978-0-521-88832-5 Hardback

Contents

Contributors

Federica Agosta, MD
Neuroimaging Research Unit,
Institute of Experimental Neurology,
Division of Neuroscience,
Scientific Institute and University Ospedale San
Raffaele,
Milan, Italy

Lakshmi Bangalore, PhD
Department of Neurology and Center for Neuroscience
and Regeneration Research,
Yale University School of Medicine,
New Haven, CT, USA;
Rehabilitation Research Center,
VA Connecticut Healthcare System,
West Haven, CT, USA

Anne Baron-Van Evercooren, PhD
Université Pierre et Marie Curie,
Centre de Recherche de l'Institut du
Cerveau et de la Moelle Epinière;
Institut de la Santé et de la Recherche Médicale;
Cnrs, UMR 7225;
Assistance Publique – Hopitaux de Paris,
Fédération de Neurologie, Paris, France

Serafin Beer, MD
Department of Neurology and Neurorehabilitation,
Rehabilitation Center,
Valens, Switzerland

Marcello Belfiore, MD
Universitá Vita Salute San Raffaele and Istituto
Scientifico San Raffaele, Milan, Italy

Joel A. Black, PhD
Department of Neurology and Center for
Neuroscience and Regeneration Research,
Yale University School of Medicine,
New Haven, CT, USA;
Rehabilitation Research Center,

VA Connecticut Healthcare System,
West Haven, CT, USA

Stefan J. Cano, PhD
Department of Clinical Neuroscience,
Peninsula College of Medicine and Dentistry,
Plymouth, UK

Michael D. Carrithers, MD PhD
Department of Neurology,
University of Wisconsin–Madison,
Madison, WI, USA

Giancarlo Comi, MD
Institute of Experimental Neurology
and Department of Neurology,
University Vita-Salute and Scientific Institute
S. Raffaele,
Milan, Italy

Anthony Feinstein, MPhil PhD FRCPC
Sunnybrook Health Sciences Centre,
Division of Neuropsychiatry,
University of Toronto, Toronto, Ontario, Canada

Mattia Ferro, MD
Universitá Vita Salute San Raffaele and Istituto
Scientifico San Raffaele,
Milan, Italy

Massimo Filippi, MD
Neuroimaging Research Unit, Institute of
Experimental Neurology,
Department of Neuroscience,
Scientific Institute and University Ospedale
San Raffaele, Milan, Italy

Clare J. Fowler, FRCP
Institute of Neurology University College London,
and Department of Uro-Neurology,

National Hospital for Neurology and Neurosurgery,
London, UK

Robin J.M. Franklin, BVetMed BSc PhD MRCVS FRCPath
MRC Centre for Stem Cell Biology and Regenerative Medicine and Department of Veterinary Medicine,
University of Cambridge,
Cambridge, UK

Roberto Furlan, MD PhD
Neuroimmunology Unit and Institute of Experimental Neurology (InSpe),
DIBIT–San Raffaele Scientific Institute,
Milan, Italy

Omar Ghaffar, MSc FRCPC
Division of Neuropsychiatry,
Sunnybrook Health Sciences Centre,
University of Toronto,
Toronto, Ontario, Canada

Angelo Ghezzi, MD
Centro Studi Sclerosi Multipla,
Ospedale di Gallarate,
Gallarate, Italy

Christian W. Hess, MD
Neurologische Universitätsklinik und Poliklinik,
Bern, Switzerland

Jürg Kesselring, MD
Department of Neurology and Neurorehabilitation,
Rehabilitation Centre,
Valeus, Switzerland

Gustav Kiss, MD
Head, Neuro-Urology Unit,
Department of Neurology,
University Hospital Innsbruck,
Austria

Clare Laing, BSc
Horizons Rehabilitation Centre,
Aberdeen, UK

Dawn W. Langdon, MD PhD CPsychol
Department of Psychology,
Royal Holloway University of London,
Egham, UK

Letizia Leocani, MD PhD
Department of Clinical Neurophysiology,
Universitá Vita Salute San Raffaele and Istituto Scientifico San Raffaele,
Milan, Italy

Per Olov Lundberg, MD PhD
Department of Neuroscience and Neurology,
University Hospital, Uppsala, Sweden

Susan L. McGowan, BSc MSc
Therapy and Rehabilitation Services,
National Hospital for Neurology and Neurosurgery,
London, UK

Antonio Malgaroli, MD
Universitá Vita Salute San Raffaele and Istituto Scientifico San Raffaele,
Milan, Italy

Gianvito Martino, MD
Neuroimmunology Unit and Institute
of Experimental Neurology (InSpe),
DIBIT–San Raffaele Scientific Institute,
Milan, Italy

Luca Muzio, PhD
Neuroimmunology Unit and Institute
of Experimental Neurology (InSpe),
DIBIT–San Raffaele Scientific Institute,
Milan, Italy

Emanuela Onesti, MD
Department of Neurological Sciences, Sapienza University of Rome,
Rome, Italy

Patrizia Pantano, MD
Section of Neuroradiology,
Department of Neurological Sciences,
Sapienza University of Rome,
Rome, Italy

Stefano Pluchino, MD PhD
Neuroimmunology Unit and Institute of Experimental Neurology (InSpe),
DIBIT–San Raffaele Scientific Institute,
Milan, Italy

Carlo Pozzilli, MD PhD
Department of Neurological Sciences,
University "La Sapienza,"
Rome, Italy

Annalisa Pulizzi, MD
Department of Neurology,
Scientific Institute and University Ospedale
San Raffaele, Milan, Italy

Eytan Raz, MD
Section of Neuroradiology,
Department of Neurological Sciences,
University "La Sapienza,"
Rome, Italy

Maddalena Ripamonti, MD
Universitá Vita Salute San Raffaele and Istituto
Scientifico San Raffaele, Milan, Italy

Julia M. Rist, PhD
MRC Centre for Stem Cell Biology and Regenerative
Medicine and Department of Veterinary Medicine,
University of Cambridge,
Cambridge, UK

Annalisa Rizzo, MD
Centro Studi Sclerosi Multipla,
Ospedale S. Antonio Abate,
Gallarate, Italy

Maria A. Rocca, MD
Neuroimaging Research Unit,
Institute of Experimental Neurology,
Division of Neuroscience,
Scientific Institute and University Ospedale
San Raffaele, Milan, Italy

Lucy Rodriguez, MA
Therapy and Rehabilitation Services,
National Hospital for Neurology and Neurosurgery,
London, UK

Kai M. Rösler, MD
Neurologische,
Bern Universitätsklinik und Poliklinik,
Switzerland

Marco Rovaris, MD
Multiple Sclerosis Center,
Scientific Institute Santa Maria Nascente – Fondazione
Don Gnocchi, and Neuroimaging Research Unit,
San Raffaele Scientific Institute and University,
Milan, Italy

Martin E. Schwab, PhD
Brain Research Institute,
University of Zurich,
Zurich, Switzerland

Alessandra Solari, MD
Unit of Neuroepidemiology,
Foundation IRCCS Neurological Institute C. Besta,
Milan, Italy

Luigi Tesio, MD
Department of Physical Medicine and Rehabilitation,
Università degli Studi and Clinical Unit and
Laboratory of Research of Neuromotor
Rehabilitation,
Istituto Auxologico Italiano,
Ospedale San Luca–IRCCS,
Milan, Italy

Alan J. Thompson, MD FRCP FRCPI
Institute of Neurology,
University College London,
London, UK

Stephen G. Waxman, MD PhD
Department of Neurology and Center for
Neuroscience and Regeneration Research,
Yale University School of Medicine,
New Haven, CT, USA;
Rehabilitation Research Center,
VA Connecticut Healthcare System,
West Haven, CT, USA

Mauro Zaffaroni, MD
Centro Studi Sclerosi Multipla,
Ospedale S. Antonio Abate,
Gallarate, Italy

Vincenzo Zimarino, MD
Universitá Vita Salute San Raffaele and Istituto
Scientifico San Raffaele,
Milan, Italy

Björn Zörner, MD
Brain Research Institute,
University of Zurich,
Zurich, Switzerland

Violetta Zujovic, MD
Université Pierre et Marie Curie,
Centre de Recherche de l'Institut du
Cerveau et de la Moelle Epinière;
Institut de la Santé de la Recherche Médicale;
Cnrs, UMR 7225;
Assistance Publique – Hopitaux de Paris,
Fédération de Neurologie,
Paris, France

Preface

For a long time neurology was considered to be a specialty with refined diagnostic possibilities but little to offer in terms of therapeutics. Therapeutic nihilism prevailed for decades. Neurological syndromes were mainly described as defects with an *alpha privativum*: A-phasia, A-lexia, A-calculia, A-taxia, even A-bulia, etc. The earlier nomenclature of the World Health Organization when classifying health conditions and diseases used terms with negative connotations: dis-ability, handicap. The new framework for classifying health conditions (such as multiple sclerosis), the International Classification of Functioning (ICF), brought a change in names and thereby in attitudes [1, 2]. This truly marks a paradigm shift and the current book attempts to describe these changes. The consequences of a disease process are further described at the level of body structures and functions as "impairment" but the focus is now on "activities" (which of course may be limited due to the disease) instead of dis-ability and on the social level the focus is more on "participation" (and its limitations) rather than on handicap. When dealing with treatment options and prognosis for an individual patient it is obvious that personal factors from his\her history and environmental factors must be considered and these factors are now fully incorporated into the classification.

Neuroplasticity in the central nervous system is the basis of adaptive changes which occur spontaneously and which may be modulated by appropriate therapies. They form the structural and functional correlates of learning. These mechanisms, as they relate to multiple sclerosis, are covered in some detal in the present book. They may be described on different levels: at the cellular level unmasking of pre-existing connections (axonal sprouting, i.e., increased arborization of neurons, changes of synaptic stability, and reorganization of synapses); at the tissue level (resorption of edema, rearrangement of sodium channels on axons,

and remyelination); at a system level as ipsilateral and contralateral excitability changes in the primary and secondary motor areas; and on a behavioral level by inducing and training novel motor and cognitive strategies. Understanding the very complex reorganization of central nervous pathways following acute lesions and chronic secondary axonal degeneration in MS is fundamental to the effective planning of rehabilitation strategies in individual patients.

These topics are covered in chapters written by leading experts in their respective fields. The editors are very grateful for their generous contributions. We are particularly grateful to Nicholas Dunton and his collaborators at Cambridge University Press who have led us through a sometimes difficult preparatory process with patience and efficiency leading to the production and distribution of our book which we consider a timely contribution to a broad and exciting new field in neurology. We hope that this book will be of interest to basic scientists studying neuroplasticity of the central nervous system as related to inflammation, demyelination, and axonal damage as well being useful to clinicians and therapists dealing with persons with multiple sclerosis and the manifold consequences of this enigmatic disease.

Jürg Kesselring
Giancarlo Comi
Alan J. Thompson

References

1. Kesselring J, Coenen M, Cieza A, Thompson A, Kostanjsek N, Stucki G. Developing the ICF core sets for multiple sclerosis to specify functioning. *Mult Scler* 2008;**14**:252–4

2. Holper L, Coenen M, Weise A, Stucki G, Cieza A, Kesselring J. Characterizing functioning in MS using the ICF. *J Neurol* 2010;**257**:103–13

Basic mechanisms

Conduction studies in multiple sclerosis

Kai M. Rösler and Christian W. Hess

Evoked potentials in the diagnosis of multiple sclerosis

The diagnosis of multiple sclerosis (MS) is based on the detection of multiple inflammatory demyelinating white matter lesions, which are disseminated in space and time. Traditionally, evoked potential (EP) studies have been employed to reveal dissemination of lesions in equivocal clinical situations. This is achieved by demonstration of clinically silent lesions. In the 1980s–1990s, a wealth of studies described the technical aspects of evoked potentials and their application in MS. Many of these studies were aimed at optimizing the yield of the EP studies, by refinement of the technical parameters or by increasing the number of stimulation modalities. These efforts resulted in sensitivities (i.e., frequencies of abnormal results) as high as 80% in some studies [1–4]. It is noteworthy that specificities (i.e., how many abnormal results are found in patients not suffering from MS) were rarely specified. Moreover, high sensitivity of a test in MS does not equal high diagnostic yield. For instance, a test that tends to confirm clinically detectable signs is not very likely to improve the diagnostic certainty in a patient, even though it might be very sensitive in terms of yielding a high proportion of abnormal results. An analysis of the diagnostic yield was done by Beer and co-workers [4], by calculating the number of patients with suspected MS who could be reclassified after the clinical examination according to the Poser Committee Criteria [5]. In their study, MRI and analysis of cerebrospinal fluid for oligoclonal banding largely outperformed EP studies (Fig. 1.1).

The introduction of magnetic resonance imaging (MRI) had a dramatic impact on the use of conduction studies in the diagnostic work-up of MS patients. Lesions and their spatial distribution in the central nervous system (CNS) can directly be demonstrated using MRI. Dissemination of lesions in time is easily assessed using serial MRIs or by demonstration of different acuity by uptake of contrast agents in a single MRI. Moreover, MRI has the advantage of being fast and painless, while EP studies are often considered cumbersome for the examiner and painful by the patient. Thus, conduction studies are not considered in the actual diagnostic criteria for MS [6], with the exception of visually evoked potentials (VEPs) in some situations with primary progressive MS, as they demonstrate subclinical lesions relatively often [4].

Despite their diminished importance in the diagnostic work-up of patients, evoked potentials may serve as **surrogate markers for the progression of the disease**, and may be of interest for the prognosis of patients. In these areas, MRI parameters have been found to be remarkably weak. The MR lesion load may not correlate with the clinical deficit of the patient [7, 8]. Furthermore, the number of gadolinium-enhancing lesions in the baseline MR scan was not found to be a strong predictive parameter for the relapse rate in the first year after diagnosis, and monthly MR scans over 6 months were not predictive of the change in the expanded disability status scale (EDSS) in the subsequent 12 and 24 months [9]. In contrast, a number of evoked potential studies demonstrated a correlation between clinical deficit and EP findings [10–12]. Evoked potentials were found useful to monitor the effect of steroid treatment of acute bouts of MS [13]. Direct comparisons between MRI parameters and EP results suggested a better relation between EP and clinical status (EDSS) than between

Multiple Sclerosis: Recovery of Function and Neurorehabilitation, eds. J. Kesselring, G. Comi, and A. J. Thompson.
Published by Cambridge University Press. © Cambridge University Press 2010.

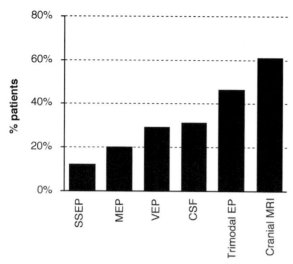

Fig. 1.1. Reclassification sensitivity (i.e., the percentage of reclassified patients according to Poser criteria) of evoked potentials studies, cerebrospinal fluid (CSF) analysis, and magnetic resonance imaging. SSEP, somatosensory evoked potentials; MEP, motor evoked potentials; VEP, visually evoked potentials. Data extracted from Beer *et al*. [4].

MRI and EDSS [10, 11]. Evoked potentials may thus serve to follow the disease during therapeutic interventions [11–13]. They may also serve as prognostic parameters: Fuhr and co-workers reported that the combined result of MEP and VEP at onset would predict the EDSS after 2 years [12].

Pathophysiology of central conduction in multiple sclerosis

Traditionally, evoked potentials have rarely been interpreted in view of the pathophysiological significance of their abnormality. Theoretically, conduction along central pathways can be altered in various ways. Acute demyelination may induce conduction block, i.e., action potentials do not propagate across the lesion. The conduction velocity across the lesion may be reduced due to myelin abnormalities. Clinically, conduction block will cause a neurological deficit (i.e., a paresis or a sensory deficit), while conduction slowing will not necessarily cause deficits and may therefore point towards a clinically silent lesion [12, 14–16]. Not only demyelination but also remyelination of a previously demyelinated axon may cause reduction of the propagation velocity. In MS, axonal damage may occur along with demyelination. While axonal death will not change conduction velocity, it will reduce the number of conducting axons, causing central conduction

failure and inducing clinical deficits. The situation may be complicated by alternative routes of transmission within the CNS, which are used to compensate for interrupted routes. Furthermore, in motor evoked potentials, a loss of central motor neurons will decrease the number of axons converging on the anterior horn cell, increasing the need for temporal summation of incoming excitatory postsynaptic potentials, resulting in an increased central conduction time [14].

Evoked potentials are most often used to measure **central conduction time**. In MS prolonged central conduction times are usually interpreted as markers of demyelination. However, this simple notion is probably not entirely true. In a retrospective study, Humm and co-workers analyzed the central motor conduction time (CMCT) in a large sample of MS patients and observed that the CMCT was mainly increased in patients with progressive forms of MS while it was normal or only slightly prolonged in patients with acute relapsing–remitting forms of MS [16]. Interestingly, this prolongation was not related to the clinical motor deficit or to the electrophysiologically measured central conduction failure, and it was not related to the duration of the disease. Hence while a patient with a relapsing–remitting form of MS would have a normal central motor conduction time, a patient with a primary (or secondary) progressive form of MS with the same disease duration would have a greatly prolonged CMCT. The finding of particularly long CMCTs in patients with progressive forms of MS was also made in a subsequent, prospective study [17]. CMCT was also found to be particularly prolonged in MS patients with marked temperature vulnerability (Uhthoff phenomenon), while it was normal in patients without temperature vulnerability [18]. Thus it appeared that a prolonged CMCT increased the likelihood of a patient to develop a transient conduction block during warming [16]. A similar observation was made using VEPs: in a study of exercise induced changes in 15 MS patients, Persson and Sachs observed an association between the degree of induced changes of visual acuity and the extent of VEP latency prolongation [19]. These observations may suggest that prolongations of CMCT are indicative for a myelin disturbance which may be typical for chronic MS, and which makes conduction vulnerable to temperature changes. Humm and co-workers speculated that these prolongations could relate to incomplete remyelination rather than to acute demyelination [16].

Assessment of central conduction failures

Theoretically, amplitudes of evoked potentials are markers of the amount of conducting fibers. Reduced amplitudes would thus indicate loss of conduction by axonal death or central conduction block within the pathway that is studied. Unfortunately, amplitudes of somatosensory evoked potentials and motor evoked potentials vary considerably between normal subjects, and therefore normal limits are broad [20, 21]. This impedes interpretation of amplitudes of evoked potential to such an extent that the only robust amplitude criterion is "lack of response." It is thus impossible with most EP protocols to demonstrate partial central conduction blocks or gradual loss of conducting axons over time. In the recent years we have developed a method to quantify central motor conduction, allowing for a meaningful interpretation of potential amplitudes. In the following, we will describe this triple stimulation technique (TST) and some of the results obtained with it.

Central motor conduction in multiple sclerosis: the triple stimulation technique

Motor evoked potentials (MEPs) are elicited by transcranial magnetic stimulation (TMS), which is a non-invasive, painless method to stimulate the human brain. Serious adverse effects were not described with single pulses. The technical implications and the basic methodology have been covered broadly and are not repeated here [22, 23]. Theoretically, the size of an MEP should reflect the number of conducting central motor neurons, but this relation is obscured, mainly by two factors. First, in healthy subjects as well as in patients, MEPs are smaller than compound muscle action potentials (CMAPs) evoked by peripheral nerve stimulation, and their size varies from one stimulus to the next and between subjects [14, 21, 24–7]. These MEP characteristics are caused by varying synchronization of the descending action potentials in response to TMS. The resulting phase cancellation phenomenon impedes direct conclusions on the number of activated motor neurons [21]. Size parameters of MEPs are thus insensitive for the detection of small to moderate central conduction failures, which may cause clinically significant deficits [2, 14, 28, 29].

To eliminate the problem of discharge desynchronization, Magistris and co-workers developed a triple stimulation technique (TST) [21]. This collision technique suppresses the effects of central action potential desynchronization, which occurs in MEPs of healthy subjects and patients. As a consequence, the TST provides a quantitative measure of the percentage of spinal motor neurons that can be brought to discharge by TMS. In healthy subjects, this percentage is always near 100%. In patients with central motor disorders, this percentage is often smaller, as a result of the corticospinal conduction failure. The term "conduction failure" is used here to describe the situation in which the brain stimulus does not lead to excitation of all motor units of the target muscle, reducing the TST amplitude ratio below normal limits. It can be due to loss of corticospinal neurons, to central axonal lesions, to conduction block, or to reduced excitability of the motor cortex to TMS.

The technical principle of TST has already been described in detail [21, 30]. It consists of a transcranial magnetic stimulus followed by two maximal electrical stimuli, one to the ulnar nerve at the wrist, and one to the brachial plexus at Erb's point, with appropriate delays. The TST test curve (TST_{test} = stimuli: brain–wrist–Erb) is compared to a TST control curve ($TST_{control}$ = stimuli: Erb–wrist–Erb). The ratio $TST_{test} : TST_{control}$ (termed "TST amplitude ratio") reflects the percentage of activated spinal motor neurons. An overview of the technique is given in Fig. 1.2. Since the original description of the technique, an adaptation has been worked out for use on the lower extremities [31]. Here, recordings are done from abductor hallucis, the distal stimulus is given to the tibial nerve at the ankle, and a proximal stimulus is given through a monopolar needle electrode placed close to the sciatic nerve [31]. Normal values and sensitivities are similar for the TST of upper and lower limbs.

Central conduction failure in multiple sclerosis

In a large collective of MS patients, Magistris *et al.* found reduced TST amplitude ratios in 106 of 221 arms, indicating central conduction failure in 48%. In the same sample of patients, prolonged central motor conduction times were only found in 48 of 221 arms (= 22%). There was a significant quantitative relationship between the TST amplitude ratio and the force

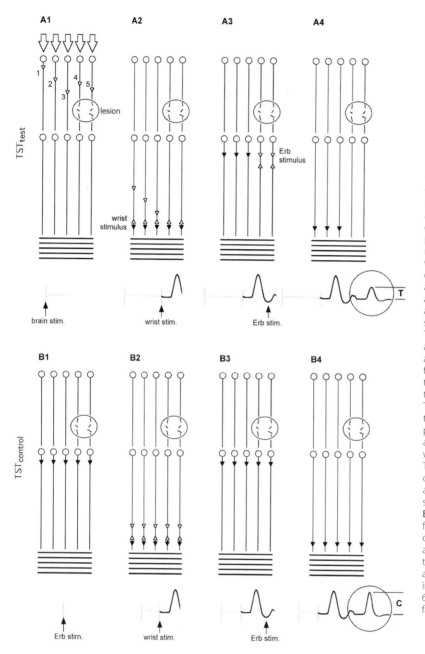

Fig. 1.2. Triple stimulation technique (TST) principle. In this scheme the motor tract is simplified to five corticospinal axons with monosynaptic connections to five peripheral axons (a simplification which does not account for complexity of corticospinal connections); horizontal lines represent the muscle fibers of the five motor units. Black arrows depict action potentials that cause a trace deflection, open arrows those that do not. Below, the trace recordings are given at each time point. **A1**: A maximal transcranial stimulation excites 100% of the axons. Action potentials (APs) are not synchronized. Conduction fails on axons 4 and 5 because of a lesion. **A2**: The APs descending on axons 1–3 excite the peripheral axons 1–3. After a delay, a maximal stimulation performed at the wrist is recorded as the first negative deflection of TST test trace. On axons 1–3, a collision occurs. On axons 4 and 5, the antidromic APs from the wrist stimulus ascend. **A3**: After a delay a maximal stimulation is performed at Erb's point. The descending APs collide on axons 4 and 5, while they continue to descend on axons 1–3. **A4**: A synchronized response from the three axons excited initially by the transcranial stimulation is recorded as the second deflection of TST test trace; T is the amplitude measured in the TST_{test} trace. **B1**: A maximal stimulation is performed at Erb's point. **B2**: After a delay a maximal stimulation performed at the wrist is recorded as the first deflection of TST control trace; antidromic APs ascend on all five axons, and collisions occur on all five axons. **B3**: After a delay a maximal stimulation is performed at Erb's point; **B4**: A synchronized response from the five axons is recorded as the second deflection of TST control trace; C is the amplitude measured in this $TST_{control}$ trace. The ratio of T:C is the TST amplitude ratio; here it is 3:5 = 60%, indicating intact central conduction on 60% of the axons, and central conduction failure on 40% of the axons.

(measured clinically using a four-step scale), and a reduction of the TST amplitude ratio was always associated with a reduction of muscle force. This suggests that muscle weakness was related to the proportion of central motor neurons that could not be activated by the transcranial stimulus as assessed by the TST [30]. Magistris and co-workers concluded that the TST was a highly sensitive method measuring

a clinically relevant conduction parameter, linked to the clinical deficit. A relation between force, signs of pyramidal dysfunction, and TST amplitude ratio was also found in a study recording from a leg muscle (Fig. 1.3) [31], confirming that the TST measures a clinically relevant parameter. Subsequently, a prospective study was conducted to monitor treatment with methylprednisolone during acute exacerbations

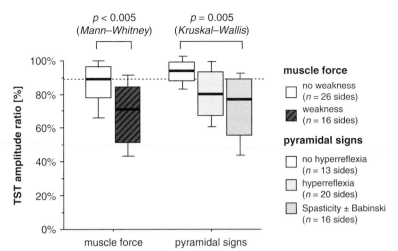

Fig. 1.3. Relation between muscle force and pyramidal signs and the TST results in 49 legs of 43 patients with MS, cervical myelopathy, or amyotropic lateral sclerosis (ALS). Muscle weakness is related to decreased TST amplitude ratio (left; ALS patients excluded because of the possibility of weakness due to lower motor neuron lesion). Presence of hyperreflexia and spasticity is associated with decreased TST amplitude ratio (right). Data extracted from Bühler *et al.* [31].

in MS [17]. The study demonstrated marked reductions of the TST amplitude ratio in MS at baseline. After 5 days of treatment with methylprednisolone, the TST amplitude increased significantly in patients with relapsing–remitting MS and secondary chronic MS, paralleled by an increase of muscle force. Methylprednisolone treatment did not improve muscle force and TST amplitude ratio in patients with primary chronic forms of MS. There was no change in CMCT with treatment in any of the three MS patient groups [17]. The increase of TST amplitude ratio during methylprednisolone treatment is most likely explained by the reduction of a central motor conduction block. As mentioned above, conduction block is an important cause of conduction failure and clinical deficit in acute demyelination [15, 32]. It can result from segmental demyelination (which would not immediately respond to steroid treatment), but may also be the consequence of edema and of inflammatory cytokines [15, 33]. Methylprednisolone has marked anti-edematous and anti-inflammatory as well as membrane stabilizing properties [34]. The lack of electroclinical improvement in patients with primary progressive MS can be attributed to the more substantial axonal loss in this patient group. Summarized, the TST allowed quantifying the functional improvement induced by treatment in this group of MS patients. It is noteworthy that a number of earlier studies concentrated mainly on measuring the CMCT, given the lack of reliable MEP amplitude measurements. Several authors have reported CMCT reductions after intravenous methylprednisolone treatment [35–37]. While these studies generally found an association between overall disease

severity and CMCT, a relationship between the improvement of the clinical motor deficit of the studied limb and of the corresponding CMCT could not be demonstrated in any of these studies.

Uhthoff phenomenon is a characteristic symptom of MS patients. It describes a worsening of deficits (or development of new deficits) after increasing the body temperature, or an amelioration of deficits by cooling. Computer model calculations [38] and animal preparations [39] suggest that the main neurophysiological mechanism underlying Uhthoff's phenomenon is a temperature-dependent central conduction block of partially demyelinated axons. Humm and co-workers immersed 20 MS patient in cold or warm water and assessed the clinical and electrophysiological consequences of this temperature manipulation [18]. They observed significant changes in TST amplitude ratio in some (but not all) patients. These changes significantly correlated with the change in walking velocity. Hence, the TST measured the conduction failure (and changes of the conduction failure) responsible for the clinical deficit of the patient. The rapid amelioration after cooling (and the rapid worsening after warming) are well compatible with transient changes of central conduction blocks, which could be quantified by using the TST. Interestingly, temperature vulnerability (as seen clinically, electrophysiologically, and in a self-assessment of the patients) was significantly more marked in patients with a prolonged CMCT [18]. These observations may suggest that prolongations of CMCT are indicative for the type of myelin disturbance that makes conduction vulnerable to temperature changes. It could be speculated that these prolongations often relate to incomplete remyelination rather than to acute demyelination. While acute demyelinization leads to conduction block, incomplete remyelination is characterized by slow and unsafe conduction, which may be more vulnerable to pertubations [15, 39].

Conclusions

Today, EP studies are largely replaced by MR imaging for the diagnostic work-up of patients with suspected MS. Magnetic resonance imaging provides an easier and more comprehensive way of assessing dissemination of lesions in space and time. EP studies may, however, be of value to follow the development of disease, since EP measurements relate better to the clinical status of the patient than imaging studies. It is of interest to analyze the pathophysiological basis of abnormal EP results. In MS, prolonged conduction times are particularly characteristic of chronic progressive forms, and prolonged conduction times are associated with increased temperature vulnerability of a patient. Both observations point to a specific type of myelin damage, possibly related to remyelination with instable and unsafe conduction. Improving the method of transcranial magnetic stimulation by the triple stimulation technique improves the detection and quantification of central conduction failures, pointing to central conduction block or loss of central neurons. The time course of conduction failure in MS patients, e.g., during methylprednisolone treatment or temperature exposure, may hint at transient central conduction block, while stable deficits may relate more to central axonal death. A refined analysis of EP results may thus allow pinpointing the abnormality of a given MS patient, and thereby provide important prognostic clues.

References

1. Chiappa K H, Ropper A H. Evoked potentials in clinical medicine (first of two parts). *N Engl J Med* 1982;**306**:1140–50

2. Mayr N, Baumgartner C, Zeitlhofer J, Deecke L. The sensitivity of transcranial cortical magnetic stimulation in detecting pyramidal tract lesions in clinically definite multiple sclerosis. *Neurology* 1991;**41**:566–9

3. Ravnborg M, Liguori R, Christiansen P, Larsson H, Sorensen P S. The diagnostic reliability of magnetically evoked motor potentials in multiple sclerosis. *Neurology* 1992;**42**:1296–301

4. Beer S, Rösler K M, Hess C W. Diagnostic value of paraclinical tests in multiple sclerosis: relative sensitivities and specificities for reclassification according to the Poser Committee criteria. *J Neurol Neurosurg Psychiatry* 1995;**59**:152–9

5. Poser C M, Paty D W, Scheinberg L, *et al.* New diagnostic criteria for multiple sclerosis: guidelines for research protocols. *Ann Neurol* 1983;**13**:227–31

6. McDonald W I, Compston A, Edan G, *et al.* Recommended diagnostic criteria for multiple sclerosis: guidelines from the International Panel on the diagnosis of multiple sclerosis. *Ann Neurol* 2001;**50**:121–7

7. Simon J H, Jacobs L D, Campion M, *et al.* Magnetic resonance studies of intramuscular interferon beta-1a for relapsing multiple sclerosis. The Multiple Sclerosis Collaborative Research Group. *Ann Neurol* 1998;**43**:79–87

8. Kappos L, Moeri D, Radue E W, *et al.* Predictive value of gadolinium-enhanced magnetic resonance imaging for relapse rate and changes in disability or impairment in multiple sclerosis: a meta-analysis. Gadolinium MRI Meta-analysis Group. *Lancet* 1999;**353**:964–9

9. Facchetti D, Mai R, Micheli A, *et al.* Motor evoked potentials and disability in secondary progressive multiple sclerosis. *Can J Neurol Sci* 1997;**24**:332–7

10. O'Connor P, Marchetti P, Lee L, Perera M. Evoked potential abnormality scores are a useful measure of disease burden in relapsing–remitting multiple sclerosis. *Ann Neurol* 1998;**44**:404–7

11. Fuhr P, Borggrefe-Chappuis A, Schindler C, Kappos L. Visual and motor evoked potentials in the course of multiple sclerosis. *Brain* 2001;**124**:2162–8

12. Brusa A, Jones S J, Plant G T. 2001; Long-term remyelination after optic neuritis: a 2-year visual evoked potential and psychophysical serial study. *Brain* 2001;**124**:468–79

13. La Mantia L, Riti F, Milanese C, *et al.* Serial evoked potentials in multiple sclerosis bouts: relation to steroid treatment. *Ital J Neurol Sci* 1994;**15**:333–40

14. Hess C W, Mills K R, Murray N M, Schriefer T N. Magnetic brain stimulation: central motor conduction studies in multiple sclerosis. *Ann Neurol* 1987;**22**:744–52

15. Smith K J, McDonald W I. The pathophysiology of multiple sclerosis: the mechanisms underlying the production of symptoms and the natural history of the disease. *Phil Trans R Soc Lond B* 1999;**354**:1649–73

16. Humm A M, Magistris M R, Truffert A, Hess C W, Rösler K M. Central motor conduction differs between acute relapsing–remitting and chronic progressive multiple sclerosis. *Clin Neurophysiol* 2003;**114**:2196–203

17. Humm A M, Z'Graggen W J, Buhler R, Magistris M R, Rösler K M. Quantification of central motor conduction deficits in multiple sclerosis patients before and after treatment of acute exacerbation by methylprednisolone. *J Neurol Neurosurg Psychiatry* 2006;**77**:345–50

18. Humm A M, Beer S, Kool J, *et al.* Quantification of Uhthoff's phenomenon in multiple sclerosis: a magnetic stimulation study. *Clin Neurophysiol* 2004;**115**:2493–501

19. Persson H E, Sachs C. Visual evoked potentials elicited by pattern reversal during provoked visual impairment in multiple sclerosis. *Brain* 1981;**104**:369–82

20. Stöhr M. Somatosensorisch evozierte Potentiale SEP. In: Maurer K, Lowitzsch K, Stöhr M, eds. *Evozierte Potentiale AEP – VEP – SEP.* Stuttgart: Ferdinand Enke Verlag, 1990;183–4

21. Magistris M R, Rösler K M, Truffert A, Myers J P. Transcranial stimulation excites virtually all motor neurons supplying the target muscle: a demonstration and a method improving the study of motor evoked potentials. *Brain* 1998;**121**(3):437–50

22. Rösler K M. Transcranial magnetic brain stimulation: a tool to investigate central motor pathways. *News Physiol Sci* 2001;**16**:297–302

23. Chen R, Cros D, Curra A, *et al.* The clinical diagnostic utility of transcranial magnetic stimulation: report of an IFCN committee. *Clin Neurophysiol* 2008;**119**:504–32

24. Amassian V E, Cracco R Q, Maccabee P J. Focal stimulation of human cerebral cortex with the magnetic coil: a comparison with electrical stimulation. *Electroencephalogr Clin Neurophysiol* 1989;**74**:401–16

25. Kiers L, Cros D, Chiappa K H, Fang J. Variability of motor potentials evoked by transcranial magnetic stimulation. *Electroencephalogr Clin Neurophysiol* 1993;**89**:415–23

26. Rösler K M, Petrow E, Mathis J, *et al.* Effect of discharge desynchronization on the size of motor evoked potentials: an analysis. *Clin Neurophysiol* 2002;**113**:1680–7

27. Rösler K M, Roth D M, Magistris M R. Trial-to-trial size variability of motor-evoked potentials: a study using the triple stimulation technique. *Exp Brain Res* 2008;**187**:51–9

28. Britton T C, Meyer B U, Benecke R. Variability of cortically evoked motor responses in multiple sclerosis. *Electroencephalogr Clin Neurophysiol* 1991;**81**:186–94

29. Zentner J, Meyer B. Diagnostic significance of MEP elicited by electrical and magnetoelectric stimulation in acute/subacute supratentorial lesions. *Electromyogr Clin Neurophysiol* 1998;**38**:33–40

30. Magistris M R, Rösler K M, Truffert A, Landis T, Hess C W. A clinical study of motor evoked potentials using a triple stimulation technique. *Brain* 1999;**122**(2):265–79

31. Bühler R, Magistris M R, Truffert A, Hess C W, Rösler K M. The triple stimulation technique to study central motor conduction to the lower limbs. *Clin Neurophysiol* 2001;**112**:938–49

32. Jones S J, Brusa A. Neurophysiological markers of relapse, remission and long-term recovery processes in MS. *Electroencephalogr Clin Neurophysiol Suppl* 1999;**50**:584–90

33. Smith K J. Conduction properties of central demyelinated and remyelinated axons, and their relation to symptom production in demyelinating disorders. *Eye* 1994;**8**(2):224–37

34. Andersson P B, Goodkin D E. Glucocorticosteroid therapy for multiple sclerosis: a critical review. *J Neurol Sci* 1998;**160**:16–25

35. Kandler R H, Jarratt J A, Davies-Jones G A, *et al.* The role of magnetic stimulation as a quantifier of motor disability in patients with multiple sclerosis. *J Neurol Sci* 1991;**106**:31–4

36. Salle J Y, Hugon J, Tabaraud F, *et al.* Improvement in motor evoked potentials and clinical course post-steroid therapy in multiple sclerosis. *J Neurol Sci* 1992;**108**:184–8

37. Fierro B, Salemi G, Brighina F, *et al.* A transcranial magnetic stimulation study evaluating methylprednisolone treatment in multiple sclerosis. *Acta Neurol Scand* 2002;**105**:152–7

38. Schauf C L, Davis F A. Impulse conduction in multiple sclerosis: a theoretical basis for modification by temperature and pharmacological agents. *J Neurol Neurosurg Psychiatry* 1974;**37**:152–61

39. Felts P A, Baker T A, Smith K J. Conduction in segmentally demyelinated mammalian central axons. *J Neurosci* 1997;**17**:7267–77

The physiopathology of multiple sclerosis

Giancarlo Comi

Introduction

Multiple sclerosis (MS) is an inflammatory disease of the central nervous system, predominantly, but not exclusively, involving the normal-appearing white matter. From an immunological point of view, chronic inflammation in MS can be thought of as an inflammatory process with a disordered resolution phase. We still do not know why inflammation in MS does not resolve, but there are several possible explanations. The persistence of inflammatory central nervous system (CNS) infiltrates could be caused by long-lasting "danger signals." Although many viruses have been implicated as possible danger signals in MS, there is no conclusive evidence that any pathogens have such a role. The most recent and perhaps attractive candidate is the Epstein–Barr virus, which has been found to be associated with MS both in children [1, 2] and in adults [3, 4]. Moreover, Aloisi and colleagues [5] found in CNS elevated numbers of B cells infected by the virus, an observation that, if confirmed, would indicate a pathogenic role of the virus.

The pathological substrates of neurological dysfunction in MS are demyelination and axonal loss [6–8]. In myelinated fibers, saltatory conduction of action potentials is determined by clustering of voltage-sensitive sodium channels within axon membranes at nodes of Ranvier and, to a much lesser extent, beneath the myelin sheaf [9]. Demyelination may produce multiple functional alterations, reported in Table 2.1. Conduction block almost invariably occurs if the length of the demyelinated area exceeds 5 mm [10]. Conduction block may also be caused by soluble mediators of inflammation, such as nitroxide, especially in demyelinated axons [11–14]. The rapid improvement of neurological deficits during an attack is in fact mostly due to the resolution of inflammation

because remyelination requires some weeks to be completed and to have functional consequences. In areas with partial demyelination, slowing of conduction velocity and a prolonged refractory period may result in failure in transmitting high-frequency impulses [10]. Moreover in multi-synaptic pathways, multifocal demyelination may induce a desynchronized afferent volley that compromises the temporal and spatial summation of synaptic potentials with a failure to elicit the next response in the pathway. Neurological dysfunction resulting from conduction block is usually transitory; however, the possibility of persistent conduction block cannot be excluded. On the other hand the functional consequences due to axonal loss are irreversible if not compensated by CNS plasticity and axonal regeneration which seems to be quite modest at the best.

Dynamic of multiple sclerosis damage

In about 85% of the MS patients, defined relapsing–remitting (RR) MS, the early phase of the disease, is marked by acute attacks characterized by unifocal (two-thirds of patients) or multifocal white matter lesions [15]; gray matter lesions are not frequent in the early phase of the disease. Attacks in the early phase of the disease are usually followed by an apparent complete recovery; however, careful neurological examination reveals deterioration of neurological functions in about a quarter of patients [16]. Intervals between attacks can be as long as 20 years or as short as a few days. Magnetic resonance imaging (MRI) has revealed the frequent occurrence of new lesions or the reactivation of old lesions during the clinically stable phases of the disease. For example in the European–Canadian clinical trial testing the efficacy of glatiramer acetate in the placebo arm, during a 9-month

Multiple Sclerosis: Recovery of Function and Neurorehabilitation, eds. J. Kesselring, G. Comi, and A. J. Thompson. Published by Cambridge University Press. © Cambridge University Press 2010.

Table 2.1 Functional effects of demyelination

Slowing of conduction

Temporal dispersion

Increased refractory period

Conduction block

Secondary axonal degeneration

period, there was a mean of 36.8 new lesions per patient compared to 0.75 relapses per patient [17]. About 90% of RRMS patients enter a progressive course of the disease, the so-called secondary progressive course (SPMS), characterized by a continuous neurological deterioration, sometimes with more or less prolonged phases of stability; relapses become rare in SPMS and also the MRI activity is substantially reduced [18–20]. In approximately 15% of patients, the disease has a progressive course from the onset, which is called primary progressive multiple sclerosis (PPMS) [18, 21]. Patients with PPMS typically have few MRI active lesions [22]. This finding may correspond to the lesser degree of inflammation seen by histopathology [23].

In a quite simplified manner the nervous damage in MS may be attributed to the white and gray matter lesions and to the diffuse white and grey matter involvement.

Lesion-related nervous damage

There is epidemiological evidence that attacks produce irreversible CNS damage. About 50% of attacks leave a residual irreversible disability [24]. The number of attacks in the first 2 years of the disease is predictive of future disability [25–28]; interestingly enough, relapses influence the speed of accumulation of disability only until the patient reaches a moderate disability (expanded disability status scale [EDSS] score of 4), the subsequent accumulation of disability (time from EDSS 4 to EDSS 6) being independent of what happened in the RR phase of the disease [26]. A recent study indicated that a shorter time from disease onset and onset of the SPMS course was associated with a faster accumulation of disability during the SPMS phase of the disease [21]. The MRI lesion load seen in the brain at the onset of disease predicts the evolution to clinically definite multiple sclerosis [17, 29, 30]. In a recent multinational study, in patients with an irreversible tissue injury first attacks

suggestive of MS were already found; macroscopic focal lesions but not "diffuse" brain damage measured by magnetization transfer ratio (MTR) resulted in an increased risk of subsequent development of definite MS in clinically isolated syndrome (CIS) patients [31]. The degree of brain MRI abnormalities seen in the early phase of the disease predicts the disability that will accumulate many years later [29, 30, 32]. In a recent long-term study, the T2 lesions seen with brain MRI in RRMS correlate strongly with brain tissue loss and with clinical disease severity 13 years later [33]. Finally, clinical trials performed in CIS and early RRMS patients have demonstrated that with reduced numbers of inflammatory lesions there was a decrease in the progression of brain atrophy [34–36]. All these observations indicate that the amount of tissue damage produced by lesions contributes to long-term disability.

Pathological studies demonstrate an important axonal transection inside the acute lesion, already occurring in the early phases of the disease [7, 37, 38]. Acute axonal loss is predominant in lesions appearing in the early phases of the disease and decreases over time [39]. The axonal transection occurs electively in the acute lesion where it is associated with large infiltration of T lymphocytes (especially CD8+ T cells) and macrophages [39] indicating a correlation between inflammation and axonal damage, a relationship also demonstrated by MRI studies. For a very long time, little attention has been paid to the occurrence of extensive axonal damage during the early phases of the disease. More recently many studies, using various MRI techniques, have shown irreversible nervous damage in CIS and early RRMS patients (Table 2.2). Magnetization transfer ratio, a measure of tissue damage, is significantly decreased in the lesions of CIS patients [40]. The same technique has been used to evaluate the longitudinal changes taking place in the white matter when a lesion occurs [41]. The appearance of the lesion is associated with a drop of MTR, due to edema, demyelination, and axonal loss variably combined. After a few days or weeks the MTR values usually increase because of the resolution of edema and remyelination [42–46]. Changes are quite variable from patient to patient and in the same patient from lesion to lesion, meaning a large intraindividual and interindividual variability of the recovery processes. Stabilization of the lesion is usually reached after 6–12 months [41, 45]; however in some lesions demyelination and remyelination, as

Table 2.2 MRI findings in CIS and early RRMS

1997 Prince *et al.*	Early spinal cord atrophy
1999 Liu *et al.*	Brain, spinal cord atrophy in RRMS
1999 De Stefano *et al.*	NAA reduced in early RRMS
1999 Rudick *et al.*	Brain atrophy in mild RRMS
2000 Simon *et al.*	Black holes in mild RRMS
2001 Iannucci *et al.*	NAWM abnormality in CIS
2001 Brex *et al.*	Brain atrophy in CIS
2003 Filippi *et al.*	NAA reduced in CIS
2004 Dalton *et al.*	Gray but not white matter atrophy in CIS
2004 Paoillo *et al.*	Brain atrophy in those with CIS who developed CDMS
2004 Filippi *et al.*	Brain atrophy in CIS partially related to inflammation
2005 Fernando *et al.*	MTR of NAWM–NAGM is abnormal in CIS

NAA, *N*-acetylaspantic acid; NAGM, normal-appearing gray matter; NAWM, normal-appearing white matter.

Table 2.3a Relation between baseline lesion characteristics and evolution to black holes at 6 months

	Characteristics	Evolution rate
Lesion size	<6 mm	35%
	>6 mm	52%
Duration of enhancement	<1	36%
	>2	54%
Re-enhancement	yes	44%
	no	43%
Type of enhancement	nodular	41%
	ring	72%

Table 2.3b Relation between location of baseline lesion characteristics and evolution to black holes at 6 months

Deep white matter	38%
Periventricular	56%
Juxtacortical	32%
Infratentorial	29%

indicated by the MTR changes, are ongoing for months and years after lesion formation [41]. The main factors influencing the residual nervous damage inside the acute lesions are lesion size, enhancement duration, and the periventricular location [47] (Tables 2.3a and 2.3b). The preferential location of MS lesions is in the periventricular area, as it is also in mice with experimental allergic encephalomyelitis (EAE) [48] (Fig. 2.1). This location could depend on the attraction of inflammatory cells in the subventricular area by chemokines, such as CXCL10 produced by multipotent stem/precursor cells (NPCs), resident in the subventricular zone [49, 50]. From the other side the recruitment of the progenitors to contribute to the reparative mechanisms orchestrated by inflammatory cells (lymphocytes and microglia) is impaired (L. Muzio, personal comunication), giving poor reparation of the new lesions occurring in this area.

Progressive brain atrophy, mostly explained by axonal loss, is already detectable in CIS patients and is significantly correlated with the number of active lesions accumulated in the same period [34, 51]. Interestingly enough, the progression of brain atrophy is only observed in patients with evolution to clinically definite MS [52]. Corpus callosum atrophy appears over a period of 1 year after a diagnosis of CIS [53]. The acute axonal damage also occurs because of the products of inflammation, such as nitric oxide and tumor necrosis factor [54]. A high electrical activity

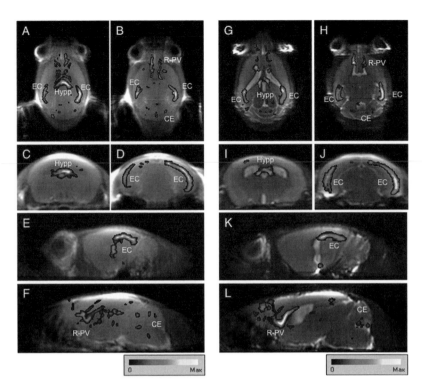

Fig. 2.1. Spatial lesion probability maps of T1 post gadolinium and T2 hyperintense brain lesions during acute chronic EAE. (With permission from Politi *et al.* [154].) (See also color plate.)

may increase the axonal degeneration at the Ranvier's nodes of partially or completely demyelinated lesions, as a consequence of the activation of glutamate receptors increasing the calcium entry into the axon [55]. Recent studies suggest that axonal damage may also be independent of demyelination [56] and be caused by antibodies against axonal antigens [57].

Experimental studies have confirmed a strong association between demyelination and axonal loss; however, in the early phases of the disease, axonal degeneration was also detected in normally myelinated axons [58]. Bitsch *et al.* [56] found that axonal injury is, at least in part, independent from demyelination and Aboul-Enein *et al.* [59] found that in acute EAE NO-related axonal degeneration can be independent of demyelination.

There is accumulating evidence that the nature of the lesions may differ between the early and the late phases of the disease. Early MS is associated with recruitment of systemically derived immune cell populations and inflammatory lesions. Late MS inflammatory responses appear to be modest, mostly at the edge of pre-existing lesions, probably locally regulated as suggested by the secondary lymphoid

organization within the Virchow–Robin spaces [60], the ectopic follicles containing B cells and plasma cells in the meninges [61], and memory B lymphocytes higher in cerebrospinal fluid (CSF) than in peripheral blood [62]. Moreover there is extensive cortical demyelination and widespread axonal injury. All these data indicate a compartmentalized immunological response in the progressive phase of the disease. Old pathological studies have shown that cortical lesions are present in the vast majority of the patients [63]. Three different types of lesions have been described, one in the context of the gray matter and the other two concerning the CSF or the white matter respectively [64, 65]. Cortical lesions have some specificities: modest lymphocyte infiltration, presence of demyelination, and microglia activation [65]. Cortical lesions are visible with MRI, particularly with high field magnets [66, 67]. They may occur in CIS, but are more frequent in progressive MS [68]. The presence of cortical lesions is associated with cognitive impairment and more severe disability [68, 69]. It is probable that these lesions are responsible for the gray matter damage observed with non-conventional MRI techniques [69].

If the acute damage caused by the occurrence of lesions is so important, why we can usually observe a full recovery in the early phases of the disease? There are at least two mechanisms that may explain these findings: the redundancy of the CNS and the recovery mechanisms. Because of the redundancy in fibers of the central nervous pathways a large number of fibers must be destroyed in order for there to be clinical manifestation. Examination of the retinal nerve fiber layer at the optic disk revealed that more than 50% of neural tissue must be lost before a visual defect is clinically evident [70].

Recovery mechanisms are of the outmost importance in MS and they are extensively discussed elsewhere in the book. Their existence is quite clear in the

Table 2.4 Factors influencing recovery after acute MS lesion

Lesion characteristics

Efficiency of remyelination

Pre-existing nervous damage

Brain plasticity

Compensatory strategies

Neurogenesis

Training of the affected limb – constraint strategy

Peripheral and central stimulation

Drugs:

- neuroprotective agents

- modulation of neurotransmitters (NE, amphetamine)

- growth factors (NGF, FGF, OP-1, BDNF, IGF)

relapsing phase of the disease because neurological deficits determined by the attacks are usually followed by a variable degree of recovery. The recovery after the relapse is apparently complete in the initial years of disease and tends to become less efficient over time. A list of the factors involved in the recovery after an acute MS lesion is given in Table 2.4. Recovery mechanisms include the resolution of acute inflammation, with the elimination of products of the inflammatory reaction which are toxic for the nerves fibers. The end of the inflammatory phase promotes remyelination [71, 72] and provides neurotrophic factors [73], very important for the restoration of the nerve function. A second key factor for recovery, which has emerged only very recently, is neuroplasticity. Neuroplasticity is immediately activated after an acute lesion, as revealed by functional imaging studies [74, 75]. Changes occurring in the brain soon after an acute lesion include the reduction/loss of function of the affected area, diaschisis or change of function of the areas functionally connected to the affected area, and changes in the excitability of homologous collateral areas, if affected areas have symmetrical organization [75, 76]. In the following days, in parallel with local reorganization of the injured tissue, there is reactivation of the perilesional regions to replace the damaged cells and start the recruitment of functionally related pathways and the formation of new pathways [77, 78]. In MS patients without signs of motor dysfunction, there is a significant correlation between enlargement of the sensorimotor cortex (in comparison to normal subjects) during a simple manual task and the degree of lesion damage [79] (Fig. 2.2), indicating that the local reorganization has been adequate

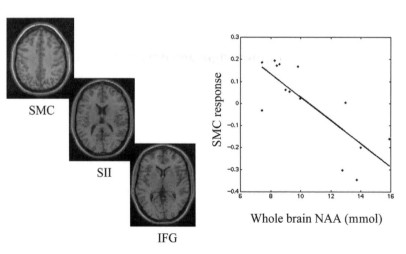

SMC

SII

IFG

Whole brain NAA (mmol)

Fig. 2.2. Functional MRI study of brain activation of simple movements of the left hand in patients with clinically isolated syndrome (right). The increased activation of the contralateral sensorimotor cortex is correlated with the decrease of NAA in the whole brain spectroscopy. (With permission from Rocca *et al.* [80].) (See also color plate.)

to compensate successfully for the tissue loss due to the new lesion. Brain plasticity is already evident in the early phases of MS, as shown by the increase of primary contralateral motor cortex activation during simple motor tasks observed in CIS patients [80]. Cortical reoganization is also important to preventing cognitive impairment in MS [81].

The contribution of neurogenesis to recovery in humans is still controversial [82–84]. The basic mechanisms operating in the restoration of function include: increased dendritic arborization [85, 86], fiber sprouting from surviving axons [87, 88], synaptogenesis [89, 90], activation and potentiation of functionally silent synaptic connections [91–93], and long-term potentiation dependent on NMDA receptors [94]. The reparative phase is usually efficient in early MS, since acute inflammation on the one hand produces relevant axonal loss, and on the other hand facilitates recovery.

As already discussed, MTR has been used to study evolution of new lesions [41, 95–97], demonstrating that changes suggestive of demyelination and remyelination are ongoing for months and years after lesion formation [41]. Longitudinal studies of the evolution of lesions in different courses of MS has revealed that tissue damage, as measured by MTR, remains stable in RRMS and increases significantly in SPMS [98, 99]. These data confirm that inside the lesions there is an ongoing process of degeneration, more pronounced in the progressive phase of the disease. Interestingly enough, a follow-up study showed that the average lesion MTR percentage change after 12 months was an independent predictor of worsening disability after 8 years [99]. In a recent MRI study, the evolution of a large lesion in the periventricular region of an SPMS patient was followed for 2 years. The reduction in the volume of a new T2 lesion during the follow-up was associated with adjacent regional white matter volume loss, which was disproportionate to concurrent diffuse atrophy in the rest of the normal appearing brain tissue and reciprocated by local ventricular expansion [100]. This observation suggests that the decrease in the volume of a new T2 lesion can result from progression of destructive/degenerative pathology in and around that lesion, which may be a long-lasting phenomenon leading to progression of atrophy.

The amount of this secondary degeneration, compared to the acute axonal loss occurring in the active lesion, is unknown. The clinical observation that

the topographic pattern of irreversible, progressive neurological deficits in MS frequently depends on the localization of the previous attacks supports the role of lesions in the progressive phase of the disease. In the same direction, there is evidence that the MRI lesion load in CIS predicts the degree of long-term disability [32, 101].

Many interpretations have been proposed for the secondary axonal degeneration that takes place in the inactive lesions. In patients in an inactive phase of the disease, unusually thick demyelinated axons with high reactivity for phosphorylated neurofilaments have been found in chronic plaques [102]. These large axons may represent a chronic axonal reaction to demyelination [103–105]. Naked, demyelinated axons may be more susceptible to degeneration because of lost trophic support from the oligodendrocyte [106–108], a hypothesis supported by the observation that remyelinated axons are protected from further damage [39]. Demyelinated axons are also more susceptible to soluble or cellular mediators present in the chronic plaque [55] and may degenerate because of the abnormal expression of sodium channel subtypes which alter the membrane excitability [109]. A mismatch between increased energy demand and decreased supply of ATP consequent to dysfunction of mitochondria may contribute to the axonal degeneration [110].

Secondary degeneration may also occur because repeated episodes of demyelination exhaust the availability of oligodendrocyte precursors or decrease their remyelinating efficiency [111]. A primary pathology of oligodendrocytes could also explain the occurrence of inefficient remyelination in some cases, an explanation that has been proposed for patients with PPMS [112].

Diffuse white and gray matter damage

Based on epidemiological, clinical, MRI, and pathological studies there is a deep ongoing debate about the existence of a primary neurodegenerative process in MS that may even be the predominant cause of CNS damage in the disease [113]. There are many clinical observations that support diffuse white and gray matter damage as the underlying pathophysiological mechanisms of the disease progression in PPMS and SPMS. In the progressive phases of MS the accumulation of disability is usually continuous and takes place in parallel in different nervous pathways – that is very difficult to explain by new lesions. The time to reach disability milestones, and the age at which these landmarks are reached, are not influenced by when they may occur, or by the initial course of the disease, whatever its phenotype [26, 27]. Patients with progressive courses accumulate irreversible disability independently from attacks or MRI activity [18] and the time course of the disability progression is identical in PPMS and SPMS [114]. Finally, anti-inflammatory treatments targeting lesions are not effective in delaying the progression of disability that occurs in PPMS and SPMS.

Pathological studies have revealed profound axonal loss in the so-called normal-appearing white matter (NAWM), which could not be fully explained by secondary degeneration of axons transected inside the lesion [38, 115–117]. Furthermore, axonal injury was also seen in inactive plaques in MS patients [38]. Using immunohistochemical staining techniques, activated microglia and a few pro-inflammatory T cells were seen in association with axonal injury detected in the NAWM [118]. The extent of such diffuse infiltration was found to be much higher in white matter tissue taken from SPMS and PPMS cases than in tissue from RRMS cases [119]. Cortical pathology is quite relevant in chronic MS [120], mostly explained by the presence of subpial, intracortical, and leukocortical lesions [65]. However, a postmortem study of brain tissue revealed a 10% cortical thinning of the normal-appearing MS cortex, but no relative changes in neuronal, glial, and synaptic densities in comparison to controls [121], suggesting that there are mechanisms contributing to cortical atrophy outside of lesions, which lead to a generalized loss of all cellular components. In the same study a more pronounced loss of neurons was found in the thalamus of chronic MS patients. Animal models of RRMS, such as encephalomyelitis in SJL mice, have shown persistent activation of microglia through the chronic disease phase leading to degeneration of cortical callosal projecting neurons [122]. These features mimic the periventricular and cortical pathology seen in chronic MS.

Studies using MRI have provided key support for the idea of the existence of a diffuse white and gray matter damage in MS. The existence of normal-appearing white and gray matter, not visible with conventional MRI techniques but detectable with new more pathology-specific MRI measures, has been used to explain the clinical/MRI paradox, that is the

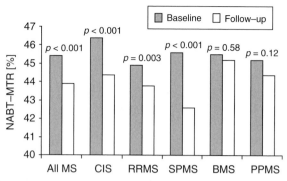

Fig. 2.3. Magnetization transfer ratio of the normal appearing white matter changes in different disease phenotypes. The largest drop in MTR is observed in SPMS patients.

weak correlation between visible lesions and disability [123]. Moreover cognitive abnormalities have been found to be more closely related to normal-appearing brain tissue damage than to the T2 or T1 lesion load [124, 125]. Magnetization transfer studies have demonstrated a decreased ratio in normal-appearing white matter (Fig. 2.3) and gray matter in patients in the early phases of the disease, increasing in magnitude with the evolution of the disease [124, 126–128]. The cervical spinal cord atrophy measured at C2 was not associated with local lesion load in RR and progressive MS [129, 130]. The mean diffusivity of the cervical spinal cord was also not associated with local lesion load [131] indicating that mechanisms other than lesion accumulation may play a role in the spinal cord lesions, such as normal-appearing white and gray matter degeneration. However, since the ascending and descending pathways are the predominant nervous tissues in the spinal cord, fiber tract degeneration at this level may also be due to lesions occurring below or above the examined spinal cord level. Moreover large spinal cord lesions are frequently associated with a corresponding focal spinal cord atrophy which can usually be seen many years after the appearance of the lesions. The absence of a strict correlation between lesion location and involvement of nervous pathways also emerged from a diffusion tensor imaging study [132] and from measurements of the progression of atrophy of the white matter fiber tracts [100].

Atrophy measures and MTR/DTI (diffusion tensor imaging) studies have shown widespread gray matter damage in MS that is already present in early phases of the disease [133–135] and more prominent than white matter damage [136, 137]. Whole brain

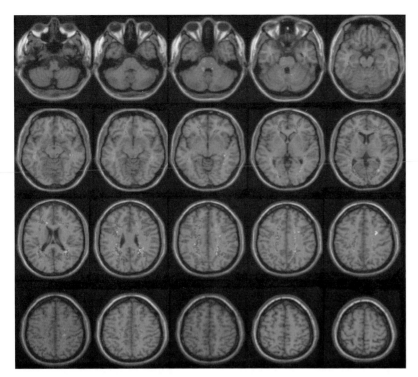

Fig. 2.4. Representative axial slices showing lesion probability maps, overlaid on a high-resolution T1-weighted image, in the different MS groups. Blue: lesion probability map of patients at presentation with clinically isolated syndromes; yellow: lesion probability map of RRMS patients; green: lesion probability map of SPMS patients; red: lesion probability map of PPMS patients. Images are in neurological convention. (See also color plate.)

atrophy and gray matter atrophy are accelerated in patients with a more advanced stage of MS; in contrast white matter atrophy remain constant across all disease categories [138]. Interestingly enough, changes in lesion volume explained partially the progression of gray matter and white matter atrophy in RRMS; however, in SPMS the correlation was found only with white matter atrophy progression. These data suggest that in the progressive phase of the disease the damage to normal-appearing white matter is still under the influence of the white matter lesions but the gray matter damage should be determined by other mechanisms, such as gray matter lesions or diffuse white matter and gray matter involvement. A recent voxel-based morphometry longitudinal study of different MS phenotypes provided new interesting information on this complex pathophysiological matter [139]. Regional gray matter atrophy varied in various phenotypes, being restricted to pre- and postcentral gyri in RRMS patients, and extended to many cortical and subcortical areas, including thalamus, in PPMS and SPMS; in all phenotypes regional gray matter loss was significantly correlated with brain T2 lesion volume. In PPMS patients there was also a strong regional correlation between gray matter atrophy and T2 lesion load. Similar results have been

found in a group of patients with a long disease duration [69]. Gray matter atrophy was found to be more predictive of disability than white matter atrophy [69, 99]. These data are in contrast with the independency of the NAWM and NAGM damage from the lesions in the progressive phase of the disease and suggest that further studies are needed.

The mechanisms responsible for the axonal degeneration seen in the normal-appearing brain tissue are debatable. Axonal loss may simply reflect the anterograde degeneration of nerve fibers transected or degenerated in the lesion: the axonal loss in the corpus callosum of progressive MS patients is significantly correlated with the lesion load in the hemispheres [140] and the longitudinal changes of the cortical gray matter are related to the subcortical lesion load (Fig. 2.4) [69, 136, 139].

Alternative mechanisms include a retrograde axonal degeneration, transsynaptic neuronal degeneration, and axonal degeneration due to low grade diffuse inflammation [141]. A very elegant postmortem study performed in 67 MS patients from different disease stages revealed that in the progressive phases of the disease the expanding lesions with T cell infiltrates at the periphery, and activated microglia in inactive lesions, cortex, and NAWM were typical findings [102]. As seen in the RR phase, in the chronic–progressive (CP) phase also axonal injury was significantly associated with inflammation [102]. Finally we should consider the extreme hypothesis that MS is a primary progressive degenerative disease, with a secondary inflammatory response. Most of the available data are not in line with this view.

Conclusions

Lesion-related damage is still a key factor in the neurological impairment observed in MS, because of the acute axonal transection occurring in the acute lesions and the late degeneration affecting the axons that survived the first attack. It is conceivable that white matter lesions, particularly those affecting the sensorimotor pathways, play a major role in physical disability, the gray matter lesions having a major role in cognitive dysfunction. We need more studies to disentangle the mechanisms of axonal degeneration in the so-called normal-appearing gray and white matter. However, there is converging evidence that inflammation is the key factor producing irreversible myelin/axonal damage. The difference between RR and CP phases, with probably a large intermediate phase, is the predominance of a T cell peripherally driven pathogenesis, mostly against white matter tissue in the early phases and a multifocal, compartmentalized, B cell and microglia driven process in the advanced phases of the disease. At present, prevention of new lesions by very early immunomodulatory and immunosuppressive drugs combined with neuroprotection by cellular therapy and neurotrophic factors for still occurring lesions seems to be the best strategy to face the disease. However, the possibility of turning down the inflammation in the chronic phases of the disease with treatments acting in the CNS compartment should soon be considered.

References

1. Alotaibi S, Kennedy J, Tellier R, Stephens D, Banwell B. Epstein–Barr virus in pediatric multiple sclerosis. *JAMA* 2004;**291**:1875–9

2. Pohl D, Krone B, Rostasy K, *et al.* High seroprevalence of Epstein–Barr virus in children with multiple sclerosis. *Neurology* 2006;**67**:2063–5

3. Delorenze G N, Munger K L, Lennette E T, *et al.* Epstein–Barr virus and multiple sclerosis: evidence of association from a prospective study with long-term follow-up. *Arch Neurol* 2006;**63**:839–44

4. Haahr S, Hollsberg P. Multiple sclerosis is linked to Epstein–Barr virus infection. *Rev Med Virol* 2006;**16**:297–310

5. Serafini B, Rosicarelli B, Franciotta D, *et al.* Dysregulated Epstein–Barr virus infection in the multiple sclerosis brain. *J Exp Med.* 2007;**204**(12):2899–912

6. Lassmann H, Wisniewski H M. Chronic relapsing experimental allergic encephalomyelitis: clinicopathological comparison with multiple sclerosis. *Arch Neurol* 1979;**36**:490–7

7. Trapp B D, Peterson J, Ransohoff R M, *et al.* Axonal transection in the lesions of multiple sclerosis. *N Engl J Med.* 1998;**338**:278–85

8. Scolding N, Franklin R. Axon loss in multiple sclerosis. *Lancet* 1998;**352**(9125);340–1

9. Ritchie J M, Rogart R B. Density of sodium channels in mammalian myelinated nerve fibers and nature of the axonal membrane under the myelin sheath. *Proc Natl Acad Sci USA* 1977;**74**(1):211–15

10. McDonald W I, Sears T A. Effect of demyelinating lesion on conduction in the central nervous system studied in single nerve fibres. *J Physiol* 1970; **207**(2):53P–54P

11. Moreau T, Coles A, Wing M, *et al.* Transient increase in symptoms associated with cytokine release in patients with multiple sclerosis. *Brain* 1996;**119**(1):225–37

12. Koller H, Siebler M, Hartung H P. Immunologically induced electrophysiological dysfunction: implications for inflammatory diseases of the CNS and PNS. *Prog Neurobiol* 1997;**52**(1):1–26

13. Smith K J, Lassmann H. The role of nitric oxide in multiple sclerosis. *Lancet Neurol* 2002;**1**(4):232–41

14. Coles A J, Cox A, Le Page E, *et al.* The window of therapeutic opportunity in multiple sclerosis: evidence from monoclonal antibody therapy. *J Neurol* 2006;**253**:98–108

15. Wingerchuk D M, Weinshenker B G. Multiple sclerosis: epidemiology, genetic, classification, natural history and clinical outcome measures. *Neuroimag Clin N Am* 2000;**10**: 611–23

16. Lublin F, Baier M, Cutter G. Effect of relapses on development of residual deficit in multiple sclerosis. *Neurology* 2003;**61**:1528–32

17. Comi G, Filippi M, Wolinsky J and The European/ Canadian Glatiramer Acetate Study Group. European/ Canadian multicenter, double-blind, randomized, placebo-controlled study of the effects of glatiramer acetate on magnetic resonance imaging-measured disease activity and burden in patients with relapsing multiple sclerosis. *Ann Neurol* 2001;**49**:290–7

18. Confavreux C, Vukus S. The clinical epidemiology of multiple sclerosis. *Neuroimag Clin N Am* 2008;**18**:589–622

19. Silver N C, Good C D, Barker G J, *et al.* Sensitivty of contrast enhancing MRI in multiple sclerosis: effects of gadolinium dose, magnetization transfer contrast and delayed imaging. *Brain* 1997;**120**:1149–61

20. Rovaris M, Confavreux C, Furlan R, *et al.* Secondary progressive multiple sclerosis: current knowledge and future challenges. *Lancet Neurol* 2006;**5**(4):343–54

21. Tremlett H, Zhao Y, Devonshire V. Natural history of secondary-progressive multiple sclerosis. *Mult Scler* 2008;**14**:314–24

22. Losseff N A, Webb S L, O'Riordan J L, *et al.* Spinal cord atrophy and disability in multiple sclerosis: a new reproducible and sensitive MRI method with potential to monitor disease progression. *Brain* 1996;**119**:701–8

23. Thompson A J, Polman C H, Miller D H, *et al.* Primary progressive multiple sclerosis. *Brain* 1997;**120**:1085–96

24. Hirst C, Ingram G, Pearson O, *et al.* Contribution of relapses to disability in multiple sclerosis. *J Neurol* 2008;**255**:280–7

25. Weinshenker B G, Bass B, Rice G P A, *et al.* The natural history of multiple sclerosis: a geographically based study: clinical course and disability. *Brain* 1989;**112**:133–46

26. Confavreux C, Vukusic S, Moreau T, Adeleine P. Relapses and progression of disability in multiple sclerosis. *N Engl J Med* 2000;**343**:1430–8

27. Confavreux C, Vukusic S. Natural history of multiple sclerosis: a unifying concept. *Brain* 2006;**129**:595–605

28. Ebers G C. Disease evolution in multiple sclerosis. *J Neurol* 2006;**253**(Suppl 6):3–8

29. Filippi M, Horsfield M A, Morrissey S P, *et al.* Quantitative brain MRI lesion load predicts the course of clinically isolated syndromes suggestive of multiple sclerosis. *Neurology* 1994;**44**:635–41

30. O'Riordan J I, Thompson A J, Kingsley D P E, *et al.* The prognostic value of brain MRI in clinically isolated syndromes of the CNS: a 10-year follow-up. *Brain* 1998;**121**:495–503

31. Rocca M A, Agosta F, Sormani M P, *et al.* A three-year, multi-parametric MRI study in patients at presentation with CIS. *J Neurol* 2008;**255**:683–91

32. Brex P A, Ciccarelli O, O'Riordan J I, *et al.* A longitudinal study of abnormalities on MRI and disability from multiple sclerosis. *N Engl J Med* 2002;**346**:158–64

33. Rudick R A, Lee J C, Simon J, Fisher E. Significance of T2 lesions in multiple sclerosis: a 13-year longitudinal study. *Ann Neurol* 2006;**60**:236–42

34. Filippi M, Rovaris M, Inglese M, *et al.* and the **ETOMS Study Group**. Interferon beta-1a for brain tissue loss in patients at presentation with syndromes suggestive of multiple sclerosis: a randomized, double-blind, placebo-controlled trial. *Lancet* 2004;**364**:1489–96

35. Rudick R A, Fisher E, Lee J C, *et al.* Brain atrophy in relapsing–remitting multiple sclerosis: relationship to relapses, EDSS, and treatment with interferon beta-1a. *Mult Scler* 2000;**6**:365–72

36. Sormani M P, Rovaris M, Valsasina P, *et al.* Measurement error of two different techniques for brain atrophy assessment in multiple sclerosis. *Neurology* 2004;**62**:1432–4

37. Ferguson B, Matyszak M K, Esiri M M, *et al.* Axonal damage in acute multiple sclerosis lesions. *Brain* 1997;**120**:393–9

38. Kornek B, Storech M K, Weissert R, *et al.* Multiple sclerosis and chronic autoimmune encephalomyelitis. *Am J Pathol* 2000;**157**:267–76

39. Kuhlmann T, Lingfeld G, Bitsch A, *et al.* Acute axonal damage in multiple sclerosis is most extensive in early disease stages and decreases over time. *Brain* 2002;**125**:2202–12

40. Rocca M A, Mezzapesa D M, Falini A, *et al.* Evidence for axonal pathology and adaptive cortical reorganization in patients at presentation with clinically isolated syndromes suggestive of multiple sclerosis. *Neuroimage* 2003;**18**:847–55

41. Chen J T, Collins D L, Atkins H L, Freedman M S, Arnold D L and the Canadian MS/BMT Study Group. Magnetization transfer ration evolution with demyelination and remyelination in multiple sclerosis. *Ann Neurol* 2008;**63**:254–62

42. Barkhof F, Bruck W, De Groot C J, *et al.* Remyelinated lesions in multiple sclerosis: magnetic resonance image appearance. *Arch Neurol* 2003;**60**:1073–81

43. Dousset V, Grossman R I, Ramer K N, *et al.* Experimental allergic encephalomyelitis and multiple sclerosis: lesion characterization with magnetization transfer imaging. *Radiology* 1992;**182**:483–91

44. Silver N C, Lai M, Symms M R, *et al.* Serial magnetization transfer imaging to characterize the early evolution of new MS lesions. *Neurology* 1998;**51**:758–64

45. Van Waesberghe J H, van Walderveen M A, Castelijns J A, *et al.* Patterns of lesion development in multiple sclerosis: longitudinal observations with T1-weighted spin-echo and magnetization transfer MR. *Am J Neuroradiol* 1998;**19**:675–83

46. Filippi M, Rocca M A, Sormani M P, *et al.* Short-term evolution of individual enhancing MS lesions studied with magnetization transfer imaging. *Magn Reson Imaging* 1999;**17**:979–84

47. Minneboo A, Uitdehaag B M, Ader H J, et al. Patterns of enhancing lesion evolution in multiple sclerosis are uniform within patients. Neurology 2005;65:56–61

48. Politi L S, Bacigaluppi M, Brambilla E, et al. Magnetic-resonance-based tracking and quantification of intravenously injected neural stem cell accumulation in the brains of mice with experimental multiple sclerosis. Stem Cells 2007;25:2583–92

49. Pluchino S, Martino G. The therapeutic plasticity of neural stem/percursor cells in multiple sclerosis. J Neurol Sci 2008;265:105–10

50. Menn B, Garcia-Verdugo J M, Yaschine C, et al. Origin of oligodendrocytes in the subventricular zone of the adult brain. J Neurosci 2006;26:7907–18

51. Paolillo A, Piattella M C, Pantano P, et al. The relationship between inflammation and atrophy in clinically isolated syndromes suggestive of multiple sclerosis. J Neurol 2004;251:432–9

52. Anderson V M, Fernando K T, Davies G R, et al. Cerebral atrophy measurement in clinically isolated syndromes and relapsing remitting multiple sclerosis: a comparison of registration-based methods. J Neuroimag 2007;17:61–8

53. Audoin B, Ibarrola D, Malikova I, et al. Onset and underpinnings of white matter atrophy at the very early stage of multiple sclerosis: a two-year longitudinal MRI/MRSI study of corpus callosum. Mult Scler 2007;13(1):41–51

54. Smith K J, Kapoor R, Felts P A. Electrically active axons degenerate when exposed to nitric oxide. Ann Neurol 2001;49:470–6

55. Kapoor R, Davied M, Blaker P A, et al. Blockers of sodium and calcium entry protect axons from nitric oxide-mediated degeneration. Ann Neurol 2003;53:174–80

56. Bitsch A, Schuchardt J, Bunkowski S, et al. Acute axonal injury in multiple sclerosis: correlation with demyelination and inflammation. Brain 2000;123:1174–83

57. Raine C, Cannella B, Hauser S, Genain C. Demyelination in primate autoimmune encephalomyelitis and acute multiple sclerosis lesions: a case for antigen-specific antibody mediation. Ann Neurol 1999;46:144–60

58. Papadopoulus D, Pham-Dinh D, Reynolds R. Axon loss is responsible for chronic neurological deficit following inflammatory demyelination in the rat. Exp Neurol 2006;197:373–85

59. Aboul-Enein F, Weiser P, Hoftberger R, Lassmann H, Bradl M. Transient axonal injury in the absence of demyelination: a correlate of clinical disease in acute experimental autoimmune encephalomyelitis. Acta Neuropathol 2006;111:539–47

60. Prineas W J, Barnard R O, Revesz T, et al. Multiple sclerosis: pathology of recurrent lesions. Brain 1993;116:681–93

61. Serafini B, Roscicarelli B, Magliozzi R, Stigliano E, Aloisi F. Detection of ectopic B-cell follicles with germinal centers in the meninges of patients with secondary progressive multiple sclerosis. Brain Pathol 2004;14:164–74

62. Corcione A, Casazza S, Ferretti E, et al. Recapitulation of B cell differentiation in the central nervous system of patients with multiple sclerosis. Proc Natl Acad Sci USA 2004;101:11 064–9

63. Lumsden C E. Properties and significance of the demyelinating antibody in multiple sclerosis. Int Arch Allergy Appl Immunol. 1969;36:(Suppl):247–75

64. Peterson J W, Bö L, Mörk S, Chang A, Trapp B D. Transected neurites, apoptotic neurons, and reduced inflammation in cortical multiple sclerosis lesions. Ann Neurol 2001;50(3):389–400

65. Bö L, Vedeler C A, Nyland H, Trapp B D, Mörk S J. Intracortical multiple sclerosis lesions are not associated with increased lymphocyte infiltration. Mult Scler 2003;9:323–31

66. Kidd D, Barkhof F, McConnell R, et al. Cortical lesions in multiple sclerosis. Brain 1999;122:17–26

67. Geurts J J, Bo L, Pouwels P J, Castelijns J A, Polman C H, Barkhof F. Cortical lesions in multiple sclerosis: combined postmortem MR imaging and histopathology. Am J Neuroradiol 2005;26:572–7

68. Calabrese M, De Stefano N, Atzori M, et al. Detection of cortical inflammatory lesions by double inversion recovery magnetic resonance imaging in patients with multiple sclerosis. Arch Neurol 2007;64(10):1416–22

69. Fisniku L K, Chard D T, Jackson J S, et al. Gray matter atrophy is related to long-term disability in multiple sclerosis. Ann Neurol 2008;64(3):247–54. Erratum in: Ann Neurol 2009;65(2):232

70. Quigley H A, Addicks E M. Quantitative studies of retinal nerve fiber layer defects. Arch Ophthalmol 1982;100(5):807–14

71. Moalem G, Leibowitz-Amit R, Yoles E, et al. Autoimmune T cells protect neurons from secondary degeneration after central nervous system axotomy. Nature Med 1999;5:49–55

72. Hohlfeld R, Kerschensteiner M, Meinl E. Dual role of inflammation in CNS disease. Neurology 2007;68(22 Suppl 3):S58–63

73. Stadelmann C, Kerschensteiner M, Misgeld T, et al. BDNF and gp145trkB in multiple sclerosis brain lesions: neuroprotective interactions between immune and neuronal cells? Brain 2002;125:75–85

74. Pantano P, Mainero C, Lenzi D, *et al.* A longitudinal fMRI study on motor activity in patients with multiple sclerosis. *Brain* 2005;**128**:2146–53

75. Ward N S. Plasticity and the functional reorganization of the human brain. *Int J Psychophysiol* 2005;**58**:158–61

76. Reddy H, Narayanan S, Woolrich M, *et al.* Functional brain reorganization for hand movement in patients with multiple sclerosis: defining distinct effects of injury and disability. *Brain* 2002;**125**: 2646–57

77. Rocca M A, Colombo B, Falini A, *et al.* Cortical adaptation in patients with MS: a cross-sectional functional MRI study of disease phenotypes. *Lancet Neurol* 2005;**4**:618–26

78. Buckle G J. Functional magnetic resonance imaging and multiple sclerosis: the evidence for neuronal plasticity. *J Neuroimag* 2005;**15**(4 Suppl):82S–93S

79. Rocca M A, Falini A, Colombo B, *et al.* Adaptive functional changes in the cerebral cortex of patients with nondisabling multiple sclerosis correlate with the extent of brain structural damage. *Ann Neurol* 2002;**51**:330–9

80. Rocca M A, Mezzapesa D M, Falini A, *et al.* Evidence for axonal pathology and adaptive cortical reorganization in patients at presentation with clinically isolated syndromes suggestive of multiple sclerosis. *Neuroimage* 2003;**18**:847–55

81. Cader S, Cifelli A, Abu-Omar Y, Palace J, Matthews P M. Reduced brain functional reserve and altered functional connectivity in patients with multiple sclerosis. *Brain* 2006;**129**:527–37

82. Magavi S S, Leavitt B R, Macklis J D. Induction of neurogenesis in the neocortex of adult mice. *Nature* 2000;**405**:951–5

83. Parent J M, Vexler Z S, Gong C, Derugin N, Ferriero D M. Rat forebrain neurogenesis and striatal neuron replacement after focal stroke. *Ann Neurol* 2002;**52**:802–13

84. Gotts J E, Chesselet M F. Migration and fate of newly born cells after focal cortical ischemia in adult rats. *J Neurosci Res* 2005;**80**:160–71

85. Belichenko P V, Dahlstrom A. Confocal laser scanning microscopy and 3-D reconstructions of neuronal structures in human brain cortex. *Neuroimage* 1995;**2**:201–7

86. Brown C H, Scott V, Ludwig M, Leng G, Bourque C W. Somatodendritic dynorphin release: orchestrating activity patterns of vasopressin neurons. *Biochem Soc Trans* 2007;**35**:1236–42

87. Johansen J, Johansen K M. Molecular mechanisms mediating axon pathway formation. *Crit Rev Eukaryot Gene Expr* 1997;**7**:95–116

88. Dancause N, Barbay S, Frost S B, *et al.* Extensive cortical rewiring after brain injury. *J Neurosci* 2005;**25**:10 167–79

89. Witte O W, Bidmon H J, Schiene K, Redecker C, Hagamann G. Functional differentiation of multiple perilesional zones after focal cerebral ischemia. *J Cereb Blood Flow Metab* 2000;**20**:1149–65

90. Centonze D, Rossi S, Tortiglione A, *et al.* Synaptic plasticity during recovery from permanent occlusion of the middle cerebral artery. *Neurobiol Dis* 2007; **27**:44–53

91. Wall P D, Egger M D. Formation of new connections in adult rat brains after partial deafferentation. *Nature* 1971;**232**:542–5

92. Wall P D. Mechanisms of plasticity of connection following damage in adult mammalian nervous system. In: Bach-y-Rita P, ed. *Recovery of Function: Theoretical Consideration for Brain Injury Rehabilitation.* Bern: Hans Huber, 1980:91–100

93. Wittenberg G F, Werhahn K J, Wassermann E M, Herscovitch P, Cohen L G. Functional connectivity between somatosensory and visual cortex in early blind humans. *Eur J Neurosci* 2004;**20**:1923–7

94. Jones T A, Schallert T. Overgrowth and pruning of dendrites in adult rats recovering from neocortical damage. *Brain Res* 1992;**581**:156–60

95. Filippi M, Rocca M A, Comi G. Magnetization transfer ratios of multiple sclerosis lesions with variable durations of enhancement. *J Neurol Sci* 1999;**159**:162–5

96. Pike G B, De Stefano N, Narayanan S, *et al.* Multiple sclerosis: magnetization transfer MR imaging of white matter before lesion appearance on T2-weighted images. *Radiology* 2000;**215**:824–30

97. Richert N D, Ostuni J L, Bash C N, *et al.* Interferon beta-1b and intravenous methylprednisolone promote lesion recovery in multiple sclerosis. *Mult Scler* 2001;**7**:49–58

98. Rocca M A, Mastronardo G, Rodegher M, Comi G, Filippi M. Long-term changes of magnetization transfer-derived measures from patients with relapsing–remitting and secondary progressive multiple sclerosis. *Am J Neuroradiol* 1999;**20**(5):821–7

99. Agosta F, Rovaris M, Pagani E, *et al.* Magnetization transfer MRI metrics predict the accumulation of disability 8 years later in patients with multiple sclerosis. *Brain* 2006;**129**:2620–7

100. Kezele I B, Arnold D L, Collins D L. Atrophy in white matter fiber tracts in multiple sclerosis is not dependent on tract length or local white matter lesions. *Mult Scler* 2008;**14**:779–85

101. Tintorè M, Rovira A, Rio J, *et al.* Baseline MRI predicts future attacks and disability in clinically isolated syndromes. *Neurology* 2006;**67**:968–72

102. Frischer J, Bramow S, Dal-Bianco A, *et al.* The relation between inflammation and neurodegeneration in multiple sclerosis brains. *Brain* 2009;**132**:1175–89

103. Waxman S G. Axonal dysfunction in chronic multiple sclerosis: meltdown in the membrane. *Ann Neurol* 2008;**63**:411–13

104. Mahad D, Ziabreva I, Campbell G, *et al.* Mitochondrial changes within axons in multiple sclerosis. *Brain* 2009;**132**:1161–74

105. Young E A, Fowler C D, Kidd G J, *et al.* Imaging correlates of decreased axonal Na^+/K^+ ATPase in chronic multiple sclerosis. *Ann Neurol* 2008;**63**:428–35

106. Griffiths I, Klugmann M, Anderson T, *et al.* Axonal swelling and degeneration in mice lacking the major proteolipid of myelin. *Science* 1998;**280**:1610–13

107. Brady S T, Witt A S, Kirkpatrick L L, *et al.* Formation of compact myelin is required for maturation of cytoskeleton. *J Neurosci* 1999;**19**:7278–88

108. Uschkureit T, Sporkel O, Stracke J, Bussow H, Stoffel W. Early onset of axonal degeneration in double (*pip-/-mag-/-*) and hypomyelinosis in triple (*pip-/-mbp-/-mag-/-*) mutant mice. *J Neurosci* 2000;**20**:5225–33

109. Waxman S G. Acquired channelopathies in nerve injury and MS. *Neurology* 2001;**56**:1621–7

110. Dutta R, McDonough J, Yin X, *et al.* Mitochondrial dysfunction as a cause of axonal degeneration in multiple sclerosis patients. *Ann Neurol* 2006; **59**:478–89

111. Linington C, Engelhardt B, Kapocs G, Lassmann H. Induction of persistently demyelinated lesions in the rat following the repeated adoptive transfer of encephalitogenic T cells and demyelinating antibody. *J Neuroimmunol* 1992;**40**:219–24

112. Lucchinetti C, Bruck W, Parisi J, *et al.* A quantitative analysis of oligodendrocytes in multiple sclerosis lesions: a study of 113 cases. *Brain* 1999;**122**:2279–95

113. Trapp B D, Nave K A. Multiple sclerosis: an immune or neurodegenerative disorder? *Annu Rev Neurosi* 2008;**31**:247–69

114. Kremenchutzky M, Rice G P, Baskerville J, *et al.* The natural history of multiple sclerosis: a geographically based study. 9: Observations on the progressive phase of the disease. *Brain* 2006;**129**:584–94

115. DeLuca G C, Williams K, Evangelou N, Ebers G C, Esiri M M. The contribution of demyelination to axonal loss in multiple sclerosis. *Brain* 2006; **129**:1507–16

116. Evangelou N, DeLuca G C, Owens T, Esiri M M. Pathological study of spinal cord atrophy in multiple sclerosis suggests limited role of local lesions. *Brain* 2005;**128**:29–34

117. Lovas G, Szilagyi N, Majtenyi K, Palkovits M, Komoly S. Axonal changes in chronic demyelinated cervical spinal cord plaques. *Brain* 2000;**123**(2):308–17

118. Kutzelnigg A, Lucchinetti C F, Stadelmann C, *et al.* Cortical demyelination and diffuse white matter injury in multiple sclerosis. *Brain* 2005;**128**:2705–12

119. Stadelmann C, Albert M, Wegner C, Bruck W. Cortical pathology in multiple sclerosis. *Curr Opin Neurol* 2008;**21**:229–34

120. Albert M, Antel J, Bruck W, Stadelmann C. Extensive cortical remyelination in patients with chronic multiple sclerosis. *Brain Pathol* 2007;**17**:129–38

121. Wegner C, Esiri M M, Chance S A, Palace J, Matthews P M. Neocortical neuronal, synaptic, and glial loss in multiple sclerosis. *Neurology* 2006;**67**:960–7

122. Rasmussen S, Wang Y, Kivisakk P, *et al.* Persistent activation of microglia is associated with neuronal dysfunction of callosal projecting pathways and multiple sclerosis-like lesions in relapsing–remitting experimental autoimmune encephalomyelitis. *Brain* 2007;**130**:2816–29

123. Barkhof, F. The clinico-radiological paradox in multiple sclerosis revisited. *Curr Opin Neurol* 2002;**15**:239–45

124. Filippi M, Inglese M, Rovaris M, *et al.* Magnetization transfer imaging to monitor the evolution of MS: a 1-year follow-up study. *Neurology* 2000;**55**:940–6

125. Deloire-Grassin M S, Brochet B, Quesson B, *et al.* In vivo evaluation of remyelination in rat brain by magnetization transfer imaging. *J Neurol Sci* 2000;**178**:10–16

126. Iannucci G, Tortorella C, Rovaris M, *et al.* Prognostic value of MR and magnetization transfer imaging findings in patients with clinically isolated syndromes suggestive of multiple sclerosis at presentation. *Am J Neuroradiol* 2001;**21**:1034–8

127. Fernando K T, Tozer D J, Miszkiel K A, *et al.* Magnetization transfer histograms in clinically isolated syndromes suggestive of multiple sclerosis. *Brain* 2005;**128**:2911–25

128. Wattjes M P, Harzheim M, Lutterbey G G, *et al.* Axonal damage but no increased glial cell activity in the normal-appearing white matter of patients with clinically isolated syndromes suggestive of multiple sclerosis using high-field magnetic resonance spectroscopy. *Am J Neuroradiol* 2007;**28**:1517–22

129. Agosta F, Benedetti B, Rocca M A, *et al.* Quantification of cervical cord pathology in primary progressive MS using diffusion tensor MRI. *Neurology* 2005;**64**:631–5

130. Agosta F, Pagani E, Caputo D, Filippi M. Associations between cervical cord gray matter damage and

disability in patients with multiple sclerosis. *Arch Neurol* 2007;**64**:1302–5

131. Valsasina P, Rocca M A, Agosta F, *et al.* Mean diffusivity and fractional anisotropy histogram analysis of the cervical cord in MS patients. *Neuroimage* 2005:**26**:822–8

132. Roosendaal S D, Geurts J J G, Vrenken H, *et al.* Regional DTI differences in multiple sclerosis patients. *Neuroimage* 2009;**44**:1397–403

133. Amato M P, Bartolozzi M L, Zipoli V, *et al.* Neocortical volume decrease in relapsing–remitting MS patients with mild cognitive impairment. *Neurology* 2004;**63**:89–93

134. Chard D T, Griffin C M, Rashid W, *et al.* Progressive grey matter atrophy in clinically early relapsing–remitting multiple sclerosis. *Mult Scler* 2004;**10**:387–91

135. Miller D H, Barkhof F, Frank J A, Parker G J, Thompson A J. Measurement of atrophy in multiple sclerosis: pathological basis, methodological aspects and clinical relevance. *Brain* 2004;**125**:1676–95

136. Dalton C M, Chard D T, Davies G R, *et al.* Early development of multiple sclerosis is associated with progressive grey matter atrophy in patients presenting with clinically isolated syndromes. *Brain* 2004;**127**:1101–7

137. Tiberio M, Chard D T, Altmann, D R, *et al.* Gray and white matter volume changes in early RRMS: a 2-year longitudinal study. *Neurology* 2005;**64**:1001–7

138. Fisher E, Lee J C, Nakamura K, Rudick R A. Gray matter atrophy in multiple sclerosis: a longitudinal study. *Ann Neurol* 2008;**64**:255–65

139. Ceccarelli A, Rocca M A, Pagani E, *et al.* A voxel-based morphometry study of grey matter loss in MS patients with different clinical phenotypes. *Neuroimage* 2008;**42**:315–22

140. Evangelou N, Konz D, Esiri M M, *et al.* Regional axonal loss in the corpus callosum correlates with cerebral white matter lesion volume and distribution in multiple sclerosis. *Brain* 2000;**123**:1845–9

141. Kutzelnigg A, Lassmann H. Cortical lesions and brain atrophy in MS. *J Neurol Sci* 2005;**233**:55–9

142. Ganter P, Prince C, Esiri M M. Spinal cord axonal loss in multiple sclerosis: a postmortem study. *Neuropathol Appl Neurobiol* 1999;**25**:459–67

143. Liu C, Edwards S, Gong Q, *et al.* Three-dimensional MRI estimates of brain and spinal cord atrophy in multiple sclerosis. *J Neurol Neurosurg Psychiatry* 1999; **66**:323–30

144. De Stefano N, Narayanan S, Matthews P M, *et al.* In vivo evidence for axonal dysfunction remote from focal cerebral demyelination of the type seen in multiple sclerosis. *Brain* 1999;**122**:1933–9

145. Rudice R A, Fisher E, Lee J C, *et al.* Use of the brain parenchymal fraction to measure whole brain atrophy in relapsing–remitting MS. *Neurology* 1999; **53**:1698–704

146. Simon J H, Lull J, Jacobs L D, *et al.* A longitudinal study of T1 hypointense lesions in relapsing MS: MSCRG trial of interferon beta-la. *Neurology* 2000; **55**:185–92

147. Iannucci G, Tortorella C, Rovaris M, *et al.* Prognostic value of MR and magnetization transfer imaging findings in patients with clinically isolated syndromes suggestive of multiple sclerosis at presentation. *Am J Neuroradiol* 2000;**21**:1034–8

148. Brex P A, Leary S M, Plant G T, Thompson A J, Miller D H. Magnetization transfer imaging in patients with clinically isolated syndromes suggestive of multiple sclerosis. *Am J Neuroradiol* 2001; **22**:947–51

149. Rocca M A, Mezzapesa D M, Falini A, *et al.* Evidence for axonal pathology and adaptive cortical reorganization in patients at presentation with clinically isolated syndromes suggestive of multiple sclerosis. *Neuroimage* 2003;**18**:847–55

150. Dalton C M, Chard D T, Davies G R, *et al.* Early development of multiple sclerosis is associated with progressive grey matter atrophy in patients presenting with clinically isolated syndromes. *Brain* 2004; **127**:1101–7

151. Paolillo A, Piattella M C, Pantano P, *et al.* The relationship between inflammation and atrophy in clinically isolated syndromes suggestive of multiple sclerosis: a monthly MRI study after triple-dose gadolinium-DTPA. *J Neurol* 2004; **251**:432–9

152. Rovaris M, Gallo A, Riva R, *et al.* An MT MRI study of the cervical cord in clinically isolated syndromes suggestive of MS. *Neurology* 2004;**63**:584–5

153. Fernando K T, Tozer D J, Miszkiel K A, *et al.* Magnetization transfer histograms in clinically isolated syndromes suggestive of multiple sclerosis. *Brain* 2005;**128**:2911–25

154. Politi L S, Bacigaluppi M, Brambilla E, *et al.* Magnetic resonance-based tracking and quantification of intravenously injected neural stem cell accumulation in the brains of mice with experimental multiple sclerosis. *Cells* 2007;**25**:2583–92

Synaptic changes in multiple sclerosis: Do they occur? How effectively can they be analyzed?

Vincenzo Zimarino, Maddalena Ripamonti, Marcello Belfiore, Mattia Ferro, and Antonio Malgaroli

Introduction

Multiple sclerosis (MS) is a chronic demyelinating disease affecting young adults and leading to significant disability. Although MS is presumed to derive from an autoimmune attack to myelin sheaths and oligodendrocytes, some evidence has recently accumulated to indicate that an axonal and synaptic pathology could accompany or even precede the central nervous system (CNS) autoimmune infiltration [1–3]; for review see Geurts & Barkhof [4]. In agreement with this idea, in chronic MS patients, together with the standard white matter lesions seen by brain imaging techniques, some degree of cortical and deep gray matter alterations have been found. The analysis of these gray matter lesions has shown a much less extensive inflammation and gliosis than in white matter lesions [5, 6]. Clearly, since gray matter is composed of neuronal cell bodies, dendrites, and synapses, these findings indicate an alteration of one or more of these neuronal structures in MS patients, which could then explain some of the contradictory clinical features of MS including the frequent association with cognitive disorders. Are these alterations of either synapses, axons, or dendrites a primary phenomenon or do they simply follow the immune attack? The former scenario would open a debate related to the real etiopathology of MS and the suitability of autoimmune myelitis as animal model of MS. The latter scenario would imply a sort of progression of the neuropathological damage initiated by the removal of myelin sheaths which alternatively might also derive from compensatory or plastic changes at the level of either upstream or downstream neuronal structures. An answer to these critical questions would depend on acquiring finer data from gray matter, from neurons and synapses at stages where the MS clinical features are not yet overt. Furthermore since at the very beginning this pathology could simply alter the functionality of neurons and synapses either dependently or independently from the immune attack to the myelin sheaths it would be important to acquire not only morphological data but also functional data on the physiological behavior of neurons and synapses. In this chapter we will review what can be done today to "image" neurons and synapses in neuronal in vitro cultures and in the intact brain of animal models of MS. These can be used to visualize morphological changes, functional alterations, and plastic rearrangements of synapses. The hope is that in the near future it will be possible to move some of this technology to human patients. We envisage that this will be the essential step towards understanding the temporal and spatial occurrence of gray matter lesions and their role in disease progression.

Synaptic plasticity in the mammalian brain

In the last few years, the study of the cellular and molecular events that form the basis of synaptic plasticity in the mammalian brain has attracted increasing interest as documented by the exponentially growing literature on this subject. The term "synaptic plasticity" was put forward by Konorski [7] to describe changes in the efficacy of synapses produced by their persistent activity. Since the work of Cajal [8] and Tanzi [9], these changes have been thought to be the basis of information storage in the brain. This hypothesis was more clearly formulated by the Canadian psychologist Donald Hebb in 1949: "when an axon of cell A is near enough to excite a cell B and

Multiple Sclerosis: Recovery of Function and Neurorehabilitation, eds. J. Kesselring, G. Comi, and A. J. Thompson. Published by Cambridge University Press. © Cambridge University Press 2010.

repeatedly or persistently takes part in firing it, some growth process or metabolic change takes place in one or both cells such that A's efficiency, as one of the cell's firing B, is increased" [10]. Each impulse arriving at a synapse initiates the release of neurotransmitter molecules, mostly glutamate, which are received at specialized postsynaptic receptor sites on the dendrites where postsynaptic receptors are located. This initiates an electrical signal in the dendritic membrane potential, the excitatory postsynaptic potential (EPSP), which tends to excite and generate further action potentials in the receiving neuron. The "volume" of the communication process, i.e., the size of the synaptic potential, will depend on the previous history of the synapse. This experimental confirmation of Hebb's postulate was found in the hippocampus by Bliss and Lomo [11] and became known as long-term potentiation (LTP). But what is LTP? LTP is a long-lasting increase in synaptic strength that occurs when synapses are strongly activated for a very brief period of time, a matter of just a few seconds. Although LTP was first described in the hippocampus, it can be easily induced in many cortical areas of many different animal species including the human brain [12]. There are a number of different forms of LTP but the best-studied is certainly the one which is triggered by the entry of Ca^{2+} into postsynaptic spines through a subtype of glutamate gated channel, the N-methyl-D-aspartate (NMDA) receptor [13]; for review see Bliss and Collingridge [14]. The NMDA-receptor-mediated LTP, displayed by many different excitatory synapses in the hippocampus (those made by perforant path, Schaffer-collateral, and commissural afferent pathways), can only be elicited by the temporal coincidence of activity in presynaptic boutons to release glutamate and a substantial depolarization of the postsynaptic membrane [14]. This feature arises from the voltage dependency of NMDA channels opening which is caused by external Mg^{2+} blocking the ionic pore of the channel at resting membrane potentials. The Mg^{2+} block can be relieved by a sustained depolarization and this renders the NMDA receptor a miniaturized coincidence detector [15]. The NMDA channel must receive two simultaneous signals: presynaptically released glutamate has to bind to NMDA receptors and, at the same time, the postsynaptic membrane must be depolarized to relieve the voltage-dependent magnesium block of the channel and allow Ca^{2+} entry. In other words, behavioral experiences produce changes in the electrical activity of the brain and these changes take place at the level of connections between neurons that are simultaneously active and these changes are initiated by the opening of NMDA receptors and Ca^{2+} entry in the postsynaptic element. The LTP features of cooperativity, input specificity, and associativity follow mainly from this property [16]. If synaptic plasticity operated only to enhance synaptic efficacy, saturation would eventually ensue. An additional mechanism allowing for activity-dependent depression of synapses should also be postulated to allow some computational flexibility of the synaptic network. It is therefore not surprising that this mechanism indeed exists and has been named long-term depression (LTD). This can be induced by prolonged low-frequency stimulation of the axonal fibers [17]. In the majority of reports, the induction of LTD in the hippocampus can be blocked by NMDA receptor blockers, although in other cortical regions this is not always the case.

In spite of major advances in understanding the mechanisms of induction of NMDA-receptor-mediated LTP and LTD, the cellular and molecular basis of maintenance are much less well understood and debate is still absorbed by the question of where the relevant changes are indeed occurring. These changes might be confined either to the presynaptic terminals, leading to an augmentation or decrement of glutamate exocytosis, or to the postsynaptic apparatus, leading to an increased or decreased sensitivity to neurotransmitter molecules, i.e., glutamate. Evidence has been obtained in support of both possibilities [14]. In addition to these two scenarios, synaptic plasticity might lead to the de novo formation of new synapses. It is envisaged that short-term changes in synaptic strength can only occur at existing synapses, but long-term changes in synaptic strength might be accompanied or fully explained by these morphological rearrangements, via neoformation and/or elimination of synapses [18]. But how long does it take to build a new synapse in the brain? And how long does it take for this newly formed synapse to become mature? Up to 10 years ago much of what was known about the time course of synaptogenesis was based on biochemical experiments from synaptic extracts of in vitro neuronal cultures. These observations led to the concept that glutamatergic synapses were formed over many days [19, 20], hence synaptogenesis could not be easily thought to contribute to the LTP–LTD phenomena. After just a few years the application of advanced brain imaging techniques based on one- or two-photon confocal imaging has shown clearly that synapses can be formed very quickly, on a timescale of just a few minutes to hours [21, 22]; for a recent review see Bhatt *et al.* [23]. Overall the recent findings strongly suggest that the formation and/or removal of individual synaptic connections in response to afferent stimulation occurs and that it is a relatively rapid process, which can contribute to late but also early time points of LTP and LTD. The functional behavior of newly formed synapses, however, depends on a slower developmental process, i.e., the arrival and clustering of specific sets of synaptic molecules at the pre- and postsynaptic specializations. Despite the availability of extraordinary techniques for the morphological imaging of synapses, we are still lacking efficient methods to monitor their activity *in situ* (see below).

Synaptic and axonal changes in multiple sclerosis

In coming to understand the occurrence of any form of synaptic distress in MS and the positive but also negative effects promoted by the activation of synaptic plasticity molecular pathways, is essential not only to appreciate the nature of the CNS degeneration but also to develop more advanced animal models of this disease. The latter are needed to establish a modern therapeutical approach aimed at curing patients but more importantly at protecting and favoring the recovery of distressed neural structures when these have already been stricken by the disease process. Indeed, in the last few years gray matter lesions in MS and in experimental autoimmune encephalomyelitis have received substantial attention despite the scarcity of available results [1, 24–28]; **for review see Geurts and Barkhof** [4]. It has been reported that an axonal pathology starts early in the course of the disease [2] and that the extent of this damage parallels the clinical symptoms of MS patients. Those reports on experimental autoimmune encephalomyelitis, at the present time the most popular animal model of MS with the characteristic autoimmune infiltration of myelin sheaths, clearly show a significant neurodegeneration of axons and synapses [1, 24–28]. This finding might be used as an argument to suggest that the immune attack of myelin sheaths and oligodendrocytes, often unnoticed at early disease stages, might produce effects that propagate at noticeable distances, therefore reaching the gray matter. Although the etiology of the axonal damage seen in MS patients could differ from that occurring in animals with experimental autoimmune encephalomyelitis, some studies suggest that excitotoxicity might contribute to the pathogenesis of both forms of pathologies [4]. In fact increased levels of glutamate have been detected in the cerebrospinal fluid of MS patients to a degree that is correlated with the disease severity. This increased glutamate level in brain tissue might originate either from the weakening of the blood–brain barrier, with brain diffusion of glutamate molecules which are highly concentrated in the blood fluid, from the enhanced activity of brain synapses, or from both phenomena. In this context CNS-infiltrating macrophages and activated microglia may also contribute because these cells can themselves release glutamate but also produce other dangerous molecules including nitric oxide which would feed back onto neurons and synapses further enhancing the release of glutamate from them.

The increased extracellular concentration of glutamate could explain the observed gray matter pathology in MS. Undeniably a brief exposure of neurons to a low concentration of glutamate or glutamate-receptor agonists such as glutamate, NMDA, or kainate (KA) has been known for a long time to result in neuronal damage, often with dramatic changes in the shape of dendrites and axonal arbors. In this respect treatment with NBQX, an AMPA-receptor antagonist, significantly reduces the severity of experimental autoimmune encephalomyelitis, including the axonal degeneration. Interestingly, in the latter condition the CNS inflammation is not diminished [6]. Emerging evidence suggests that with more severe excitotoxic insults the primary site of damage resides in the synaptic structures themselves. Glutamate and the other molecules released in the extracellular space might induce damage per se, a likely scenario when a high concentration of these molecules is reached, but they could also activate the synaptic plasticity cascades we have already described. The activation of this pathway would lead to an augmentation of glutamate exocytosis from synapses located in the area of initial damage. The glutamate release by plastic potentiation of synapses would sum with glutamate molecules already present in the extracellular environment. On one hand more and more synapses would be recruited by this process and on the other hand this positive feedback process might bring glutamate concentration to toxic levels, hence spreading the area of damage in the gray matter. In other words, some of the pathological alterations seen in the brain of MS patients may reflect not simply the primary pathological process but an overcompensatory change of brain tissue propagated by the inflated activation of synaptic plasticity processes. In this respect it is important to consider that the activated cascade could belong to the LTP process described above, but also to another interesting form of synaptic plasticity, the so-called synaptic homeostasis or synaptic scaling [29]. This phenomenon is a form of adaptation of synaptic strength to the global level of network activity sensed over a prolonged period of time. This process might act in a negative but more importantly for us in a positive homeostatic manner: neurons that experience a general low activity can upregulate their synaptic strength while cells that experience an increased stimulation might downregulate these weights. These two forms of plasticity work together, in the sense that individual synaptic weights are regulated by LTP/LTD, while the synaptic volume of all the synapses of an individual neuron are modified by synaptic scaling which does not modify the relative strength of individual terminals [30]. Both depend on similar features of synapses such as their size and previous history of activity. The increase in extracellular glutamate concentration in gray matter of MS brains would certainly trigger both types of plasticity processes and depending on the relative contribution this might alter the stability of the synaptic circuits in the affected areas. While at the beginning of this process relative synaptic weights are likely to be altered, at later time points morphological changes must dominate the picture. In the long term, coordination between these functional and morphological changes of axons and synapses would introduce multiplicative effects on downstream effector circuits, further amplifying the damage.

How can axons and synapses and their plastic changes be assayed in vivo? Recent technical advances

In recent years, the development of one- and two-photon confocal microscope technologies has represented a significant advance for brain imaging. These technologies have allowed unprecedented high-resolution three-dimensional imaging within brain tissue. The one-photon confocal microscope was developed to collect light only from the focal plane, stopping the acquisition of light from other regions located below and above the focal plane. This was achieved by using a laser point source and by collecting the emitted fluorescence through a spatial filter, a pinhole, which corresponds exactly to this focal spot. By scanning on the X–Y–Z axes this illuminated point within the image, an optical section of the brain tissue can be reconstructed. Although one-photon confocal microscopes can generate very high-resolution three-dimensional images, the high intensity of the excitation can produce some tissue damage and also destruction of the fluorescent molecules (photobleaching). These caveats impede the use of confocal microscopes for long-term in vivo imaging of the brain tissue. More recently a further advancement for in vivo brain imaging has been achieved. This is represented by the two-photon confocal microscope [31, 32]. In a two-photon microscope, a fluorescent molecule is excited by a high-intensity laser which is chosen in the infrared spectrum, invisible to the human eye. The light wavelength is selected to be twice the excitation wavelength of the fluorescent molecule of interest. The fluorophore molecule in the focal spot can be pushed to absorb two of these infrared photons simultaneously. Since each of these photons provides half of the necessary excitation energy, the sum of two can fully excite one fluorophore molecule. This excitation event occurs only in the focal spot because its probability depends on the square of the intensity which drops off rapidly away from the focal point. This sharp localization of the excitation and therefore emission produces a sort of optical voxel. If one thinks about the modern radiological brain imaging techniques, where the voxel is in the order of a few square millimeters, then two-photon imaging provides an optical voxel which is below 1 square micrometer, thus reaching a spatial resolution which is 1 billion times greater than those nowadays obtainable by magnetic resonance and other radiological technologies. This technique provides several other advantages [32]. Among these is the fact that infrared radiation penetrates much deeper into brain tissue than visible light, because longer-wavelength photons are less energetic and therefore scatter more weakly. More importantly, infrared radiation is less energetic, and hence causes much less photodamage to brain structures. These factors have permitted extended live imaging over several months of the brain and its synapses in vivo with an unprecedented spatial and time resolution; for review see Svoboda and Yasuda [33], Pan and Gan [34], and Bhatt et al. [23].

But to understand if MS produces any primary or secondary morphological alteration of axons and synapses, how can we effectively use these optical techniques? Also, to visualize potential damage to axons and synapses and to study the relevance and the time course of adaptive plastic changes it would be important to monitor synaptic weights inside the gray matter, before and after the initiation of the disease process. Could this be achieved? If this is not feasible yet for the human brain, can we envisage approaches to the analysis of these issues in the brains of laboratory animals with experimental autoimmune encephalomyelitis? Clearly the application of optical techniques such as those described above would require the neuronal structures to be rendered fluorescent. Therefore, we must ask how can we make axons and synapses fluorescent? It is well known that early in vivo imaging of axons required invasive labeling with vital dyes, such as lipophilic carbocyanide dyes or fluorescent dextrans. Nowadays, thanks to the green fluorescent proteins (GFP) and GFP-based markers this task has been simplified [35]. These GFP molecules can be be attached to specific axonal and synaptic constituents, expressed in defined populations of neuronal cells, and used to visualize in a very simple manner living axons and synapses. Once these neuronal structures are rendered fluorescent, fine analysis of the morphology of axons and synapses, in specific brain areas, before and after the induction of experimental autoimmune encephalomyelitis should be quite straightforward.

What about activity? At early stages of disease synapses might look normal in number and morphology, while there could still be some clear malfunctioning. Synapses release neurotransmitter molecules which are stored in synaptic vesicles, the first step of neuronal communication. These molecules bind to postsynaptic receptors thus generating the postsynaptic potentials. Either the pre- or the postsynaptic events might be altered in animal models of MS. In the last 20 years many novel methodologies have become available that enable the presynaptic aspects of transmission to be studied more directly. Some of these are based on use-dependent labeling or unlabeling of synapses with dyes (for example FM1–43) and antibodies but also smaller peptidic molecules

targeted at intraluminal epitopes of synaptic vesicle proteins. In fact, release of neurotransmitters is achieved by coalescence of the synaptic vesicle membrane with the plasma membrane of the synaptic terminal, i.e., exocytosis, a process that is quickly reversed by endocytosis, i.e., surface membrane withdrawal. These two processes, exocytosis and endocytosis, are supposedly coupled and their balance maintains a stable number of functional synaptic vesicles. Many molecules, including FM1–43 [36], can be introduced in synapses via this endocytic step and used to report presynaptic activity with high fidelity. FM1–43 is an amphiphilic styrylpyridinium molecule, with a lipophilic tail and a positively charged head. The lipophilic tail allows FM1–43 to partition in the plasma membrane but the molecule cannot cross the lipid bilayer of the synaptic vesicle due to the large cationic head. Once incorporated in the membrane, interaction with lipid molecules causes a large increase in brightness with a strong fluorescent staining of the surface of all exposed cells. During release of neurotransmitter through exocytosis, synaptic vesicles briefly expose their internal face to the outside world and FM1–43 stains these membranes before they are recycled back. Because of this, FM1–43 gets trapped inside the synaptic vesicles and stains the nerve terminal. In some experiments, FM1–43 is utilized as a tool to visualize the number and location of living synaptic boutons but, most importantly, FM1–43 has been extensively used for the investigation of the presynaptic activity levels. Similarly antibodies and small peptides can be used to study presynaptic aspects of synaptic transmission. During synaptic communication internal components of synaptic vesicles are briefly exposed at the surface of the presynaptic terminals. Vesicular constituents are then quickly sorted, to exclude protein contaminants of plasma membrane origin, and the efficiency of the recovery process is so high that a few seconds after the vesicle fusion event, these antigens are again fully segregated. On these grounds, in the past we have developed a ratiometric approach to directly monitor changes in presynaptic activity which takes advantage of this cycling exposure of synaptic antigens [37]. Vesicular fusion and recycling are detected by the uptake of a specific antibody directed against the luminal epitope of synaptotagmin-I, an integral component of synaptic vesicles; this epitope is exposed when synaptic communication occurs, i.e., when the synaptic vesicle releases neurotransmitter molecules through exocytosis. Using this assay, levels of activity during two sequential experimental epochs can be monitored separately using two different antibodies followed by independent detection with indirect immunofluorescence. When neurons are exposed to these antibodies for periods ranging from a few minutes to a few hours, synapses take up these molecules and the amount of antibody uptake follows the level of synaptic activity, i.e., of the amount of synaptic communication that has occurred during that period of time. These antibodies can be independently detected using species-specific, fluorescently tagged anti-immunoglobulin secondary antibodies, and synapses can then be watched using a standard one- or two-photon fluorescent confocal microscope. In this way sites of uptake (synapses) can be identified as fluorescent puncta and the relative amount of activity at each individual synapse easily quantified. The spatial resolving power of this method is very valuable in addressing the effects of LTP on presynaptic function but also in the mapping of patterns of stably expressed potentiation in complex neural networks. Comparison of the relative amounts of antibody uptake during consecutive periods provides a means for visualizing changes in synaptic activity in reference to prior basal activity at the same synaptic site. This procedure can be used to address the effect of physiological manipulation, drugs, and toxicants. For example this technique has been extremely useful for examining presynaptic correlates of a long-lasting synaptic potentiation allowing for the first time the direct visualization of an enhancement of presynaptic activity in association with synaptic memory [38]. A major advantage of the present method is its ability to detect changes at the level of single synapses. This offers a way of analyzing synaptic plasticity against a background of great variability within a large population of synapses. Indeed, we found for example that the degree of synaptic memorization is highly heterogeneous, varying inversely with the initial level of activity at individual nerve terminals, as if synapses behave as a sort of quasi-digital devices, with synapses with low or high basal activity that attain a common ceiling upon experience memorization. In order to extend this technology to the intact brain we are now developing a set of functional smaller molecules of greatly reduced size that can penetrate into organized tissue. We hope that soon these molecules will be fully characterized to be used for the investigation of synaptic changes in MS using the various imaging techniques here described.

Conclusions

The approach presented here can provide information that is clearly distinct from that obtained with standard techniques. Such an experimental strategy seems most promising for revealing early changes in gray matter that could lead to the identification of modulators of synaptic connectivities and to the identification of drugs that could promote damage repair. To conclude, we must underline that a valuable goal in neurology is to arrive at a better understanding of how specific neuronal cell types, specific subsets of axons and synapses, do perform *in situ*. Unfortunately this presupposes the ability to track synapses and axons deep in the brain tissue and to reveal their functional behavior in living conditions, before and after the initiation of the MS pathology. We hope that in the near future it will be possible to apply the non-invasive methods described here to the study of MS, thus providing important information on the functional state of synapses in this brain disease and helping to reveal if their possible alterations reflect a primary phenomenon or more simply follow the immune attack.

References

1. Vercellino M, Plano F, Votta B, *et al*. Grey matter pathology in multiple sclerosis. *J Neuropathol Exp Neurol* 2005;**64**:1101–7

2. Dutta R, Trapp B D. Pathogenesis of axonal and neuronal damage in multiple sclerosis. *Neurology* 2007;**68**:S22–S31.

3. Chard D, Miller D. Grey matter pathology in clinically early multiple sclerosis: evidence from magnetic resonance imaging. *J Neurol Sci* 2009;**282**:5–11

4. Geurts J J, Barkhof F. Grey matter pathology in multiple sclerosis. *Lancet Neurol* 2008;**7**:841–51

5. Peterson J W, Bo L, Mork S, *et al*. Transected neurites, apoptotic neurons, and reduced inflammation in cortical multiple sclerosis lesions. *Ann Neurol* 2001;**50**:389–400

6. Bo L, Vedeler C A, Nyland H. Intracortical multiple sclerosis lesions are not associated with increased lymphocyte infiltration. *Mult Scler* 2003;**9**:323–31

7. Konorski J. Conditioned reflexes and neuron organization. Cambridge: Cambridge University Press, 1948.

8. Cajal y Ramón S. Nuevo concepto de la histología de los centros nerviosos. *Rev Ciencias Méd Barcelona* 1892;**18**:361–76, 457–76, 505–20, 529–41

9. Tanzi G. I fatti i le indizioni nell'odierna istologi del sistema nervoso. *Riv Sper Freniatr* 1893;**19**:419–72

10. Hebb D O. The organization of behavior. New York: Wiley, 1949.

11. Bliss T V P, Lomo T. Long-lasting potentiation of synaptic transmission in the dentate area of the anaesthetized rabbit following stimulation of the perforant path. *J Physiol* 1973;**232**:331–56

12. Cooke S F, Bliss T V. Plasticity in the human central nervous system. *Brain* 2006;**129**:1659–73

13. Collingridge G L, Kehl S J, McLennan H. The antagonism of amino acid-induced excitations of rat hippocampal CA1 neurones in vitro. *J Physiol* 1983;**334**:19–31

14. Bliss T V, Collingridge G L. A synaptic model of memory: long-term potentiation in the hippocampus. *Nature* 1993;**361**:31–9

15. Bailey C H, Kandel E R. Structural changes accompanying memory storage. *Annu Rev Physiol* 1993;**55**:397–426

16. Collingridge G L, Kehl S J, McLennan H. The antagonism of amino acid-induced excitations of rat hippocampal CA1 neurones in vitro. *J Physiol* 1983;**334**:19–31

17. Dudek S M, Bear M F. Homosynaptic long-term depression in area CA1 of hippocampus and the effects of NMDA receptor blockade. *Proc Natl Acad Sci USA* 1992;**89**:4363–7

18. Mayer M L, Westbrook G L, Guthrie P B. Voltage-dependent block by $Mg2+$ of NMDA responses in spinal cord neurones. *Nature* 1984;**309**:261–3

19. Lee S H, Sheng M. Development of neuron–neuron synapses. *Curr Opin Neurobiol* 2000;**10**:125–31

20. Rao A, Kim E, Sheng M, Craig A M. Heterogeneity in the molecular composition of excitatory postsynaptic sites during development of hippocampal neurons in culture. *J Neurosci* 1998;**18**:1217–29

21. Ziv N E, Smith S J. Evidence for a role of dendritic filopodia in synaptogenesis and spine formation. *Neuron* 1996;**17**:91–102

22. Lendvai B, Stern E A, Chen B, Svoboda K. Experience-dependent plasticity of dendritic spines in the developing rat barrel cortex in vivo. *Nature* 2000;**404**:876–81

23. Bhatt D H, Zhang S, Gan W B. Dendritic spine dynamics. *Annu Rev Physiol* 2009;**71**:261–82

24. Zhu B, Luo L, Moore G R, Paty D W, Cynader M S. Dendritic and synaptic pathology in experimental autoimmune encephalomyelitis. *Am J Pathol* 2003;**162**:1639–50

25. Marques K B, Santos L M, Oliveira A L. Spinal motoneuron synaptic plasticity during the course of an animal model of multiple sclerosis. *Eur J Neurosci* 2006;**24**:3053–62

26. Jovanova-Nesic K, Shoenfeld Y. MMP-2, VCAM-1 and NCAM-1 expression in the brain of rats with experimental autoimmune encephalomyelitis as a trigger mechanism for synaptic plasticity and pathology. *J Neuroimmunol* 2006;**181**:112–21

27. Wegner C, Esiri M M, Chance S A, Palace J, Matthews P M. Neocortical neuronal, synaptic, and glial loss in multiple sclerosis. *Neurology* 2006;**67**:960–7

28. Vercellino M, Merola A, Piacentino C, *et al.* Altered glutamate reuptake in relapsing–remitting and secondary progressive multiple sclerosis cortex: correlation with microglia infiltration, demyelination, and neuronal and synaptic damage. *J Neuropathol Exp Neurol* 2007;**66**:732–9

29. Turrigiano G G, Leslie K R, Desai N S, Rutherford L C, Nelson S B. Activity-dependent scaling of quantal amplitude in neocortical neurons. *Nature* 1998;**391**:892–6

30. Denk W, Strickler J H, Webb W W. Two-photon laser scanning fluorescence microscopy. *Science* 1990;**248**:73–6

31. Turrigiano G G. AMPA receptors unbound: membrane cycling and synaptic plasticity. *Neuron* 2000;**26**:5–8

32. Helmchen F, Denk W. New developments in multiphoton microscopy. *Curr Opin Neurobiol* 2002;**12**:593–601

33. Svoboda K, Yasuda R. Principles of two-photon excitation microscopy and its applications to neuroscience. *Neuron* 2006;**50**:823–39

34. Pan F, Gan W B. Two-photon imaging of dendritic spine development in the mouse cortex. *Dev Neurobiol* 2008;**68**:771–8

35. Tsien R Y. The green fluorescent protein. *Annu Rev Biochem* 1998;**67**:509–44

36. Betz W J, Bewick G S. Optical anlysis of synaptic vesicle recycling at the frog neuromuscular junction. *Science* 1992;**255**:200–3

37. Malgaroli A, Ting A E, Wendland B, *et al.* Presynaptic component of long-term potentiation visualized at individual hippocampal synapses. *Science* 1995;**268**:1624–8

Chapter

4

Sodium channel expression and function in multiple sclerosis

Lakshmi Bangalore, Joel A. Black, Michael D. Carrithers, and Stephen G. Waxman

Introduction

Multiple sclerosis (MS) is a disease in which damage to and ultimately loss of myelin within the central nervous system (CNS) leaves axons incapable of securely transmitting nerve impulses. Demyelination also causes axons to become vulnerable to irreversible degeneration and may possibly trigger degeneration of their neuronal cell bodies, and thus sets the stage for disease worsening. As might be expected from lesion dissemination, MS is characterized by multiple neurological deficits. It is also characterized by a highly variable pattern of disease progression with some patients displaying a relapsing–remitting course and others displaying a progressive course. In recent years, there has been growing recognition of the role of voltage-gated sodium (Na^+) channels in multiple aspects of MS pathophysiology including remissions, axonal degeneration, immune modulation, and possibly in the abnormal firing of Purkinje neurons and cerebellar dysfunction. Modulation of the expression and activity of Na^+ channels has therefore emerged as a potential approach toward the development of therapies to prevent or limit neurological damage and disability in MS. In this chapter, we discuss Na^+ channel plasticity and the multiple roles of Na^+ channels in the pathophysiology of MS.

Ion channels in myelinated axons

Unlike the slow, continuous, wave-like transmission of action potentials along non-myelinated axons, action potentials in myelinated axons travel in a "saltatory" manner, leaping from one node of Ranvier to another, at remarkable rates of meters per second. Such rapid transmission of action potentials by myelinated axons is due to their molecular and structural specialization. Unlike non-myelinated axons which have uniform properties along their length [1], the molecular architecture of myelinated axons is complex and heterogeneous. While compacted spirals of myelin encase internodal segments of CNS axons and confer a capacitative shield upon them [2], clusters of voltage-gated Na^+ channels with densities in the range of 1000 per μm^2 are present at the nodes of Ranvier where inward transmembrane currents underlie action potential electrogenesis [3, 4]. Interestingly, similar clusters of Na channels are present along the intraretinal portions of the axons of retinal ganglion cells, proximal to the zone (within the optic nerve) where they become myelinated [5]. The high concentration of Na^+ channels at the nodes of Ranvier, in contrast to their meager distribution of less than 25 Na^+ channels per μm^2 along the internodal and paranodal regions beneath the myelin sheath [3, 4, 6], enables the rapid production and transmission of action potentials from one node to another along a myelinated axon. This arrangement also ensures less energy expenditure since the amount of Na^+/K^+ ions that need to be pumped to restore resting ionic concentration is limited due to action potential electrogenesis being confined to the nodes of Ranvier. There are nine subtypes of voltage-gated Na^+ channels known to exist in mammals, and one isoform, namely Na^+ channel Nav1.6, is known to be expressed at high levels along myelinated axons at the nodes of Ranvier (Fig. 4.1) [7].

Na^+ channel plasticity in demyelinated axons

The dense clustering of Na^+ channels at the nodes of Ranvier, and their relative scarcity along the axonal

Multiple Sclerosis: Recovery of Function and Neurorehabilitation, eds. J. Kesselring, G. Comi, and A. J. Thompson.
Published by Cambridge University Press. © Cambridge University Press 2010.

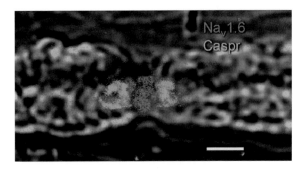

Fig. 4.1. Distribution of Na$^+$ channels in myelinated axons. Of the nine isoforms of voltage-gated Na$^+$ channels known to exist in mammals, one isoform, namely Nav1.6, is clustered at the nodes of Ranvier. Image shows clustering of Nav1.6 channels (red) at a node of Ranvier, and expression of Caspr (green) to mark the paranodal boundary. Expression of Na$^+$ channels is sparse along the paranodal and internodal axon membranes beneath the myelin. Fluorescence and differential contrast images are merged to reveal the myelin sheath. Scale bar = 5 μm. (See also color plate.)

membrane beneath the myelin, has important implications for axonal pathophysiology following demyelination. The low density of Na$^+$ channels in the exposed internodal membrane results in a low density of inward Na$^+$ current that is insufficient for secure action potential electrogenesis, and this interferes with the conduction of action potentials after demyelination [8]. Impedance mismatch further contributes to impaired impulse conduction [9]. Because demyelination is not an all-or-none process, and can range from minimal damage to loss of the entire myelin sheath, it can manifest in a spectrum of conduction abnormalities. These abnormalities, although confined to zones of demyelination with apparently normal conduction in regions proximal and distal to the area of demyelination, can range from slowed and desynchronized conduction, to failure to transmit high-frequency trains of action potentials, to complete blockade of conduction [10, 11].

Endogenous remyelination can occur in MS but it is scarce. However, spontaneous remissions are common, and can occur in the context of persistent demyelination. For example, some patients retain or recover functional visual acuity even while extensive demyelination encompasses extensive territories (>1 cm) of many myelin segments along the entire population of axons within the optic nerve [12, 13]. Recovery of function in such cases can not be supported by mechanisms such as synaptic plasticity or utilization of alternative conduction pathways, and requires restoration of secure action potential

conduction along at least some of the demyelinated axons. Early studies revealed that some chronically demyelinated axons can recover the ability to conduct action potentials in a continuous manner [14], and that, after demyelination, the denuded axon membrane can develop higher-than-normal densities of Na$^+$ channels [15]. Saxitoxin-binding studies also demonstrated a fourfold increase in the number of Na$^+$ channels within demyelinated lesions from MS patients [16]. Subsequent immunocytochemical studies using pan-specific Na$^+$ channel antibodies confirmed the appearance of increased numbers of Na$^+$ channels in experimentally demyelinated axons [17, 18], even though they did not reveal the molecular identity of the Na$^+$ channels along demyelinated axon regions that were previously Na$^+$ channel poor.

Axonal degeneration: Na$^+$ channels as therapeutic targets

Although MS is primarily viewed as a demyelinating disease, it has been recognized for over a century that axons degenerate in MS, and that disease progression, namely, acquisition of persistent, nonremitting neurological deficits, may be due in large part to such degeneration [19, 20]. Studies during the past decade have focused new attention on axonal degeneration in MS, and have underscored its high frequency in both chronic and early lesions, as well as in normal-appearing and peri-plaque white matter [21–24]. Importantly, such studies demonstrated that axonal degeneration produces permanent, non-remitting neurological deficits both in animal models of MS and in human MS [25, 26]. While a number of mechanisms have been proposed to account for axonal degeneration in MS, there is growing evidence that Na$^+$ channels play an important role in the cascade of cellular events that lead to axonal injury.

Early studies on anoxic white matter tracts in vitro indicated that sustained Na$^+$ influx through Na$^+$ channels drives the Na$^+$–Ca^{2+} exchanger to operate in reverse, providing a route for injurious levels of Ca^{2+} to enter the axons where it triggers dissolution of the axonal cytoskeleton and axonal degeneration [27, 28]. The timing of Na$^+$ influx and the prolonged effect of tetrodotoxin (TTX) suggest the involvement of a persistent (non-inactivating) Na$^+$ conductance, and in fact a TTX-sensitive persistent conductance can be measured along the trunks of optic nerve axons [29]. Electron microscopy analysis has demonstrated a continuous rise in intra-axonal Na^+ which is paralleled by a rise in Ca^{2+} levels within anoxic myelinated axons [28].

Energy insufficiency, unrestrained Na^+ influx, and escalation of neuronal damage

A number of studies have demonstrated that an energy-deficient state may arise in MS such that ATP levels within axons become diminished. Nitric oxide (NO) which is present at increased concentrations within acute MS lesions [30] has a negative effect on mitochondria [31, 32]. Kapoor *et al.* [33] proposed that NO-induced damage of mitochondria reduces ATP levels and thereby causes a gradual rundown of Na^+/K^+ ATPase which in turn limits the ability of axons to extrude Na^+. Such a proposal would predict that blockers of Na^+ entry would protect axons from NO-induced injury, and Kapoor *et al.* showed that this is indeed the case. Further support for the idea that Na^+ influx after exposure to NO strains the ability of ATP-dependent mechanisms for Na^+ extrusion comes from studies in which TTX application was shown to preserve ATP levels with concomitant protection of white matter axons from NO-induced injury [34].

Another link to energy failure has been provided by a recent study of gene expression levels in postmortem brain tissue from MS patients which demonstrated decreased mRNA levels for nuclear-encoded mitochondrial genes in MS lesions [32]; notably, the activities of respiratory gene complexes I and III (membrane-bound redox carriers within mitochondria that have essential roles in electron transport and thereby in ATP production) were decreased in this tissue, suggesting that the changes could have functional significance in MS. This study also revealed fragmented neurofilaments, depolymerized microtubules, and reduced organelle content within residual demyelinated axons, suggestive of Ca^{2+}-mediated axonal injury. On the basis of these results, the authors of the study proposed that an inadequate axonal ATP supply contributes to the degeneration of demyelinated axons in MS because it impairs Na^+/K^+ ATPase activity, and thereby limits or prevents extrusion of axoplasmic Na^+ [32].

Identity of Na^+ channels along myelinated and demyelinated axons

Recent studies using isoform-specific antibodies have shown that both the Nav1.2 and Nav1.6 isoforms of channels are expressed in the CNS along normal myelinated axons and their premyelinated precursors, but that each isoform is present at different stages of development. During early development, before glial ensheathment, a low density of Na^+ channels [35], identified as Nav1.2 channels [36, 37], is present along the entire length of premyelinated central axons where they support action potential propagation prior to myelination [38, 39]. Nav1.2 channels are also expressed diffusely along mature non-myelinated CNS axons [36, 40, 41]. As myelination proceeds, there is a gradual loss of Nav1.2 channels and an aggregation of Nav1.6 channels at mature nodes of Ranvier [36, 37], such that mature myelinated axons contain few if any Nav1.2 channels, with Nav1.6 being the predominant Na^+ channel isoform at fully formed nodes of Ranvier [7]. Immunocytochemical studies in experimental autoimmune encephalomyelitis (EAE) [42] and in rapid postmortem MS tissue from acute lesions [43] have demonstrated that Nav1.2 Na^+ channels are diffusely distributed along extensive lengths of some demyelinated axons, and Nav1.6 along extensive lengths of other demyelinated axons (Fig. 4.2).

Nav1.2 and Nav1.6 in experimental autoimmune encephalomyelitis

Experimental autoimmune encephalomyelitis (EAE) is a commonly used model of MS in which animals are inoculated with components of the white matter to induce an inflammatory disorder that includes demyelination and axonal degeneration. The Na^+ channel isoforms expressed along demyelinated axons in EAE have recently been identified in studies that used subtype-specific antibodies. These studies revealed upregulated expression of Nav1.2 and Nav1.6 over long stretches of demyelinated CNS axons in EAE, with domains of Nav1.2 or Nav1.6 immunoreactivity extending for tens of micrometers along tracts such as the optic nerve and dorsal columns. Increased levels of Nav1.2 channel mRNA within retinal ganglion cells, the cell bodies of optic nerve axons, indicated that neuronal transcription of the gene encoding Nav1.2 channels was upregulated [42].

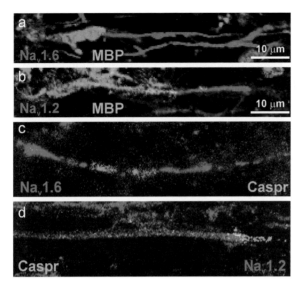

Fig. 4.2. Expression of Nav1.6 and Nav1.2 channels along demyelinated axons in active MS lesions within spinal cord tissue. Residual damaged myelin (green) can be seen next to extensive regions of diffuse expression of Nav1.6 channels (red; a) and Nav1.2 channels (red; b). Such regions of Nav1.6 channel (red; c) or Nav1.2 channel (red; d) expression in some axons are bounded by contactin-associated protein (Caspr; green), without overlap, consistent with the expression of Nav1.6 and Nav1.2 channels in the demyelinated axon membrane. (Reproduced with permission from Craner *et al.* [43] © 2004 National Academy of Sciences.) (See also color plate.)

Studies have also shown an extensive distribution of Nav1.2 channels, for tens of micrometers along demyelinated but apparently uninjured axons in EAE [44], a pattern that is similar to the diffuse distribution of Nav1.2 channels along premyelinated axons [36] and non-myelinated axons in the CNS [40, 45, 46]. Action potential conduction is known to occur along these fibers [38, 39], suggesting that Nav1.2 might support this function. Nav1.2 channels display activation and availability (steady-state inactivation) properties that are more depolarized than for Nav1.6 channels so that Nav1.2 channels show less inactivation with modest depolarization. Nav1.2 channels, however, show greater accumulation of inactivation, and thus are less available to open and contribute to action potentials at high frequencies (20–100 Hz) [47].

These observations suggest that Nav1.2 channels might support action potential conduction along demyelinated axons even in the context of any depolarization that occurs in the fibers as a result of injury, but that conduction in these axons would be limited to lower frequencies. Importantly, Nav1.6

channels produce a larger persistent current than Nav1.2 channels [47]. Therefore, demyelinated axons expressing Nav1.6 would be expected to be subjected to a larger sustained Na^+ influx, a factor that could encourage their degeneration, as has been observed and described below in immunohistochemical studies of EAE and MS [43, 44].

Several lines of evidence suggest a link between aberrant Nav1.6 expression and axonal injury in EAE. As described above, sustained Na^+ influx through Na^+ channels can trigger Ca^{2+}-dependent mechanisms of white matter injury by driving the reverse operation of Na^+–Ca^{2+} exchanger [48]. Since Nav1.6 channels produce a larger persistent current than Nav1.2 channels [47], co-expression of Nav1.6 channels and the Na^+–Ca^{2+} exchanger would be expected to predispose demyelinated axons to import injurious levels of Ca^{2+}. To determine whether Nav1.6 channels and the Na^+–Ca^{2+} exchanger are, in fact, co-expressed in degenerating axons in EAE, Craner *et al.* [44] immunolocalized these molecules and β-amyloid precursor protein (β-APP), a marker of axonal injury, in spinal cord axons from mice with EAE. They showed that 92% of β-APP-positive axons in EAE express Nav1.6 (either alone [56%] or co-expressed with Nav1.2 [36%]); by contrast, less than 2% of β-APP-positive axons express Nav1.2 in the absence of Nav1.6. Co-expression of Nav1.6 and the Na^+–Ca^{2+} exchanger was seen in 74% of β-APP-positive axons, in contrast to only 4% of β-APP-negative axons. Thus, Nav1.6 and the Na^+–Ca^{2+} exchanger are co-expressed in injured CNS axons in EAE (Fig. 4.3A).

Nav1.2 and Nav1.6 in multiple sclerosis

Although direct analysis of human tissue is necessary for improved understanding of MS, it is challenging because brain tissue is rarely biopsied in patients with MS or suspected MS and because the time lag of usually at least a few hours between death and removal of tissue for postmortem study limits the utility of postmortem tissue for molecular analysis. Further complications are introduced by lesion-to-lesion variability, both between patients and within patients [49]. Nevertheless, some clues can be gleaned from a recent analysis of spinal cord and optic nerve tissue obtained by rapid autopsy of patients who died with a disabling secondary progressive MS [43].

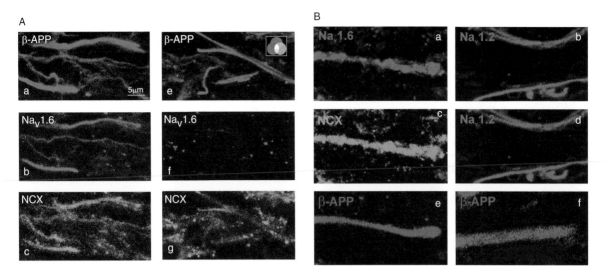

Fig. 4.3. (a) Co-expression of the sodium–calcium exchanger (NCX) and Nav1.6 along extensive regions of spinal cord axons that are immunopositive for β-APP, a marker of neuronal injury, in EAE. These digital images of immunostaining reveal β-APP (blue; a, e), sodium channel Nav1.6 (red; b) or Nav1.2 (red; f) and NCX (green; c, g) immunostaining in EAE spinal cord axons. Panels a, b, and c show co-expression of Nav1.6, NCX with β-APP, a marker of axonal injury. In contrast, panels e, f, and g demonstrate β-APP- and NCX-positive profiles but absence of Nav1.2 immunostaining (magnification 1800×). (Modified with permission from Craner *et al.* [44] © 2004 Oxford University Press.) (B) Co-expression of NCX and Nav1.6 along extensive regions of β-APP-positive spinal cord axons in acute MS lesions. These digital immunofluroscent images of axons in MS spinal cord white matter reveal the presence of β-APP (e and f; blue), Nav1.6 (a; red) or Nav1.2 (b; red) and NCX (c and d; green). Panels a, c, and e show co-expression of Nav1.6 and NCX in axons displaying β-APP. In contrast, panels b, d, and f demonstrate NCX-positive immunostaining but the absence of Nav1.2 immunostaining within β-APP-positive axons, and the co-expression of NCX and Nav1.2 in β-APP-negative axons. (Modified with permission from Craner *et al.* [43] © 2004 National Academy of Sciences.) (See also color plate.)

Acute MS lesions in this study displayed a pattern of Na$^+$ channel expression similar to that seen in EAE. Control white matter showed foci of Nav1.6 expression at the nodes of Ranvier, but not in the internodes. In contrast, acute MS lesions (which could be identified on the basis of attenuated myelin basic protein (MBP) immunostaining, evidence of inflammation, and recent phagocytosis of myelin) displayed Nav1.6 and Nav1.2 expression along extensive regions of demyelinated axons, often in the order of tens of micrometers (Fig. 4.2). Zones of Nav1.6 or Nav1.2 channel immunostaining in some cases were bounded by damaged myelin or contactin associated protein (Caspr), a constituent of paranodal domains [50], confirming the identity of these profiles as axons in which myelin was damaged. Thus, Nav1.6 and Nav1.2 were identified as the Na$^+$ channel isoforms expressed along demyelinated axons in both EAE and MS.

This study also examined Na$^+$ channel expression in β-APP-positive axons in these MS lesions and found that almost all β-APP immunopositive axons in MS lesions were associated with stretches of Nav1.6 expression; by contrast, few β-APP immunopositive axons expressed Nav1.2 immunostaining [43]. Nav1.6 and the Na$^+$–Ca^{2+} exchanger tended to be co-localized in β-APP-positive axons within the MS lesions that were studied (Fig. 4.3B). Thus, as in EAE, Nav1.6 and the Na$^+$–Ca^{2+} exchanger appear to be co-expressed in injured axons in MS.

The findings described above have led to the examination of therapeutic strategies that employ Na$^+$ channel blockers, inhibitors of the Na$^+$–Ca^{2+} exchanger, and inhibitors of downstream calcium-dependent proteases that target various elements of the cascade of axonal destruction. Tetrodotoxin (TTX) [27], quaternary and tertiary local anesthetics such as QX-314, QX-222, lidocaine, and procaine [51], phenytoin, carbamezepine [52], and mexilitine [53] have been shown to protect white matter myelinated axons from anoxic injury in vitro.

The Na$^+$ channel blockers phenytoin [54], flecainaide [55], and lamotrigine [56] have been shown to have a protective effect in experimental rodent models of MS, i.e., EAE, where they prevent degeneration of CNS axons, maintain impulse conduction,

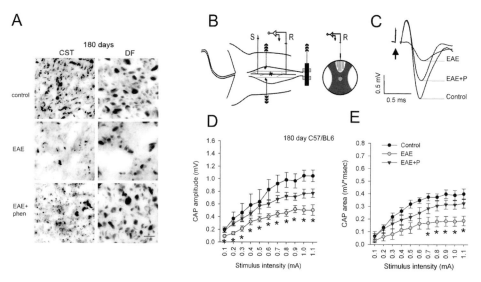

Fig. 4.4. Phenytoin is neuroprotective when administered for 180 days to mice with EAE. Neurofilament staining of dorsal CST and DF from normal (A; top), EAE (A; middle) and EAE+phenytoin (A; bottom) C57/BL6 mice at 180 days after myelin oligodendrocyte glycoprotein (MOG) injection reveals substantial loss of axons in cerebrospinal tract (CST) and dorsal funiculus (DF) in EAE compared with normal animals. Phenytoin-treated EAE (EAE+phen) show significantly more axons in the CST and DF than the untreated controls. Panel B shows a schematic of spinal cord recording configuration with stimulating (S) and recording (R) electrodes placed at L1–L2 and T4–T5, respectively; schematic to the right shows a cross-section of the spinal cord with the recording electrode at the surface of the dorsal median funiculus, overlying the dorsal columns. Panel C shows superimposed CAP recordings elicited with 1.1 mA stimulus intensity from representative normal, EAE, and EAE+phenytoin (EAE+P) C57/BL6 mice at 180 days post-MOG injection; arrow indicates stimulus artifact. Panel D shows CAP amplitudes elicited by stimulus intensities of 0.1–1.1 mA for normal, EAE, and EAE+phenytoin in C57/BL6 mice at 180 days post-MOG injection. Panel E shows CAP areas elicited by stimulus intensity of 0.1–1.1 mA for normal, EAE, and EAE+phenytoin in C57/BL6 mice at 180 days post-MOG injection. Significant differences ($p < 0.05$) between EAE and EAE+P animals are indicated by asterisks. (Reproduced, with permission, from Black *et al.* [57] © 2006 Oxford University Press.)

and improve clinical outcome as long as their administration continues, for as long as 180 days in some studies [57]. For example, continuous administration of phenytoin reduces the loss of dorsal corticospinal axons from 63% to 25% and of cuneate fasciculus axons from 43% to 17% as assessed 28–30 days after disease onset [54]. Electrophysiological recordings show that axonal conduction is maintained in a significant fraction of the surviving axons (Fig. 4.4). Importantly, animals treated with these Na^+ channel blockers display improved clinical outcome. Recent studies [57] have shown that the protective effect of phenytoin on axons and clinical improvement persists when administration of phenytoin is continued for as long as 180 days following treatment.

An unexpected effect of Na^+ channel blockade, however, was introduced by the observation in C57/BL6 mice with MOG-induced EAE that sudden withdrawal of phenytoin could result in clinical exacerbation associated with increased inflammatory activity. In these experiments abrupt withdrawal of phenytoin on day 28 post-EAE

induction, after a period of continuous treatment (with plasma levels within the human therapeutic range, during which there was less inflammatory activity, less axonal loss, and improved clinical status, compared to untreated mice with EAE), was followed by rapid clinical worsening including death of more than 50% of mice in the first week post-withdrawal (Fig. 4.5A), together with significantly increased inflammatory (macrophages/microglia, and T lymphocytes) infiltrate (Fig. 4.5B) [58]. Exacerbation of this type was not seen after abrupt withdrawal of phenytoin from healthy (no EAE) mice [58] or after gradual withdrawal (7-day taper) of phenytoin from mice with EAE (Black and Waxman, unpublished observations). Black *et al.* [58] also demonstrated that the Na^+ channel blocker carbamazepine exerts a protective effect in EAE, as long as it is given, but that, as with phenytoin, abrupt withdrawal of carbamazepine from mice with EAE induced by myelin oligodendrocyte glycoprotein (MOG) was accompanied by acute exacerbation, associated with a significantly increased CNS inflammatory infiltrate including

A

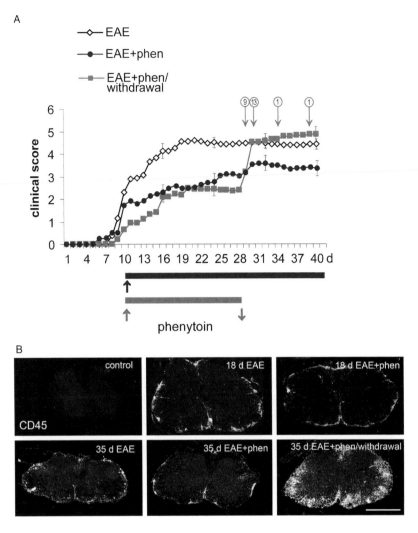

Fig. 4.5. Abrupt withdrawal of phenytoin worsens clinical status in EAE. Panel A shows mean clinical scores for C57/BL6 mice with untreated EAE (diamonds), EAE+phenytoin (circles), and EAE+phenytoin/withdrawal (squares). Phenytoin treatment is indicated by black (continuous treatment) and gray (withdrawal) bars. Phenytoin-treated mice (EAE+phenytoin) exhibit significantly lower clinical scores when compared with untreated mice on all days after day 12 (asterisks omitted for clarity). Abrupt withdrawal of phenytoin, at day 28, results in rapid deterioration of clinical scores. Numbers above the arrows indicate deaths at each post-withdrawal time period. No deaths occurred in untreated EAE and EAE+phenytoin mice from days 28 to 40. Standard error bars are shown only for days 16, 24, 32, and 40 for clarity, but they are representative. Panel B shows cross-sections through lumbar spinal cords labeled for CD45 in control, EAE 18 days after MOG injection (18 d EAE), EAE+phenytoin 18 days after injection (18 d EAE+phen), EAE 35 days after injection (35 d EAE), and 35-day EAE+phenytoin/withdrawal (35 d EAE+phen/withdrawal) mice. Withdrawal of phenytoin is accompanied by a substantial CD45+infiltrate into the spinal cord; the immune infiltrate is significantly greater after phenytoin withdrawal compared with untreated EAE at 18 or 35 days after injection. Scale bar = 500 μm. (Reproduced, with permission, from Black *et al.* [58], © 2007 American Neurological Association.)

activated macrophages/microglia in addition to T lymphocytes. There were no adverse effects of withdrawal of carbamazepine from healthy mice without EAE.

Na⁺ channels and immune modulation

Although a direct neuroprotective effect of Na⁺ channel blockers on axons is well established, the findings outlined above suggest the possibility that Na⁺ channel blockers may also be protective in neuroinflammatory disorders via an immunomodulatory action. While Na⁺ channels have been extensively studied as "neuronal" molecules, there is emerging evidence that they are present in, and may regulate the activity of,

microglia and macrophages [59, 60], two types of immune cells that contribute to CNS injury in EAE and MS. Microglia and macrophages are closely associated with degenerating axons in MS [21, 22, 61], and produce axonal injury by multiple mechanisms, including induction of CD4+ T cell proliferation [62], production of pro-inflammatory cytokines [63] and NO [64, 65], antigen presentation [66], and phagocytosis [67]. Immunocytochemical studies by Craner *et al.* [59] have shown that Nav1.6 channels are indeed present in microglia, and that their levels are increased during activation in EAE. Their studies on Nav1.6 also demonstrated that it is upregulated within microglia and macrophages in acute lesions of MS patients compared with control patients without neurological disease.

Control   **EAE**   **EAE-Phenytoin**

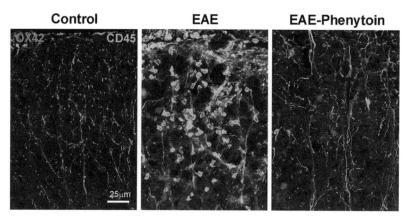

Fig. 4.6. Phenytoin treatment reduces inflammatory response in EAE. Digital images of control, EAE, and phenytoin-treated EAE spinal cord immunostained for anti-CD45 (green), anti-OX42 (blue). Middle panel (EAE) shows a significant increase in the number of immune cells (CD45 and/or OX42 immunopositive) compared with untreated control (left). Administration of phenytoin to EAE mice results in a significant reduction of inflammatory infiltrate (right). (Modified with permission from Craner *et al.* [59] © 2005 Wiley-Liss, Inc.) (See also color plate.)

To test whether Na^+ channels are important for the function of macrophages and microglia, Craner *et al.* [59] examined the effect of Na^+ channel blockade on the activity of these cells, and found a 40% reduction in phagocytic activity of cultured microglia following exposure to TTX and a 75% decrease in the number of inflammatory cells in EAE during treatment with phenytoin (Fig. 4.6). They also found that activation of microglia harvested from med mice (which lack functional Nav1.6) is reduced compared with wild-type mice (in which Nav1.6 is present), and showed that the suppressing effect of TTX on microglial activation is not present in med mice, confirming a role for Nav1.6 in microglial activation. Craner *et al.* [59] also found that treatment with phenytoin substantially reduced the inflammatory cell infiltrate in EAE, a finding that has been confirmed for both phenytoin and carbamazepine by Black *et al.* [58]. Bechtold *et al.* [55] also noted a protective effect of flecainide on neurological symptoms early in the course of EAE (10–13 days post disease induction) and suggested a possible immunmodulatory effect.

More recent studies by Carrithers *et al.* [60] on human macrophages have demonstrated the presence of Nav1.5 channels on endosomes, (but not the plasma membrane) of these cells (Fig. 4.7), and have shown that these endosomal Nav1.5 channels provide a route for Na^+ efflux that is associated with endosomal acidification, thus regulating phagocytosis in primed macrophages (Fig. 4.8). Nav1.6 channels are also present intracellularly within macrophages, where they are associated with cytoskeletal structures such as actin stress fibers and the intermediate filament vimentin [60].

The mechanism(s) underlying the rebound exacerbation after sudden withdrawal of sodium channel blockers in MOG-induced EAE in C57/BL6 mice are not yet understood, nor is it known whether these results can be extrapolated to other models of EAE, or to human MS, or other Na^+ channel blockers. While a substantial number of MS patients have been treated (e.g., for trigeminal neuralgia) with carbamezepine and phenytoin and there have been no reports of apparent adverse events following withdrawal of these drugs in these patients, the possibility of more subtle long-term changes in their immune status has not been examined. Irrespective of the underlying mechanisms, the data available thus far suggest that, in addition to assessing the neuroprotective actions, the potential long-term effects of Na^+ channel blockers, and their withdrawal, should be considered in the design of trials of these agents in neuroinflammatory disorders.

Nav1.8 in the cerebellum in multiple sclerosis

Although demyelination and axonal degeneration are considered primary causes of the many clinical abnormalities observed in MS, some observations suggest that molecular pathology of intact neurons, i.e., dysregulation of ion channel expression that leads to mistuning of intact neurons, may contribute to some clinical abnormalities [68]. Clinical abnormalities in MS due to cerebellar dysfunction are unusual in that they tend to be persistent, even early in the course of the disease, in contrast to other types of clinical deficits which tend to be remitting [69]. Cerebellar dysfunction is also occasionally observed in patients with MS in whom demyelinated lesions in the cerebellum cannot be visualized through neuroimaging. In addition, occasional patients with MS have

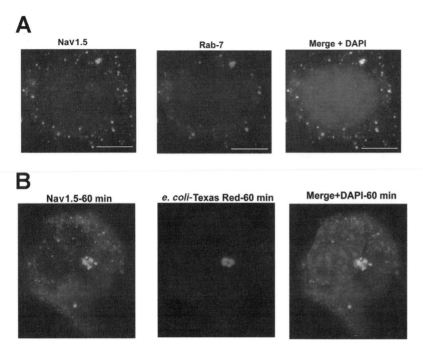

Fig. 4.7. Co-localized expression of Nav1.5 with late endosomal marker Rab-7 (A) and with internalized Texas Red-labeled *E. coli* (B). Nav1.5-positivity (A and B; left panels; green) in differentiated THP-1 cells primed with INF-γ and LPS co-localizes with late endosomal marker Rab-7 (A, middle panel; red) and with internalized Texas Red-labeled *E. coli* 60 minutes following bacterial challenge. Merged images are shown on the right, with DAPI (4′,6′-diamidino-2-phenylindole) stained nuclei (blue). (Modified with permission from Carrithers *et al.* [60] © 2007 by The American Association of Immunologists, Inc.) (See also color plate.)

paroxysmal bouts of ataxia similar to those seen in the episodic ataxias, a group of disorders caused by hereditary channelopathies, and the paroxysmal attacks have been reported to respond favorably to treatment with Na^+ channel blockers such as carbamazepine [70, 71].

Black *et al.* investigated the deployment of abnormal repertoires of ion channels that could alter the electrical signaling capability of cerebellar neurons and demonstrated an upregulated expression of Na^+ channel Nav1.8 within the cerebellar Purkinje cells of the Taiep rat [72], a dysmyelinating model in which myelin ensheaths CNS axons but subsequently degenerates due to an inherited abnormality of the oligodendrocytes. They subsequently employed *in situ* hybridization and immunocytochemical methods to examine the cerebellum of mice with EAE and humans with progressive MS, and observed the presence within Purkinje cells of Nav1.8 mRNA and protein, which are not present in normal Purkinje neurons (Fig. 4.9A) [73]. They showed that annexin II/p11, a protein that binds to the amino (N)-terminus of Nav1.8 and facilitates insertion of functional Nav1.8 channels into the neuronal cell membrane [74], is also upregulated within Purkinje cells in EAE and MS, and colocalizes with Nav1.8 (Fig. 4.9A) [75]. The coordinated upregulation of Nav1.8 and its binding partner annexin II/p11 suggest that functional

Nav1.8 channels could be inserted into Purkinje cell membranes in MS and its animal models.

Na^+ channel Nav1.8 was initially termed SNS, or Sensory Neuron Specific, because it is selectively expressed in the dorsal root ganglion neurons of the healthy nervous system. Nav1.8 is different from other Na^+ channels in that it is relatively resistant to TTX, and displays a steady-state inactivation with voltage dependence that is more depolarized than for other Na^+ channel isoforms – a property that enables these channels to remain open even when the cell membrane is depolarized to an extent where other Na^+ channel isoforms are inactivated [76, 77]. Another unique feature of Nav1.8 is its rapid recovery from inactivation [78, 79], a feature that enables it to activate repetitively in a pattern that can support high-frequency action potential activity. Nav1.8 produces most of the current underlying the depolarizing upstroke of the action potential in cells in which it is expressed [80, 81], and supports repetitive firing even when depolarization inactivates the other Na^+ channels present in these cells [80].

Action potential electrogenesis in Purkinje neurons is strongly dependent on the activity of Na^+ channels [82–84]. Mutations in Na^+ channels that are normally expressed within Purkinje neurons produce substantial changes in the patterns of firing in these cells, which can result in clinical cerebellar

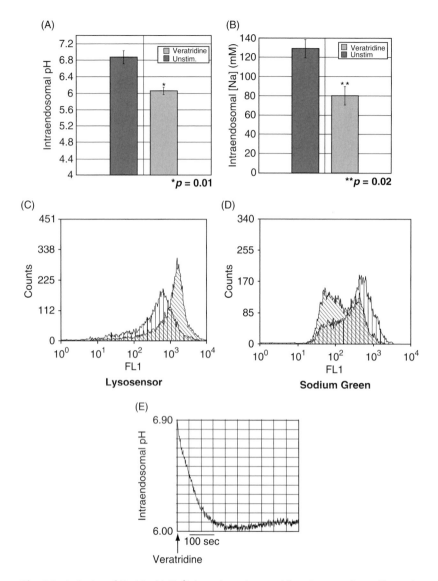

Fig. 4.8. Activation of Nav1.5 with Na$^+$ channel agonist veratridine triggers sodium efflux and protein influx in purified endosomes derived from THP-1 cells, a human monocyte cell line. Panels A and B show intraendosomal pH and [Na] as determined by flow cytometry with dyes Lysosensor Green DND-189 (1 μM) and Sodium Green (4 μM). The endosome gate was deteremined with 0.5 μM fluorescent beads before each experiment. Following stimulation with veratridine (100 μM) for 30 mins, the intraendosomal pH declined from 6.89 ± 0.16 to 6.05 ± 0.85 ($p = 0.01$, $n = 6$) (panel A), and the intraendosomal [Na] decreased from 129 ± 9.5 mM in the unstimulated condition to 80.3 ± 9.6 mM ($p = 0.02$, $n = 3$). Panels C–E, isolated endosomes were equilibrated in K$^+$-free intracellular buffer (140 mM CsF, 10 mM NaCl, 1 mM EGTA, and 10 mM HEPES) by dialysis and then loaded with functional dyes for 30 min. C, endosomes were loaded with the pH-sensitive dye Lysosensor Green DND-189 (1 μM) and subsequently analyzed in the presence or absence of veratridine (100 μM). Stimulation for 30 min resulted in a mean fluorescent shift from a fluorescent intensity of 608 (unstimulated, dark vertical lines) to 1540 (stimulated, light diagonal lines), demonstrating decreased intraendosomal pH. D, in endosomes loaded with Sodium Green (4 μM), veratridine stimulation caused decreased fluorescence (decreased intraendosomal sodium). Mean fluorescence was 535 in unstimulated condition (light diagonal lines). E, time-resolved fluorometry demonstrated that the effect of veratridine in acidification occurs very rapidly in isolated endosomes. (Modified with permission from Carrithers *et al.* [60] © 2007 by The American Association of Immunologists, Inc.)

dysfunction, including ataxia [84, 85]. Electrophysiological recordings from Purkinje neurons transfected with Nav1.8 in vitro [86] indicate that expression of Nav1.8 can substantially alter their pattern of firing, and in vivo recordings suggest that similar changes occur in Purkinje cells in mice with EAE [87]. The

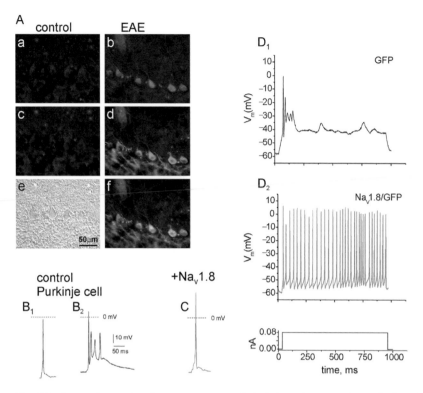

Fig. 4.9. Abnormal expression of sensory neuron specific Na$^+$ channel Nav1.8 within cerebellar Purkinje neurons in MS and EAE. Nav1.8 channel (red, Ab), and annexinII/p11 (Ad), a binding partner which facilitates the insertion of functional Nav1.8 channels into the cell membrane, exhibit co-localized expression (merged image, yellow, Af) in the Purkinje cells of EAE mice. Neither molecule can be detected within control Purkinje neurons (Aa, Ac, Ae). Nav1.8 expression alters action potential electrogenesis in Purkinje neurons as shown in B$_1$, B$_2$, and C. Current clamp recordings show spontaneous action potentials in control Purkinje neurons lacking Nav1.8 (B$_1$, B$_2$), and 2 days after transfection with Nav1.8 (C). Action potentials in control Purkinje neurons lacking Nav1.8 (B$_1$) show less overshoot (dotted lines indicate 0 mV) and tend to be conglomerate, consisting of two or more spikes in 62% of cells (B$_2$). By contrast, conglomerate action potentials contain fewer spikes and are far less common (15%) in Purkinje cells that express Nav1.8 (C). Purkinje neurons transfected with Nav1.8 show sustained repetitive firing (D$_2$; middle), not present in the absence of Nav1.8 (D$_1$; top), in response to the injection of a depolarizing current (D, bottom). GFP, green fluorescent protein; Vm, membrane potential. (Panels Aa–Af reproduced, with permission, from Craner *et al.* [75] © (2003) Lippincott, Williams & Wilkins. Panels B–D reproduced, with permission, from Renganathan *et al.* [86] © (2003) Elsevier Science.) (See also color plate.)

firing patterns of Purkinje neurons that are transfected in vitro with Nav1.8 are altered in several ways [86]: first, by increased action potential duration and amplitude; second, by fewer action potentials that consist of multiple spikes and a reduction in the number of spikes in these conglomerate action potentials; and third, by the generation of sustained, pacemaker-like impulse trains in response to depolarization, which are not seen in the absence of Nav1.8 (Fig. 4.9, panels B and C). Unit recordings suggest that similar changes in firing patterns of Purkinje cells occur in mice with EAE [87].

The trigger for abnormal expression of Nav1.8 within Purkinje cells in MS and its animal models is not known. Interestingly, levels of nerve growth factor (NGF), which is known to activate transcription of the Nav1.8 gene [88, 89], are increased in humans with MS [90] and in animal models of MS, and there is a concomitant increase in the expression of the neurotrophin receptor p75 [91]. Reasoning that NGF might trigger the abnormal expression of Nav1.8 in Purkinje cells in EAE and MS, Damarjian *et al.* [92] examined the relationship between upregulation of Nav1.8 and expression of the NGF receptors p75 and TrkA in the cerebellum in EAE. Consistent with previous studies [93, 94], they observed low levels of p75 and TrkA in control Purkinje neurons; they also observed a significant upregulation of p75 within Purkinje cells in EAE, with a high level of expression of p75 in Purkinje cells that expressed Nav1.8. These observations suggest that NGF could trigger abnormal expression of Nav1.8 within Purkinje cells in EAE and MS.

Some support for this hypothesis is provided by the observation that antisense knockdown of p75 reduces disease severity in EAE [95].

Clinical cerebellar deficits (e.g., cerebellar ataxia, intention tremor) tend not to remit, and can be disabling. On the basis of the results described above, it has been suggested that Na^+ channel blockers, especially blockers that target Nav1.8, may provide symptomatic relief for cerebellar dysfunction in MS [68]. Because expression of Nav1.8 is confined to dorsal root ganglion neurons, dose-limiting side effects would be limited to sensory abnormalities and would not be expected to include cardiac or CNS depression. When Nav1.8-specific blockers become available (an event that has become increasingly likely because of the important role of Nav1.8 in pain), a conservative strategy would be first to examine their effects on Purkinje neurons transfected with Nav1.8 in vitro [86], and then to examine their effects on firing patterns of Purkinje cells in EAE [87]. If this approach was shown to be efficacious in these in vitro and whole animal models, carefully controlled studies could then be carried out in MS patients with cerebellar deficits.

References

1. Black J A, Foster R E, Waxman S G. Freeze-fracture ultrastructure of rat CNS and PNS nonmyelinated axolemma. *J Neurocytol* 1981;**10**:981–93

2. Waxman S G, Swadlow H A. Ultrastructure of visual callosal axons in the rabbit. *Exp Neurol* 1976;**53**(1):115–27

3. Ritchie J M, Rogart R B. The density of sodium channels in mammalian myelinated nerve fibers and the nature of the axonal membrane under the myelin sheath. *Proc Natl Acad Sci USA* 1977;**74**:211–15

4. Waxman S G. Conduction in myelinated, unmyelinated, and demyelinated fibers. *Arch Neurol* 1977;**34**:585–90

5. Hildebrand C, Waxman S G. Regional node-like membrane specializations in non-myelinated axons of rat retinal nerve fiber layer. *Brain Res* 1983;**258**:23–32

6. Shrager P. Sodium channels in single demyelinated mammalian axons. *Brain Res* 1989;**483**:149–54

7. Caldwell J H, Schaller K L, Lasher R S, Peles E, Levinson S R. Sodium channel Na(v)1.6 is localized at nodes of ranvier, dendrites, and synapses. *Proc Natl Acad Sci USA* 2000;**97**(10):5616–20

8. Waxman S G. Current concepts in neurology: membranes, myelin and the pathophysiology of multiple sclerosis. *New Engl J Med* 1982;**306**:1529–33

9. Waxman S G, Brill M H. Conduction through demyelinated plaques in multiple sclerosis: computer simulations of facilitation by short internodes. *J Neurol Neurosurg Psychiatry* 1978;**41**:408–17

10. McDonald W I. The effects of experimental demyelination on conduction in peripheral nerve: a histological and electrophysiological study – electrophysiological observations. *Brain* 1963;**86**:501–24

11. McDonald W I, Sears T A. The effects of experimental demyelination on conduction in the central nervous system. *Brain* 1970;**93**:583–98

12. Ulrich J, Groebke–Lorenz W. The optic nerve in multiple sclerosis: a morphological study with retrospective clinicopathological correlation. *Neurol Ophthalmol* 1983;**3**:149–59

13. Wisniewski H M, Oppenheimer D, McDonald W E. Relation between myelination and function in MS and EAE. *J Neuropathol Exp Neurol* 1976;**35**:327

14. Bostock H, Sears T A. The internodal axon membrane: electrical excitability and continuous conduction in segmental demyelination. *J Physiol Lond* 1978;**280**:273–301

15. Foster R E, Whalen C C, Waxman S G. Reorganization of the axonal membrane of demyelinated nerve fibers: morphological evidence. *Science* 1980;**210**:661–3

16. Moll C, Mourre C, Lazdunski M, Ulrich J. Increase of sodium channels in demyelinated lesions of multiple sclerosis. *Brain Res* 1991;**556**:311–16

17. England J D, Gamboni F, Levinson S R. Increased numbers of sodium channels form along demyelinated axons. *Brain Res* 1991;**548**:334–7

18. Novakovic S D, Levinson S R, Schachner M, Shrager P. Disruption and reorganization of sodium channels in experimental allergic neuritis. *Muscle Nerve* 1998;**21**(8):1019–32

19. Charcot J. Histologie de la sclérose en plaque. *Gaz Hospital (Paris)* 1848;**41**:554–66

20. Kornek B, Lassmann H. Axonal pathology in multiple sclerosis: a historical note. *Brain Pathol* 1999;**4**:651–6

21. Trapp B, Peterson J, Ransohoff R, *et al.* Axonal transection in the lesions of multiple sclerosis. *N Engl J Med* 1998;**338**(5):323–5

22. Ferguson B, Matyszak M, Esiri M, Perry V. Axonal damage in acute multiple sclerosis lesions. *Brain* 1997;**120**:393–9

23. Evangelou N, Esiri M, Smith S, Palace J, Matthews P. Quantitative pathological evidence for axonal loss in

normal appearing white matter in multiple sclerosis. *Ann Neurol* 2000;**47**(3):391–5

24. Kuhlmann T, Lingfeld G, Bitsch A, Schuchardt J, Bruck W. Acute axonal damage in multiple sclerosis is most extensive in early disease stages and decreases over time. *Brain* 2002;**125**:2202–12

25. Davie C, Barker G, Webb S, *et al.* Persistent functional deficit in multiple sclerosis and autosomal dominant cerebellar ataxia is associated with axon loss. *Brain* 1996;**124**:1052–3

26. Wujek J, Bjartmar C, Richer E, *et al.* Axon loss in the spinal cord determines permanent neurological disability in an animal model of multiple sclerosis. *J Neuropathol Exp Neurol* 2002;**61**:23–32.

27. Stys P K, Waxman S G, Ransom B R. Ionic mechanisms of anoxic injury in mammalian CNS white matter: role of Na^+ channels and $Na^{(+)}$–Ca^{2+} exchanger. *J Neurosci* 1992;**12**(2):430–9

28. Waxman S G, Black J A, Stys P K, Ransom B R. Ultrastructural concomitants of anoxic injury and early post-anoxic recovery in rat optic nerve. *Brain Res* 1992;**574**(1–2):105–19

29. Stys P K, Sontheimer H, Ransom B R, Waxman S G. Noninactivating, tetrodotoxin-sensitive Na^+ conductance in rat optic nerve axons. *Proc Natl Acad Sci USA* 1993;**90**(15):6976–80

30. Smith K, Lassmann H. The role of nitric oxide in multiple sclerosis. *Lancet Neurol* 2002;**1**(4):232–41

31. Brown G, Bal-Price A. Inflammatory neurodegeneration mediated by nitric oxide, glutamate, and mitochondria. *Mol Neurobiol* 2003;**27**(3):325–55

32. Dutta R, McDonough J, Yin X, *et al.* Mitochondrial dysfunction as a cause of axonal degeneration in multiple sclerosis patients. *Ann Neurol* 2006;**59**(3):478–89

33. Kapoor R, Davies M, Blaker P, Hall S, Smith K. Blockers of sodium and calcium entry protect axons from nitric oxide-mediated degeneration. *Ann Neurol* 2003;**53**(2):174–80

34. Garthwaite G, Goodwin D A, Batchelor A M, Leeming K, Garthwaite J. Nitric oxide toxicity in CNS white matter: an *in vitro* study using rat optic nerve. *Neuroscience* 2002;**109**(1):145–55

35. Waxman S G, Black J A, Kocsis J D, Ritchie J M. Low density of sodium channels supports action potential conduction in axons of neonatal rat optic nerve. *Proc Natl Acad Sci USA* 1989;**86**:1406–10

36. Boiko T, Rasband M N, Levinson S R, *et al.* Compact myelin dictates the differential targeting of two sodium channel isoforms in the same axon. *Neuron* 2001;**30**(1):91–104

37. Kaplan M R, Cho M, Ullian E M, *et al.* Differential control of clustering of the sodium channels na(v)1.2 and na(v)1.6 at developing CNS nodes of Ranvier. *Neuron* 2001;**30**(1):105–19

38. Foster R E, Connors B W, Waxman S G. Rat optic nerve: electrophysiological, pharmacological, and anatomical studies during development. *Dev Brain Res* 1982;**3**:361–76

39. Rasband M N, Peles E, Trimmer J S, *et al.* Dependence of nodal sodium channel clustering on paranodal axoglial contact in the developing CNS. *J Neurosci* 1999;**19**(17):7516–28

40. Westenbroek R E, Merrick D K, Catterall W A. Differential subcellular localization of the RI and RII Na^+ channel subtypes in central neurons. *Neuron* 1989;**3**(6):695–704

41. Boiko T, Van Wart A, Caldwell J H, *et al.* Functional specialization of the axon initial segment by isoform-specific sodium channel targeting. *J Neurosci* 2003;**23**(6):2306–13

42. Craner M J, Lo A C, Black J A, Waxman S G. Abnormal sodium channel distribution in optic nerve axons in a model of inflammatory demyelination. *Brain* 2003;**126**(7):1552–61

43. Craner M J, Newcombe J, Black J A, *et al.* Molecular changes in neurons in multiple sclerosis: altered axonal expression of Nav1.2 and Nav1.6 sodium channels and Na^+/Ca^{2+} exchanger. *Proc Natl Acad Sci USA* 2004;**101**(21):8168–73

44. Craner M J, Hains B C, Lo A C, Black J A, Waxman S G. Co-localization of sodium channel Nav1.6 and the sodium–calcium exchanger at sites of axonal injury in the spinal cord in EAE. *Brain* 2004;**127**(2):294–303

45. Gong B, Rhodes K J, Bekele-Arcuri Z, Trimmer J S. Type I and type II Na^+ channel alpha-subunit polypeptides exhibit distinct spatial and temporal patterning, and association with auxiliary subunits in rat brain. *J Comp Neurol* 1999;**412**(2):342–52

46. Whitaker W R, Clare J J, Powell A J, *et al.* Distribution of voltage-gated sodium channel alpha-subunit and beta- subunit mRNAs in human hippocampal formation, cortex, and cerebellum. *J Comp Neurol* 2000;**422**(1):123–39

47. Rush A M, Dib-Hajj S D, Waxman S G. Electrophysiological properties of two axonal sodium channels, Nav1.2 and Nav1.6, expressed in mouse spinal sensory neurons. *J Physiol* 2005;**564**(3):803–15

48. Stys P K, Waxman S G, Ransom B R. Reverse operation of the Na^+ – Ca^{2+} exchanger mediates Ca^{2+} influx

during anoxia in mammalian CNS white matter. *Ann NY Acad Sci* 1992;**639**:328–32

49. Lassmann H. Pathology of neurons in multiple sclerosis. Amsterdam: Elsevier, 2005.

50. Bhat M A, Rios J C, Lu Y, *et al*. Axon–glia interactions and the domain organization of myelinated axons requires neurexin iv/caspr/paranodin. *Neuron* 2001; **30**(2):369–83

51. Stys P K, Ransom B R, Waxman S G. Tertiary and quaternary local anesthetics protect CNS white matter from anoxic injury at concentrations that do not block excitability. *J Neurophysiol* 1992; **67**(1):236–40

52. Fern R, Ransom B R, Stys P K, Waxman S G. Pharmacological protection of CNS white matter during anoxia: actions of phenytoin, carbamazepine and diazepam. *J Pharmacol Exp Therapeut* 1993;**266**(3):1549–55

53. Stys P K, Lesiuk H. Correlation between electrophysiological effects of mexiletine and ischemic protection in central nervous system white matter. *Neuroscience* 1996;**71**(1):27–36

54. Lo A C, Saab C Y, Black J A, Waxman S G. Phenytoin protects spinal cord axons and preserves axonal conduction and neurological function in a model of neuroinflammation *in vivo*. *J Neurophysiol* 2003; **90**(5):3566–71

55. Bechtold D A, Kapoor R, Smith K J. Axonal protection using flecainide in experimental autoimmune encephalomyelitis. *Ann Neurol* 2004; **55**(5):607–16

56. Bechtold D, Miller S, Dawson A, *et al*. Axonal protection achieved in a model of multiple sclerosis using lamotrigine. *J Neurol* 2006;**253**(12):1542–51

57. Black J, Liu S, Hains B, Saab C, Waxman S. Long-term protection of central axons with phenytoin in monophasic and chronic-relapsing EAE. *Brain* 2006;**129**(12):3196–208

58. Black J A, Liu S, Carrithers M, Carrithers L M, Waxman S G. Exacerbation of experimental autoimmune encephalomyelitis after withdrawal of phenytoin and carbamazepine. *Ann Neurol* 2007; **62**(1):21–33

59. Craner M J, Damarjian T G, Liu S, *et al*. Sodium channels contribute to microglia/macrophage activation and function in EAE and MS. *Glia* 2005; **49**(2):220–9

60. Carrithers M, Dib-Hajj S D, Carrithers L, *et al*. Expression of the voltage-gated sodium channel NaV1.5 in the macrophage late endosome regulates endosomal acidification. *J Immunol* 2007;**178**(12):7822–32

61. Kornek B, Storch M, Weissert R, *et al*. Multiple sclerosis and chronic autoimmune encephalomyelitis: a comparative quantitative study of axonal injury in active, inactive, and remyelinated lesions. *Am J Pathol* 2000;**157**(1):267–76

62. Cash E, Rott O. Microglial cells qualify as the stimulators of unprimed CD4+ and CD8+ T lymphocytes in the central nervous system. *Clin Exp Immunol* 1994;**98**(2):313–18

63. Renno T, Krakowski M, Piccirillo C, Lin J, Owens T. TNF-alpha expression by resident microglia and infiltrating leukocytes in the central nervous system of mice with experimental allergic encephalomyelitis: regulation by Th1 cytokines. *J Immunol* 1995;**154**(2):944–53

64. Hooper D, Bagasra O, Marini J, *et al*. Prevention of experimental allergic encephalomyelitis by targeting nitric oxide and peroxynitrite: implications for the treatment of multiple sclerosis. *Proc Natl Acad Sci USA* 1997;**94**(6):2528–33

65. De Groot C, Ruuls S, Theeuwes J, Dijkstra C, Van der Valk P. Immunocytochemical characterization of the expression of inducible and constitutive isoforms of nitric oxide synthase in demyelinating multiple sclerosis lesions. *J Neuropathol Exp Neurol* 1997;**56**(1):10–20

66. Matsumoto Y, Ohmori K, Fujiwara M. Immune regulation by brain cells in the central nervous system: microglia but not astrocytes present myelin basic protein to encephalitogenic T cells under *in vivo*-mimicking conditions. *Immunology* 1992;**76**(2):209–16

67. Li H, Cuzner M, Newcombe J. Microglia-derived macrophages in early multiple sclerosis plaques. *Neuropathol Appl Neurobiol* 1996;**22**(3):207–15

68. Waxman S G. Cerebellar dysfunction in multiple sclerosis: evidence for an acquired channelopathy. *Prog Brain Res* 2004;**148**:353–65

69. Matthews W B, Compston A, Allen I V, Martyn C N. *McAlpine's Multiple Sclerosis*. New York: Churchill Livingstone, 1991

70. Andermann F, Cosgrove J, Lloyd-Smith D, Walters A. Paroxysmal dysarthria and ataxia in multiple sclerosis: a report of two unusual cases. *Neurology* 1959;**9** (4):211–15

71. Espir M, Watkins S, Smith H. Paroxysmal dysarthria and other transient neurological disturbances in disseminated sclerosis. *J Neurol Neurosurg Psychiatry* 1966;**29**(4):323–30

72. Black J A, Fjell J, Dib-Hajj S, *et al*. Abnormal expression of SNS/PN3 sodium channel in cerebellar Purkinje cells following loss of myelin in the taiep rat. *Neuroreport* 1999;**10**(5):913–18

73. Black J A, Dib-Hajj S, Baker D, *et al.* Sensory neuron-specific sodium channel SNS is abnormally expressed in the brains of mice with experimental allergic encephalomyelitis and humans with multiple sclerosis. *Proc Natl Acad Sci USA* 2000; **97**(21):11 598–602

74. Okuse K, Malik-Hall M, Baker M D, *et al.* Annexin II light chain regulates sensory neuron-specific sodium channel expression. *Nature* 2002; **417**(6889):653–6

75. Craner M J, Lo A C, Black J A, *et al.* Annexin II/p11 is up-regulated in Purkinje cells in EAE and MS. *Neuroreport* 2003;**14**(4):555–8

76. Akopian A N, Sivilotti L, Wood J N. A tetrodotoxin-resistant voltage-gated sodium channel expressed by sensory neurons. *Nature* 1996;**379**(6562):257–62

77. Sangameswaran L, Delgado S G, Fish L M, *et al.* Structure and function of a novel voltage-gated, tetrodotoxin-resistant sodium channel specific to sensory neurons. *J Biol Chem* 1996;**271**(11):5953–6

78. Elliott A A, Elliott J R. Characterization of TTX-sensitive and TTX-resistant sodium currents in small cells from adult rat dorsal root ganglia. *J Physiol Lond* 1993;**463**:39–56

79. Dib-Hajj S D, Ishikawa K, Cummins T R, Waxman S G. Insertion of a SNS-specific tetrapeptide in S3–S4 linker of D4 accelerates recovery from inactivation of skeletal muscle voltage-gated Na channel μ1 in HEK293 cells. *FEBS Lett* 1997;**416**(1):11–14

80. Renganathan M, Cummins T R, Waxman S G. Contribution of Nav1.8 sodium channels to action potential electrogenesis in DRG neurons. *J Neurophysiol* 2001;**86**(2):629–40

81. Blair N T, Bean B P. Roles of tetrodotoxin (TTX)-sensitive Na$^+$ current, TTX-resistant Na$^+$ current, and Ca^{2+} current in the action potentials of nociceptive sensory neurons. *J Neurosci* 2002;**22**(23):10 277–90

82. Llinas R, Sugimori M. Electrophysiological properties of *in vitro* Purkinje cell somata in mammalian cerebellar slices. *J Physiol Lond* 1980;**305**:171–95

83. Stuart G, Hausser M. Initiation and spread of sodium action potentials in cerebellar Purkinje cells. *Neuron* 1994;**13**(3):393–404

84. Raman I M, Sprunger L K, Meisler M H, Bean B P. Altered subthreshold sodium currents and disrupted firing patterns in Purkinje neurons of Scn8a mutant mice. *Neuron* 1997;**19**(4):881–91

85. Kohrman D C, Smith M R, Goldin A L, Harris J, Meisler M H. A missense mutation in the sodium channel Scn8a is responsible for cerebellar ataxia in the mouse mutant jolting. *J Neurosci* 1996;**16**(19):5993–9

86. Renganathan M, Gelderblom M, Black J A, Waxman S G. Expression of Na(v)1.8 sodium channels perturbs the firing patterns of cerebellar Purkinje cells. *Brain Res* 2003;**959**(2):235–42

87. Saab C Y, Craner M J, Kataoka Y, Waxman S G. Abnormal Purkinje cell activity *in vivo* in experimental allergic encephalomyelitis. *Exp Brain Res* 2004;**158**:1–8

88. Black J A, Langworthy K, Hinson A W, Dib-Hajj S D, Waxman S G. NGF has opposing effects on Na$^+$ channel III and SNS gene expression in spinal sensory neurons. *NeuroReport* 1997;**8**(9–10):2331–5

89. Dib-Hajj S D, Black J A, Cummins T R, *et al.* Rescue of alpha-SNS sodium channel expression in small dorsal root ganglion neurons following axotomy by *in vivo* administration of nerve growth factor. *J Neurophysiol* 1998;**79**:2668–76

90. Laudiero L, Aloe L, Levi-Montalcini R, *et al.* Multiple sclerosis patients express increased levels of beta-nerve growth factor in cerebrospinal fluid. *Neurosci Lett* 1992;**147**(1):9–12

91. De Simone R, Micera A, Tirassa P, Aloe L. mRNA for NGF and p75 in the central nervous system of rats affected by experimental allergic encephalomyelitis. *Neuropathol Appl Neurobiol* 1996;**22**(1):54–9

92. Damarjian T G, Craner M J, Black J A, Waxman S G. Upregulation and colocalization of p75 and Na(v)1.8 in Purkinje neurons in experimental autoimmune encephalomyelitis. *Neurosci Lett* 2004;**369**(3):186–90

93. Muragaki Y, Timothy N, Leight S, *et al.* Expression of trk receptors in the developing and adult human central and peripheral nervous system. *J Comp Neurol* 1995;**356**(3):387–97

94. Yan Q, Johnson E J. An immunohistochemical study of the nerve growth factor receptor in developing rats. *J Neurosci* 1988;**8**(9):3481–98

95. Soilu-Hanninen M, Epa R, Shipham K, *et al.* Treatment of experimental autoimmune encephalomyelitis with antisense oligonucleotides against the low affinity neurotrophin receptor. *J Neurosci Res* 2000;**59**(6):712–21

Chapter 5

Basic mechanisms of functional recovery

Björn Zörner and Martin E. Schwab

In multiple sclerosis (MS), inflammatory and immunomediated processes cause local destruction of glial and neuronal components of the central nervous system (CNS). Accordingly, MS is a chronic inflammatory and neurodegenerative disorder. Symptoms in patients are due to the formation of disseminated focal lesions or so-called MS plaques in the gray and white matter of the brain and spinal cord. Neuropathological characteristics of such lesions are destruction of oligodendrocytes, demyelination of axons, axon degeneration, axon loss, and neuronal damage [1, 2]. Functional impairments during the inflammatory episodes and subsequent irreversible neurological disabilities are due to variable degrees of nervous tissue damage and differentially affected cell types, but neither clinical nor pathological criteria are currently predictive of the extent of recovery during the course of MS. Nevertheless, recession of the causative pathological processes, repair of and substitution for damaged nervous tissue as well as substantial compensatory reorganization of neuronal networks are thought to be strategies utilized by the CNS to re-establish function.

For the development of effective therapies it is essential to understand MS etiology, pathology, and, in particular, endogenous recovery strategies. It is likely that the fundamental mechanisms responsible for functional recovery from lesions associated with diseases such as MS or traumatic CNS injuries share common characteristics. Therefore, in this chapter we summarize recent concepts of functional recovery after CNS damage focusing on insights obtained from animal models and human studies of demyelinating disorders and traumatic injuries to the CNS.

Recession of pathophysiological processes

Local inflammatory activity has been linked to the emergence and remission of many of the functional impairments in MS patients. Local endothelial damage due to inflammation or mechanical stress causes breakdown of the blood–brain barrier (BBB). Increased BBB permeability can impede neuronal function through a number of mechanisms. Extravasation of fluid leads to myelin swelling, edema formation, tissue compression, and metabolic disturbances. Therefore, restitution of BBB integrity and subsequent edema resolution can contribute to improvements observed in the acute phase of recovery.

A short-lasting, reversible inhibition of axonal impulse conduction can be observed in MS patients and after traumatic CNS injury, e.g., spinal cord injury, and is associated with transient neurological symptoms in patients. The underlying mechanisms leading to conduction block and its disappearance are currently unknown; however, a potential role for nitric oxide, several cytokines, and ionic disequilibrium has been postulated [3, 4].

Repair of damaged nervous tissue

In rodent models of experimentally induced demyelination, significant spontaneous remyelination can be observed 3 weeks post-lesion [5]. By contrast, spontaneous myelin repair in humans is limited and often restricted to the margins of lesions. However, in MS patients, a few areas of extensive remyelination can be found in the white matter. These remyelinated regions, referred to as shadow plaques, are sharply circumscribed and characterized by thin myelin

Multiple Sclerosis: Recovery of Function and Neurorehabilitation, eds. J. Kesselring, G. Comi, and A. J. Thompson. Published by Cambridge University Press. © Cambridge University Press 2010.

sheets and gliosis [6]. In addition to remyelination, the compensatory reassembly of sodium channels along demyelinated axons can contribute, at least partially, to functional recovery in the subacute phase after injury [7]. A prerequisite for remyelination is the availability of axon-myelinating oligodendrocytes at the site of the lesion. Thus, one line of experimental therapeutic attempts to enhance remyelination currently focuses on optimizing the recruitment of endogenous oligodendrocytes or their precursors [8]. A second approach is based on cell transplantation strategies which will be discussed below.

Replacement of lost nervous tissue

Permanent functional deficits seen in progressive MS or following traumatic CNS injury have been ascribed to irreversible neuronal and axonal degeneration. Encouragingly, recent findings in stem cell research suggest that some replacement of lost or degenerated cells by newly born cells might be feasible at least in some regions of the adult CNS. Multipotent neural stem cells reside especially in specific germinal regions in the brain including the subventricular zone of the lateral ventricles and the subgranular zone of the hippocampal dentate gyrus [9, 10]. In addition, in other parts of the CNS, e.g., the spinal cord, dividing cells that show in vitro multipotency are also present [11]. These endogenous stem cell pools are a potential source of cellular replacement following injury [12, 13]. After induction of local axon demyelination in the CNS of adult rats endogenous progenitor cells were shown to proliferate and to differentiate into mature oligodendrocytes which have the ability to remyelinate axons [8]. Increased proliferation of progenitor cells as well as migration of these cells from germinal regions towards lesioned areas has been reported after CNS injury in various animal models [14, 15]. However, it is evident clinically that after severe insults newly generated cells derived from endogenous stem cells are insufficient to compensate entirely for lost CNS tissue.

Transplantation of embryonic or adult stem cells has been considered as an alternative strategy to substitute for damaged CNS tissue [16]. Despite promising results obtained in animal studies, where migration and differentiation of transplanted stem cells has been demonstrated, this approach faces a number of key challenges and safety issues with

regards to clinical translation [13, 16, 17]. Crucial prerequisites for successful transplantation in human trials include identification of the most appropriate stem cell type and transplantation paradigm, adequate cell survival and immunological tolerance by the host tissue, precise control of proliferation, and region-specific differentiation of grafted cells. In multifocal CNS diseases, such as MS, the feasibility of multiple stem cell injections into lesion sites is limited. Systemic applications of cells into the bloodstream or the cerebrospinal fluid might overcome this problem [17, 18]. Whether these cells are eventually able to migrate to their appropriate target tissue ("specific homing") or become distributed to other organs is an open question. In addition, many underlying mechanisms for the reported beneficial effects are unknown; for example grafted stem cells could act as a source of trophic factors or differentiate into glial cells or neurons which might be integrated into neuronal networks. Finally, it should be considered that only a few studies have conclusively demonstrated that effects observed following transplantation are directly linked to functional recovery [19, 20]. Therefore, whereas pharmacological manipulation of endogenous stem cell pools or transplantation of stem cell grafts might provide therapeutic options in the future, more basic research in this field is required before clinical application becomes safe and feasible.

Regeneration of damaged axons

A strict definition of "successful axonal regeneration" might include the following: the lesioned axon has (1) to form growth cones and sprouts close to the transection site; (2) to elongate long distances past the lesion and to reach the denervated areas; and (3) to be integrated into functional neuronal circuitries (Fig. 5.1A–C). Since central networks can be plastic and undergo structural adaptations that contribute to functional recovery after CNS lesion (see below), one has to consider that the original local circuitries might experience major changes before regrowth of axons is accomplished.

Axonal damage is a common feature in MS and traumatic CNS injury

In MS, injured axons are not only present within, and adjacent to, the plaques but can also be found in normal-appearing white matter [21]. The precise

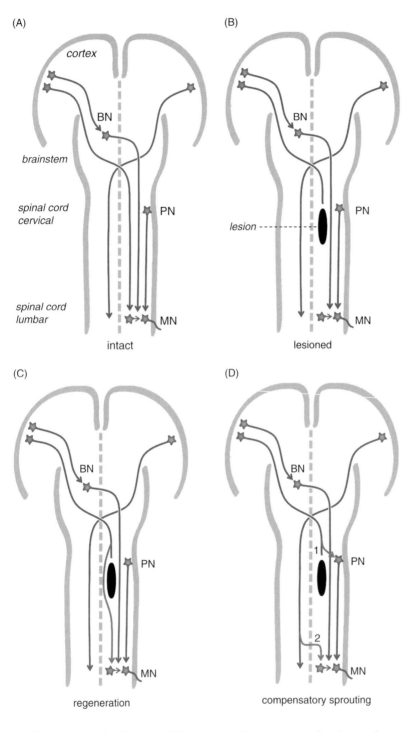

Fig. 5.1. Focal damage to the corticospinal tract (CST) in the adult CNS leads to compensatory anatomical changes which are accompanied by functional recovery after injury. Neurons in the cortex, brainstem, and propriospinal interneurons project to spinal circuitries in the lumbar spinal cord and are important for hindlimb control (A). After selective transection of hindlimb CST fibers at the midthoracic level of the spinal cord, spontaneous regeneration of lesioned fibers is restricted by growth inhibitory factors in the adult mammalian CNS, but some control of hindlimb function is maintained via spared bulbospinal and propriospinal pathways (B). Application of antibodies against the growth inhibitory protein Nogo-A promotes regeneration of the injured axons. Lesioned fibers show enhanced regenerative sprouting rostral to the lesion site and are able to bypass it to reinnervate lumbar circuitries (C). In addition, damaged axons can spontaneously form detour pathways by contacting spared descending propriospinal interneurons rostral to the lesion site which relay cortical control to lumbar neuronal networks (D, 1). After Nogo-A neutralization, intact contralateral CST fibers show collateral sprouting at spinal levels, cross the midline, and contact lumbar motoneurons and interneurons in the partially deafferented hemicord (D, 2). BN, brainstem neuron; PN, propriospinal (inter)neuron; MN, motoneuron.

mechanisms involved in axonal damage in MS are not well understood, whereas processes following traumatic injury have been characterized in more detail [22]. After transection, central axons undergo a series of time-dependent modifications. In the acute phase after lesion the proximal part of the axon retracts up to several millimeters, a process referred to as "axonal die-back," eventually resulting in the formation of a retraction bulb. The section of the axon separated from its cell body is subject to Wallerian degeneration. Interestingly, lesioned central fibers can show a transient growth response which is associated with the upregulation of cytoskeletal and growth-associated proteins (e.g. GAP-43) in injured cell bodies [23]; however, this response subsides after 7–14 days [22]. Axons can form growth-cone-like structures at the lesion site, but are not capable to grow beyond it, illustrating the limited potential of axons to regenerate in the adult mammalian CNS [22]. Therefore, in contrast to the situation in the peripheral nervous system or during CNS development, regeneration of axons has traditionally not been considered to contribute to functional recovery after CNS injury [24]. Given that premise, several questions arise such as, why do central axons fail to regenerate? What are the underlying mechanisms of this failure? And, how can we, by inducing axonal regeneration, improve functional recovery after CNS injury?

First insights into the answers for these questions arose from experiments performed by Tello in 1911 and Aguayo in the early 1980s suggesting that adult central neurons have some regenerative potential [24, 25]. In adult rabbits or rats, peripheral nerve grafts were transplanted into the CNS, e.g., the cortex or spinal cord. Axons that entered the graft grew over long distances, i.e. several centimeters, thereby demonstrating that damaged central axons are able to regrow in the presence of a growth-promoting environment. Thus, growth inhibitory factors were postulated to be present in the adult CNS [26]. Components of central myelin were found to impede axonal outgrowth and, eventually, the existence of myelin-associated, growth-restricting proteins was demonstrated [27]. Antibodies raised against the most important one of these, Nogo-A, were shown to block its inhibitory activity in vitro [28] and to promote axonal regeneration in vivo (Fig. 5.2) [29, 30]. To date, six to eight additional molecules with some neurite growth-restricting properties in vitro have been identified [31–34]. This group of central growth inhibitors comprises ephrins, semaphorins, proteoglycans, and myelin proteins such as myelin-associated glycoprotein (MAG) and oligodendrocyte myelin glycoprotein (OMgp). Whether axonal regeneration can be induced by blocking these molecules in vivo is still unclear [35].

The Nogo-A signaling pathway

The transmembrane protein Nogo-A is expressed predominantly on the surface of oligodendrocytes and some subpopulations of central neurons [36–39]. Growth inhibition is attributed to at least two regions within the Nogo-A protein; one located close to the C-terminus, the so-called Nogo-66 region, and the other termed the Nogo-A specific domain [40]. Nogo-66, present in all Nogo isoforms, exerts its inhibitory potential via a specific binding site in the neuronal membranes, the Nogo-66 receptor (NgR) [41, 42]. Interestingly, binding of MAG and OMgp to NgR has also been demonstrated in vitro [33, 43]. For signal transmission NgR interacts with several co-receptors (Lingo-1, TROY, and the low-affinity neurotrophin receptor p75) leading to activation of the small intracellular GTPase RhoA [44, 45]. Downstream targets of RhoA, which eventually transmit the growth inhibitory signal to the cytoskeleton and induce growth arrest and growth cone collapse, are kinases like ROCK and LimK and the actin-binding protein cofilin [46, 47]. Enhanced axonal regeneration accompanied by functional improvements has been reported after *nogo* gene deletions (Nogo-A knockout mice) [48], blockade of different components of the Nogo-66 receptor complex [49, 50] and downstream messengers in rodent models of spinal cord injury [51].

Effects of Nogo-A inactivation after CNS injury

For blocking Nogo-A activity in vivo, monoclonal antibodies against Nogo-A can be applied to the cerebrospinal fluid. These antibodies bind to and mask their molecular targets and are, together with Nogo-A, then internalized from the cell surface decreasing the Nogo-A tissue levels [52]. By using this approach in different animal models of CNS injury enhanced regenerative sprouting and fiber growth has been demonstrated and was shown to be closely associated with enhanced functional recovery (Fig. 5.2) [29, 53, 54]. For example, after transection of the corticospinal tract (CST) at thoracic level, adult rats were either treated with anti-Nogo-A or control antibodies [53]. Motor recovery was tested in various behavior tasks at different post-lesional time points. Sensory testing demonstrated that there were no severe malfunctions such as hypersensitivity or increased pain that might be a result of aberrant fiber sprouting. Animals that received a Nogo-A neutralizing antibody showed a faster and more complete hindlimb motor recovery, e.g., during running over a horizontal ladder or a narrow beam, but

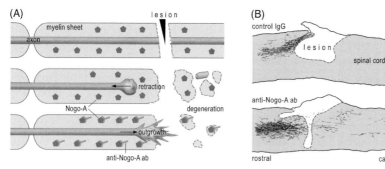

Fig. 5.2. Treatment with anti-Nogo-A antibodies after CNS injury promotes axonal regeneration in vivo. The growth-inhibitory protein Nogo-A is expressed mainly by oligodendrocytes which form the myelin sheets surrounding central axons. Nogo-A signaling leads to retraction of the proximal section of the axon which is still connected to its cell body whereas the separated distal section undergoes Wallerian degeneration. Application of Nogo-A-neutralizing antibodies leads to the formation of growth cones and axonal outgrowth after CNS lesion (A). After experimental spinal cord injury in rats, anti-Nogo-A antibodies delivered via an intrathecal catheter induce regenerative sprouting and long-distance elongation of lesioned CST fibers (labeled in black) whereas axonal regeneration is absent after treatment with control antibodies. Regenerating fibers bypass the lesion site in spared tissue bridges and extend caudally on an irregular course up to 5 mm in the spinal cord as demonstrated by camera lucida reconstructions of the spinal cord. In addition, massive sprouting of CST fibers and growth cone formation rostral to the lesion site can be observed in anti-Nogo-A antibody-treated animals. The growth response after blocking Nogo-A signaling was accompanied by substantial functional recovery in several behaviour tests. (Adapted with kind permission from *Annals of Neurology* (2005) Vol. 58, No. 5, pp. 706–719, © 2005 Wiley-Liss, Inc.)

also of precision movements, e.g., skilled reaching, while pain and allodynia were absent [53, 54]. Quantification of regenerative sprouts rostral to and regenerated fibers caudal to the lesion site revealed a massive increase of CST branches and fibers in anti-Nogo-A antibody-treated animals. Most importantly, profound long-distance regeneration of lesioned CST axons was only present after Nogo-A neutralization. By using spared tissue bridges as scaffolds, these fibers grew irregularly around the lesion site, elongated, and arborized up to 5 mm caudal to the lesion (Fig. 5.2). Similarly, a proof-of-concept study in adult macaque monkeys demonstrated that application of anti-Nogo-A antibodies delivered intrathecally over a period of 4 weeks after unilateral cervical spinal cord' injury resulted in enhanced recovery of manual dexterity and was found to promote regrowth of CST fibers. Again, CST axons bypassed the lesion site and grew into the denervated hemicord [54]. These preclinical findings implicate a major role for Nogo-A Nogo-receptor signaling in restriction of neurite regeneration and neuronal plasticity in the adult CNS and suggest what remains to be proven in the currently ongoing clinical trials: Nogo-A neutralization might be a novel medical strategy to enhance axonal regeneration in humans with the potential to substantially alleviate the patient's suffering from CNS injury.

Reorganization and neuronal plasticity in damaged and spared systems

Cortical neuronal networks and representational maps are subject to permanent modifications in the adult CNS [55, 56]. After injury, compensatory adaptations in intact and damaged neuronal networks have been shown to contribute to functional recovery [57–59]. The potential of the CNS to change and adapt is described as "neuronal plasticity." Neuronal plasticity can occur at different levels ranging from intracellular to neuroanatomical alterations. Modifications of synaptic transmission include changes in neurotransmitter release, receptor number and function, and second-messenger cascades. Activity-dependent changes in synaptic strength can be short- or long-lasting. Long-term potentiation (LTP) and long-term depression (LTD) are examples of activity-dependent alterations in synaptic connectivity important for memory formation. It has been suggested that synaptic plasticity and changes in the balance between inhibition and excitation in cortical horizontal connections, i.e., connections between neurons in different subregions of the motor cortex, are responsible for rapid reorganization of cortical maps after lesion [60]. Single synapses or entire dendritic spines can be newly generated, remodeled, or eliminated [61]. Finally, whole neuronal circuitries have been shown to be plastic. Anatomical or structural plasticity involves sprouting, outgrowth, and pruning of axonal or dendritic processes leading to the reorganization and formation of new networks.

Spontaneous anatomical plasticity at different CNS levels has been extensively documented in animal models of spinal cord injury and stroke and is thought to be a major mechanism accounting for functional improvements at later stages in the recovery process [57, 60]. Neutralization of the growth-inhibitory protein Nogo-A facilitates axonal outgrowth, compensatory sprouting of lesioned and intact fibers, and anatomical rearrangements after CNS injury [62, 63]. Axons lesioned at the midthoracic level of the spinal cord, which ordinarily project to the lumbar spinal cord, can show spontaneous collateral sprouting into the cervical spinal cord [64]. Such sprouts can contact unlesioned propriospinal neurons, which bypass the lesion site, and form functional detour pathways. Formation of detour circuits was observed after traumatic spinal cord injury and in MS models, i.e. experimental autoimmune encephalomyelitis (EAE) [65, 66]. In the presence of Nogo-A blocking antibodies collateral sprouts of lesioned axons cross the midline at the brainstem level to innervate contralateral nuclei [67]. Therefore, injured neurons are able to retain motor control by collateral sprouting and the formation of new supraspinal and intraspinal circuits relaying cortical input to spinal targets (Fig. 5.1D). In addition, reactive collateral sprouting after CNS injury is present in spared fiber tracts. Following unilateral stroke or transection of CST fibers and anti-Nogo-A treatment, contralateral unlesioned CST fibers sprout and cross the midline at spinal levels to innervate the deafferented hemicord. These midline-crossing fibers show topographically appropriate innervation patterns and are functionally integrated into local spinal circuitries indicated by improved behavioral outcome [62]. After stroke, neurons of the intact cortex form new axonal projections to contralateral subcortical targets, e.g., the striatum or the red nucleus, resulting in a bilateral corticofugal innervation pattern [68–71]. These findings suggest that descending projections emanating from cortical regions contralateral to the lesion site are able to compensate for functions lost due to injury (Fig. 5.1D). How far activity drives these changes, e.g., by training of the impaired limb, is currently subject to intense investigation.

Several descending fiber tracts are important for motor functions, i.e., the corticospinal, rubrospinal, vestibulospinal, and reticulospinal system as well as serotonergic and dopaminergic projections from the brainstem. Each system is considered to be partially specialized for motor control, whereby some degree of functional overlap and parallel processing can be assumed. Both the red nucleus and the motor cortex share common features with regard to target neurons in the spinal cord and also function, i.e., control of skilled movements. Interestingly, after bilateral CST transection, rubrospinal projections sprout into de-afferented spinal regions in the presence of Nogo-A neutralizing antibodies and this is correlated with functional recovery [72]. This demonstrates that parallel, anatomically separate systems are able to compensate, at least partially, for the loss of another system. One could hypothesize that relearning of motor tasks in the rehabilitation phase after CNS injury is partially based on the functional switch between neuronal systems. In patients, physical training during rehabilitation is crucial and might contribute to activity-dependent fine-tuning of newly formed neural circuitries.

Here, we have emphasized that ample evidence has been provided for anatomical reorganization of neuronal networks in the cortex, subcortical systems, and the spinal cord after CNS injury in animals. Studies performed in MS and stroke patients using functional magnetic resonance imaging or transcranial magnetic stimulation techniques have demonstrated that functionally relevant adaptive changes and processes of reorganization can also occur in the human CNS [73, 74]. However, patients with large or progressive CNS lesions often show only limited functional recovery, a clinical observation that might be explained by the concept of "reserve capacity" [66]. According to this, functional recovery continues as long as a sufficient number of plastic pathways exist that are capable of functionally compensating for lost neurons or entire neuronal networks. By enhancing the plastic potential of the CNS, e.g., by suppression of growth-inhibitory proteins like Nogo-A, and by the incorporation of additional neuronal networks in the recovery process, new therapeutic approaches might be able to increase the endogenous reserve capacity.

Conclusion

Recession, repair, replacement, regeneration, and reorganization are basic repair strategies of the adult CNS in order to achieve functional recovery after injury. It is not only the absolute number of neurons and fibers spared or repaired after lesion that accounts for functional outcome, but the capability of the CNS to adapt, reorganize, and establish new neural networks that also play a key role in functional improvements. Knowledge about spontaneous mechanisms of functional recovery is crucial for the identification of therapeutic targets and for the development of new therapies. Interventions can support the recovery process but could also interfere with inherent mechanisms of recovery. Therapies that have proven efficient in animal models face the hurdle of secure translation to human patients, but recent progress in this field gives hope that we will be able to substantially support the damaged CNS in its efforts to repair itself in the future.

References

1. Dutta R, Trapp B D. Pathogenesis of axonal and neuronal damage in multiple sclerosis. *Neurology* 2007;**68**(22 Suppl 3):S22–31; discussion S43–54

2. Dhib-Jalbut S. Pathogenesis of myelin/oligodendrocyte damage in multiple sclerosis. *Neurology* 2007; **68**(22 Suppl 3):S13–21; discussion S43–54

3. Moreau T, Coles A, Wing M, *et al.* Transient increase in symptoms associated with cytokine release in patients with multiple sclerosis. *Brain* 1996;**119**(1): 225–37

4. Kapoor R, Davies M, Smith K J. Temporary axonal conduction block and axonal loss in inflammatory neurological disease: a potential role for nitric oxide? *Ann NY Acad Sci* 1999;**893**:304–8

5. Radtke C, Spies M, Sasaki M, Vogt P M, Kocsis J D. Demyelinating diseases and potential repair strategies. *Int J Dev Neurosci* 2007;**25**(3):149–53

6. Bruck W, Kuhlmann T, Stadelmann C. Remyelination in multiple sclerosis. *J Neurol Sci* 2003;**206**(2):181–5

7. Waxman S G. Demyelinating diseases: new pathological insights, new therapeutic targets. *N Engl J Med* 1998;**338**(5):323–5

8. Gensert J M, Goldman J E. Endogenous progenitors remyelinate demyelinated axons in the adult CNS. *Neuron* 1997;**19**(1):197–203

9. Alvarez-Buylla A, Temple S. Stem cells in the developing and adult nervous system. *J Neurobiol* 1998;**36**(2):105–10

10. Gage F H. Mammalian neural stem cells. *Science* 2000;**287**(5457):1433–8

11. Shihabuddin L S, Ray J, Gage F H. FGF-2 is sufficient to isolate progenitors found in the adult mammalian spinal cord. *Exp Neurol* 1997;**148**(2):577–86

12. Martino G, Pluchino S. The therapeutic potential of neural stem cells. *Nat Rev Neurosci* 2006;**7**(5):395–406

13. Miller R H. The promise of stem cells for neural repair. *Brain Res* 2006;**1091**(1):258–64

14. Gould E, Tanapat P. Lesion-induced proliferation of neuronal progenitors in the dentate gyrus of the adult rat. *Neuroscience* 1997;**80**(2):427–36

15. Picard-Riera N, Decker L, Delarasse C, *et al.* Experimental autoimmune encephalomyelitis mobilizes neural progenitors from the subventricular zone to undergo oligodendrogenesis in adult mice. *Proc Natl Acad Sci USA* 2002;**99**(20):13 211–16

16. Lassmann H. Stem cell and progenitor cell transplantation in multiple sclerosis: the discrepancy between neurobiological attraction and clinical feasibility. *J Neurol Sci* 2005;**233**(1–2):83–6

17. Magnus T, Rao M S. Neural stem cells in inflammatory CNS diseases: mechanisms and therapy. *J Cell Mol Med* 2005;**9**(2):303–19

18. Pluchino S, Furlan R, Martino G. Cell-based remyelinating therapies in multiple sclerosis: evidence from experimental studies. *Curr Opin Neurol* 2004;**17** (3):247–55

19. McDonald J W, Liu X Z, Qu Y, *et al.* Transplanted embryonic stem cells survive, differentiate and promote recovery in injured rat spinal cord. *Nat Med* 1999;**5**(12):1410–12

20. Cummings B J, Uchida N, Tamaki S J, *et al.* Human neural stem cells differentiate and promote locomotor recovery in spinal cord-injured mice. *Proc Natl Acad Sci USA* 2005;**102**(39):14 069–74

21. Kutzelnigg A, Lucchinetti C F, Stadelmann C, *et al.* Cortical demyelination and diffuse white matter injury in multiple sclerosis. *Brain* 2005;**128** (11):2705–12

22. Kerschensteiner M, Schwab M E, Lichtman J W, Misgeld T. In vivo imaging of axonal degeneration and regeneration in the injured spinal cord. *Nat Med* 2005;**11**(5):572–7

23. Plunet W, Kwon B K, Tetzlaff W. Promoting axonal regeneration in the central nervous system by enhancing the cell body response to axotomy. *J Neurosci Res* 2002;**68**(1):1–6

24. Ramón y Cajal S. *Degeneration and Regeneration of the Nervous System.* New York: Hafner, 1928

25. David S, Aguayo A J. Axonal elongation into peripheral nervous system "bridges" after central nervous system injury in adult rats. *Science* 1981;**214** (4523):931–3

26. Schwab M E, Thoenen H. Dissociated neurons regenerate into sciatic but not optic nerve explants in culture irrespective of neurotrophic factors. *J Neurosci* 1985;**5**(9):2415–23

27. Caroni P, Schwab M E. Two membrane protein fractions from rat central myelin with inhibitory properties for neurite growth and fibroblast spreading. *J Cell Biol* 1988;**106**(4):1281–8

28. Caroni P, Schwab M E. Antibody against myelin-associated inhibitor of neurite growth neutralizes nonpermissive substrate properties of CNS white matter. *Neuron* 1988;**1**(1):85–96

29. Schnell L, Schwab M E. Axonal regeneration in the rat spinal cord produced by an antibody against myelin-associated neurite growth inhibitors. *Nature* 1990;**343** (6255):269–72

30. Schwab M E. Nogo and axon regeneration. *Curr Opin Neurobiol* 2004;**14**(1):118–24

31. Mukhopadhyay G, Doherty P, Walsh F S, Crocker P R, Filbin M T. A novel role for myelin-associated glycoprotein as an inhibitor of axonal regeneration. *Neuron* 1994;**13**(3):757–67

32. Niederost B P, Zimmermann D R, Schwab M E, Bandtlow C E. Bovine CNS myelin contains neurite growth-inhibitory activity associated with chondroitin sulfate proteoglycans. *J Neurosci* 1999;**19**(20):8979–89

33. Wang K C, Koprivica V, Kim J A, *et al.* Oligodendrocyte-myelin glycoprotein is a Nogo receptor ligand that inhibits neurite outgrowth. *Nature* 2002;**417**(6892):941–4

34. Benson M D, Romero M I, Lush M E, *et al.* Ephrin-B3 is a myelin-based inhibitor of neurite outgrowth. *Proc Natl Acad Sci USA* 2005;**102**(30):10 694–9

35. Bartsch U, Bandtlow C E, Schnell L, *et al.* Lack of evidence that myelin-associated glycoprotein is a major inhibitor of axonal regeneration in the CNS. *Neuron* 1995;**15**(6):1375–81

36. Chen M S, Huber A B, van der Haar M E, *et al.* Nogo-A is a myelin-associated neurite outgrowth inhibitor and an antigen for monoclonal antibody IN-1. *Nature* 2000;**403**(6768):434–9

37. GrandPre T, Nakamura F, Vartanian T, Strittmatter S M. Identification of the Nogo inhibitor of axon regeneration as a Reticulon protein. *Nature* 2000;**403** (6768):439–44

38. Prinjha R, Moore S E, Vinson M, *et al.* Inhibitor of neurite outgrowth in humans. *Nature* 2000;**403** (6768):383–4

39. Wang X, Chun S J, Treloar H, *et al.* Localization of Nogo-A and Nogo-66 receptor proteins at sites of axon-myelin and synaptic contact. *J Neurosci* 2002;**22** (13):5505–15

40. Oertle T, van der Haar M E, Bandtlow C E, *et al.* Nogo-A inhibits neurite outgrowth and cell spreading with three discrete regions. *J Neurosci* 2003;**23**(13):5393–406

41. Fournier A E, GrandPre T, Strittmatter S M. Identification of a receptor mediating Nogo-66 inhibition of axonal regeneration. *Nature* 2001;**409** (6818):341–6

42. Fournier A E, GrandPre T, Gould G, Wang X, Strittmatter S M. Nogo and the Nogo-66 receptor. *Prog Brain Res* 2002;**137**:361–9

43. Liu B P, Fournier A, GrandPre T, Strittmatter S M. Myelin-associated glycoprotein as a functional ligand for the Nogo-66 receptor. *Science* 2002;**297** (5584):1190–3

44. Buchli A D, Schwab M E. Inhibition of Nogo: a key strategy to increase regeneration, plasticity and functional recovery of the lesioned central nervous system. *Ann Med* 2005;**37**(8):556–67

45. Yiu G, He Z. Glial inhibition of CNS axon regeneration. *Nat Rev Neurosci* 2006;**7**(8):617–27

46. Alabed Y Z, Grados-Munro E, Ferraro G B, Hsieh S H, Fournier A E. Neuronal responses to myelin are mediated by rho kinase. *J Neurochem* 2006;**96**(6):1616–25

47. Hsieh S H, Ferraro G B, Fournier A E. Myelin-associated inhibitors regulate cofilin phosphorylation and neuronal inhibition through LIM kinase and Slingshot phosphatase. *J Neurosci* 2006;**26**(3):1006–15

48. Dimou L, Schnell L, Montani L, *et al.* Nogo-A-deficient mice reveal strain-dependent differences in axonal regeneration. *J Neurosci* 2006;**26**(21):5591–603

49. GrandPre T, Li S, Strittmatter S M. Nogo-66 receptor antagonist peptide promotes axonal regeneration. *Nature* 2002;**417**(6888):547–51

50. Ji B, Li M, Wu W T, *et al.* LINGO-1 antagonist promotes functional recovery and axonal sprouting after spinal cord injury. *Mol Cell Neurosci* 2006;**33** (3):311–20

51. McKerracher L, Higuchi H. Targeting Rho to stimulate repair after spinal cord injury. *J Neurotrauma* 2006;**23** (3–4):309–17

52. Weinmann O, Schnell L, Ghosh A, *et al.* Intrathecally infused antibodies against Nogo-A penetrate the CNS and downregulate the endogenous neurite growth inhibitor Nogo-A. *Mol Cell Neurosci* 2006;**32**(1–2):161–73

53. Liebscher T, Schnell L, Schnell D, *et al.* Nogo-A antibody improves regeneration and locomotion of spinal cord-injured rats. *Ann Neurol* 2005;**58**(5):706–19

54. Freund P, Schmidlin E, Wannier T, *et al.* Nogo-A-specific antibody treatment enhances sprouting and functional recovery after cervical lesion in adult primates. *Nat Med* 2006;**12**(7):790–2

55. Nudo R J, Milliken G W, Jenkins W M, Merzenich M M. Use-dependent alterations of movement representations in primary motor cortex of adult squirrel monkeys. *J Neurosci* 1996;**16**(2):785–807

56. Johansson B B. Brain plasticity and stroke rehabilitation. The Willis Lecture. *Stroke* 2000;**31**(1):223–30

57. Payne B R, Lomber S G. Reconstructing functional systems after lesions of cerebral cortex. *Nat Rev Neurosci* 2001;**2**(12):911–19

58. Ward N S, Cohen L G. Mechanisms underlying recovery of motor function after stroke. *Arch Neurol* 2004;**61**(12):1844–8

59. Bradbury E J, McMahon S B. Spinal cord repair strategies: why do they work? *Nat Rev Neurosci* 2006;**7**(8):644–53

60. Raineteau O, Schwab M E. Plasticity of motor systems after incomplete spinal cord injury. *Nat Rev Neurosci* 2001;**2**(4):263–73

61. Holtmaat A J, Trachtenberg J T, Wilbrecht L, *et al.* Transient and persistent dendritic spines in the neocortex in vivo. *Neuron* 2005;**45**(2):279–91

62. Thallmair M, Metz G A, Z'Graggen W J, *et al.* Neurite growth inhibitors restrict plasticity and functional recovery following corticospinal tract lesions. *Nat Neurosci* 1998;**1**(2):124–31

63. Emerick A J, Neafsey E J, Schwab M E, Kartje G L. Functional reorganization of the motor cortex in adult rats after cortical lesion and treatment with monoclonal antibody IN-1. *J Neurosci* 2003;**23**(12):4826–30

64. Fouad K, Pedersen V, Schwab M E, Brosamle C. Cervical sprouting of corticospinal fibers after thoracic spinal cord injury accompanies shifts in evoked motor responses. *Curr Biol* 2001;**11**(22):1766–70

65. Bareyre F M, Kerschensteiner M, Raineteau O, *et al.* The injured spinal cord spontaneously forms a new intraspinal circuit in adult rats. *Nat Neurosci* 2004;**7**(3):269–77

66. Kerschensteiner M, Bareyre F M, Buddeberg B S, *et al.* Remodeling of axonal connections contributes to recovery in an animal model of multiple sclerosis. *J Exp Med* 2004;**200**(8):1027–38

67. Blochlinger S, Weinmann O, Schwab M E, Thallmair M. Neuronal plasticity and formation of new synaptic contacts follow pyramidal lesions and neutralization of Nogo-A: a light and electron microscopic study in the pontine nuclei of adult rats. *J Comp Neurol* 2001;**433**(3):426–36

68. Wenk C A, Thallmair M, Kartje G L, Schwab M E. Increased corticofugal plasticity after unilateral cortical lesions combined with neutralization of the IN-1 antigen in adult rats. *J Comp Neurol* 1999;**410**(1):143–57

69. Lee J K, Kim J E, Sivula M, Strittmatter S M. Nogo receptor antagonism promotes stroke recovery by enhancing axonal plasticity. *J Neurosci* 2004;**24**(27):6209–17

70. Seymour A B, Andrews E M, Tsai S Y, *et al.* Delayed treatment with monoclonal antibody IN-1 1 week after stroke results in recovery of function and corticorubral plasticity in adult rats. *J Cereb Blood Flow Metab* 2005;**25**(10):1366–75

71. Cafferty W B, Strittmatter S M. The Nogo–Nogo receptor pathway limits a spectrum of adult CNS axonal growth. *J Neurosci* 2006;**26**(47):12 242–50

72. Raineteau O, Fouad K, Noth P, Thallmair M, Schwab M E. Functional switch between motor tracts in the presence of the mAb IN-1 in the adult rat. *Proc Natl Acad Sci USA* 2001;**98**(12):6929–34

73. Cifelli A, Matthews P M. Cerebral plasticity in multiple sclerosis: insights from fMRI. *Mult Scler* 2002;**8**(3):193–9

74. Ward N S. Functional reorganization of the cerebral motor system after stroke. *Curr Opin Neurol* 2004;**17**(6):725–30

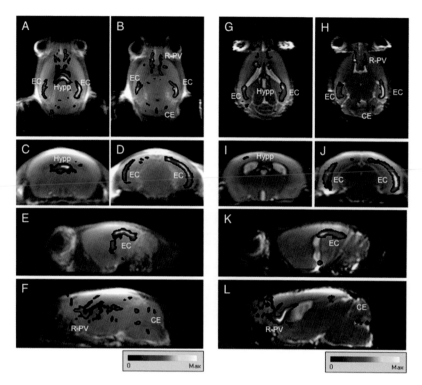

Fig. 2.1 Spatial lesion probability maps of T1 post gadolinium and T2 hyperintense brain lesions during acute chronic EAE. (With permission from Politi *et al.* [154].)

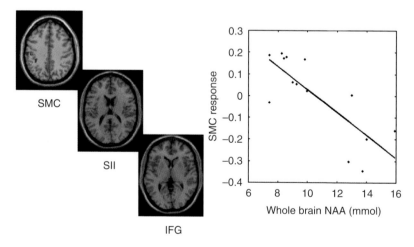

Fig. 2.2 Functional MRI study of brain activation of simple movements of the left hand in patients with clinically isolated syndrome (right). The increased activation of the contralateral sensorimotor cortex is correlated with the decrease of NAA in the whole brain spectroscopy. (With permission from Rocca *et al.* [80].)

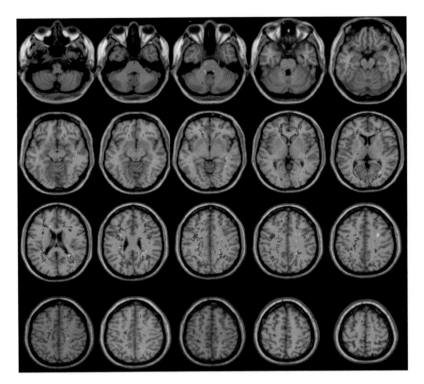

Fig. 2.4 Representative axial slices showing lesion probability maps, overlaid on a high-resolution T1-weighted image, in the different MS groups. Blue: lesion probability map of patients at presentation with clinically isolated syndromes; yellow: lesion probability map of RRMS patients; green: lesion probability map of SPMS patients; red: lesion probability map of PPMS patients. Images are in neurological convention.

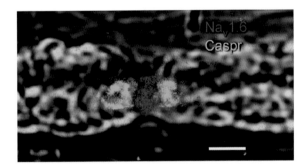

Fig. 4.1 Distribution of Na$^+$ channels in myelinated axons. Of the nine isoforms of voltage-gated Na$^+$ channels known to exist in mammals, one isoform, namely Nav1.6, is clustered at the nodes of Ranvier. Image shows clustering of Nav1.6 channels (red) at a node of Ranvier, and expression of Caspr (green) to mark the paranodal boundary. Expression of Na$^+$ channels is sparse along the paranodal and internodal axon membranes beneath the myelin. Fluorescence and differential contrast images are merged to reveal the myelin sheath. Scale bar = 5 μm.

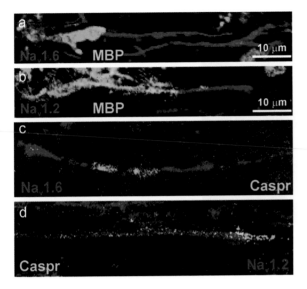

Fig. 4.2 Expression of Nav1.6 and Nav1.2 channels along demyelinated axons in active MS lesions within spinal cord tissue. Residual damaged myelin (green) can be seen next to extensive regions of diffuse expression of Nav1.6 channels (red; a) and Nav1.2 channels (red; b). Such regions of Nav1.6 channel (red; c) or Nav1.2 channel (red; d) expression in some axons are bounded by contactin-associated protein (Caspr; green), without overlap, consistent with the expression of Nav1.6 and Nav1.2 channels in the demyelinated axon membrane. (Reproduced with permission from Craner et al. [43] © 2004 National Academy of Sciences.)

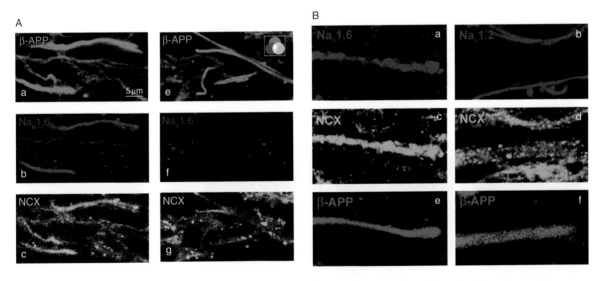

Fig. 4.3 (a) Co-expression of the sodium–calcium exchanger (NCX) and Nav1.6 along extensive regions of spinal cord axons that are immunopositive for β-APP, a marker of neuronal injury, in EAE. These digital images of immunostaining reveal β-APP (blue; a, e), sodium channel Nav1.6 (red; b) or Nav1.2 (red; f) and NCX (green; c, g) immunostaining in EAE spinal cord axons. Panels a, b, and c show co-expression of Nav1.6, NCX with β-APP, a marker of axonal injury. In contrast, panels e, f, and g demonstrate β-APP- and NCX-positive profiles but absence of Nav1.2 immunostaining (magnification 1800×). (Modified with permission from Craner et al. [44] © 2004 Oxford University Press.) (B) Co-expression of NCX and Nav1.6 along extensive regions of β-APP-positive spinal cord axons in acute MS lesions. These digital immunofluroscent images of axons in MS spinal cord white matter reveal the presence of β-APP (e and f; blue), Nav1.6 (a; red) or Nav1.2 (b; red) and NCX (c and d; green). Panels a, c, and e show co-expression of Nav1.6 and NCX in axons displaying β-APP. In contrast, panels b, d, and f demonstrate NCX-positive immunostaining but the absence of Nav1.2 immunostaining within β-APP-positive axons, and the co-expression of NCX and Nav1.2 in β-APP-negative axons. (Modified with permission from Craner et al. [43] © 2004 National Academy of Sciences.)

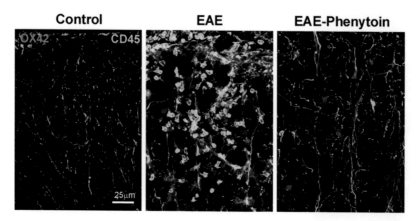

Fig. 4.6 Phenytoin treatment reduces inflammatory response in EAE. Digital images of control, EAE, and phenytoin-treated EAE spinal cord immunostained for anti-CD45 (green), anti-OX42 (blue). Middle panel (EAE) shows a significant increase in the number of immune cells (CD45 and/or OX42 immunopositive) compared with untreated control (left). Administration of phenytoin to EAE mice results in a significant reduction of inflammatory infiltrate (right). (Modified with permission from Craner *et al.* [59] © 2005 Wiley-Liss, Inc.)

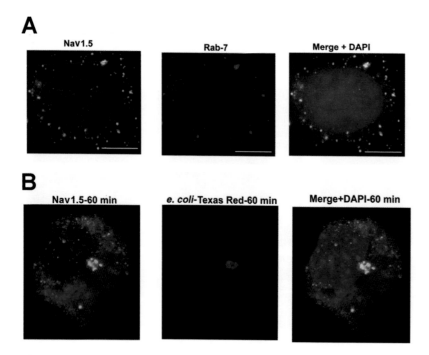

Fig. 4.7 Co-localized expression of Nav1.5 with late endosomal marker Rab-7 (A) and with internalized Texas Red-labeled *E. coli* (B). Nav1.5-positivity (A and B; left panels; green) in differentiated THP-1 cells primed with INF-γ and LPS co-localizes with late endosomal marker Rab-7 (A, middle panel; red) and with internalized Texas Red-labeled-*E. coli* 60 minutes following bacterial challenge. Merged images are shown on the right, with DAPI (4′,6′-diamidino-2-phenylindole) stained nuclei (blue). (Modified with permission from Carrithers *et al.* [60] © 2007 by The American Association of Immunologists, Inc.)

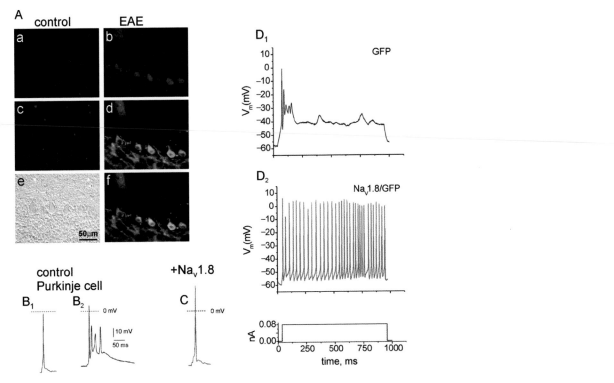

Fig. 4.9 Abnormal expression of sensory neuron specific Na$^+$ channel Nav1.8 within cerebellar Purkinje neurons in MS and EAE. Nav1.8 channel (red, Ab), and annexinII/p11 (Ad), a binding partner which facilitates the insertion of functional Nav1.8 channels into the cell membrane, exhibit co-localized expression (merged image, yellow, Af) in the Purkinje cells of EAE mice. Neither molecule can be detected within control Purkinje neurons (Aa, Ac, Ae). Nav1.8 expression alters action potential electrogenesis in Purkinje neurons as shown in B$_1$, B$_2$, and C. Current clamp recordings show spontaneous action potentials in control Purkinje neurons lacking Nav1.8 (B$_1$, B$_2$), and 2 days after transfection with Nav1.8 (C). Action potentials in control Purkinje neurons lacking Nav1.8 (B$_1$) show less overshoot (dotted lines indicate 0 mV) and tend to be conglomerate, consisting of two or more spikes in 62% of cells (B$_2$). By contrast, conglomerate action potentials contain fewer spikes and are far less common (15%) in Purkinje cells that express Nav1.8 (C). Purkinje neurons transfected with Nav1.8 show sustained repetitive firing (D$_2$; middle), not present in the absence of Nav1.8 (D$_1$; top), in response to the injection of a depolarizing current (D, bottom). GFP, green fluorescent protein; Vm, membrane potential. (Panels Aa–Af reproduced, with permission, from Craner *et al.* [75] © (2003) Lippincott, Williams & Wilkins. Panels B–D reproduced, with permission, from Renganathan *et al.* [86] © (2003) Elsevier Science.)

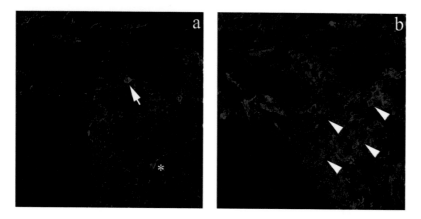

Fig. 7.1 Inflammation in experimental autoimmune encephalomyelitis (EAE) affects CNS (germinal) areas where neural stem/precursor cells (NPCs) reside. The figure shows infiltrating microglia in the SVZ of EAE and healthy control mice (HC). Coronal sections from brains of HC (panel a) and myelin oligodendrocyte glycoprotein (MOG)35–55-induced EAE (panel b) mice are stained for Iba1 (macrophage/microglia marker, red staining) and DAPI (nuclear marker, blue staining). In HC mice, few ramified Iba1[+] cells are located within the dorsolateral SVZ (arrow in panel a) while resting Iba1[+] ramified cells are sparse throughout the CNS parenchyma (asterisk in panel a). In EAE mice 20 days post-immunization, many Iba1[+] cells are found within the dorsolateral SVZ (arrowheads in panel b) and appear more hyperthophic than those found in HC.

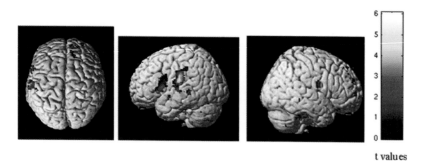

Fig. 11.2 Areas showing increased activations in patients with BMS in comparison with healthy controls during the analysis of the Stroop facilitation condition (random effect interaction analysis, ANOVA, $p < 0.05$ corrected for multiple comparisons). The BMS patients had increased activations of several areas located in the frontal and parietal lobes, bilaterally, including the anterior cingulate cortex, the superior frontal sulcus, the inferior frontal gyrus, the precuneus, the secondary sensorimotor cortex, the bilateral visual cortex, and the cerebellum, bilaterally. Note that the color-encoded activations have been superimposed on a rendered brain and normalized into standard Statistical Parametric Mapping (SPM) space (neurological convention).

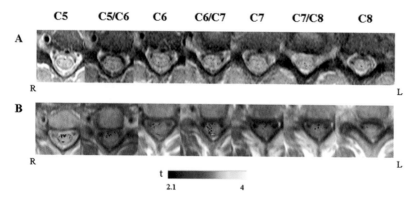

Fig. 11.3 Illustrative activation maps (color coded for t values) of cervical cord on axial proton density-weighted spin-echo images from C5 to C8, from a healthy control (A) and a patient with MS (B) during a tactile stimulation of the palm of the right hand. Right (R) and left (L).

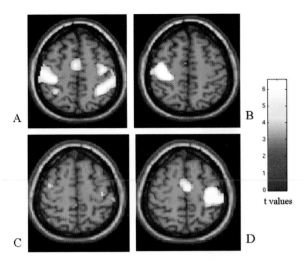

Fig. 11.4 Longitudinal evolution of cortical activations in the primary sensorimotor cortex (SMC), bilaterally, during task performance with impaired hand compared to unimpaired hand in one patient with good clinical recovery during follow-up (A and B), and in one patient with poor/absent clinical recovery (C and D). Scans obtained during a left-hand motor task have been flipped in order to keep the left hemisphere contralateral to movement. At baseline, both patients showed increased activation of the primary SMC of the unaffected (ipsilateral) hemisphere (A and C). During follow-up, the patient with good clinical recovery showed an increased recruitment of the primary SMC of the affected hemisphere (B), while the patient with poor/absent clinical recovery continued to show an increased recruitment of the primary SMC of the unaffected hemisphere (D). Note that the activations are color-coded according to their t values.

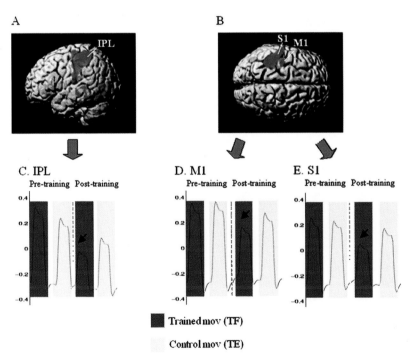

Fig. 11.5 Three-dimensional rendering (A and B) of task-specific reductions of activations in contralateral inferior parietal lobule (IPL) (BA 40; A and C), primary motor cortex (M1) (B and D), and primary somatosensory cortex (S1) (B and E) in healthy volunteers after training. Panels C, D, and E illustrate average signal intensities in voxels representing cluster maxima in IPL (BA 40), M1, and S1 for 30-s blocks of thumb flexion (trained movement, gray bars), extension (control movement, blue bars), and rest. Note that training led to a decrease in signal intensity predominantly for the trained movement (black arrows). Images are in neurological convention. (Reproduced from Morgen *et al.* [49] Training-dependent plasticity in patients with multiple sclerosis. *Brain* 2004;**127**:2506–17, by permission of Oxford University Press and the Guarantors of *Brain*.)

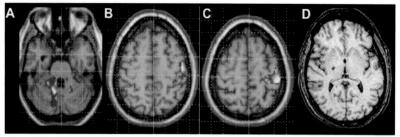

Fig. 12.1 Results obtained in a randomized, cross-over, double-blind study on ten patients with pure motor hemiparesis following a subcortical lacunar infarct. Patients were randomly assigned in two counterbalanced groups and underwent two fMRI examinations a week apart, after donepezil and after placebo. During each fMRI session, patients performed an active motor task consisting of a finger flexion–extension of the paretic hand. A single dose of donepezil induced a significantly reduced activation in sensorimotor areas (sensorimotor cortex of the healthy hemisphere: B and C) and contralateral cerebellum (A) compared to placebo, associated with a significant motor skill improvement of the affected hand. (From Tombari et al. [27]).

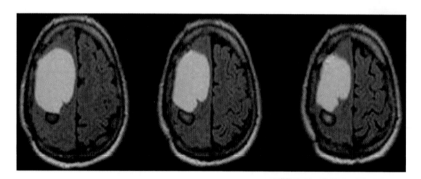

Fig. 12.2 Motor fMRI in a patient with a large neuroepithelial cyst in the right rolandic region in the pre-surgical planning: fMRI during left-hand finger-tapping showed a cortical activation area posteriorly dislocated by the lesion.

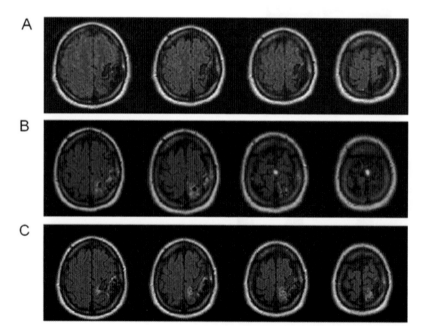

Fig. 12.3 Example of cortical plasticity in a case of arteriovenous malformation (AVM). Motor fMRI in a patient with an AVM located in the left rolandic region during flexo-extension of the last four fingers of the right hand: fMRI was performed at baseline (A), 2 days (B), and 2 months (C) after endovascular embolization. Following embolization, the patient showed a mild motor deficit of the right upper limb which completely recovered in the following weeks. (A) Before embolization: fMRI showed contralateral activation of the sensorimotor cortex located anteriorly to the AVM. (B) 2 days after embolization, in association with the mild right motor deficit: fMRI showed a bilateral activation of sensorimotor cortex and of the supplementary motor area. (C) 2 months after embolization, in association with clinical recovery: fMRI showed the return to a normal activation pattern. (With permission from Raz et al. [40]).

The adult human oligodendrocyte precursor cell: a key player in myelin repair

Julia M. Rist and Robin J. M. Franklin

Oligodendrocyte precursor cells (OPCs) are the cells that generate oligodendrocytes, the myelinating cells of the central nervous system (CNS). They do so not only during development, but persist in the adult CNS throughout life, ensuring homeostasis of glial cells in the normal white matter, and replacing lost oligodendrocytes following injury. Cells of the oligodendrocyte lineage are amongst the best-understood lineages in the vertebrate CNS and the oligodendrocyte precursor cells have been extensively characterized in vitro and in vivo.

In this chapter, we give an overview of the development and properties of OPCs and discuss their role in remyelination. We will review what is known about the well-characterized rodent OPCs and compare them to human OPCs, which are less well understood.

Oligodendrocyte precursor cell biology in rodents

Development and properties of oligodendrocyte precursor cells

Oligodendrocyte precursor cells in rodents can be identified by their expression of the cell surface markers NG2 (chondroitin sulfate proteoglycan), platelet-derived growth factor α receptor (PDGFαR) as well as gangliosides recognized by the monoclonal antibody A2B5. They depend on a number of growth factors that can modulate their survival, proliferation, and differentiation. The literature on the actions of these different growth factors on OPCs is complex, but a consensus view is that platelet-derived growth factor A (PDGF-A) and fibroblast growth factor (FGF) are each potent mitogens for OPCs, while combination of PDGF-A/FGF inhibits differentiation.

Insulin-like growth factor (IGF-1) on the other hand is recognized as an inducer of differentiation of OPCs.

The nomenclature of these cells has changed over the years. Initially, they were identified as bipotential precursor cells that can give rise to oligodendrocytes as well as type II astrocytes in vitro [1], and were therefore referred to as O2A progenitor cells. But evidence discussed later in this chapter suggests that this cell retains more plasticity and competence than previously thought.

The cells of the oligodendrocyte lineage are – like most other neural cell types of the CNS – derived from cells of the neural tube. The patterning of the neural tube generates restricted progenitor cell domains. During embryonic development, cells of the oligodendroglial lineage are specified in the pMN domain via activation of Olig2 by ventrally (floor-plate) derived Sonic hedgehog (Shh) signaling. In contrast, dorsally (roof-plate) derived bone morphogenic proteins (BMPs) and Wnt signals have been shown to antagonize oligodendrocyte development. The relative intensities of Shh, BMP, and Wnt signals are the critical determinant of early glial specification. These ventral OPCs then migrate out and populate the entire neural tube. Besides this ventral origin of OPCs, cells of the oligodendrocyte lineage can also have dorsal origin during fetal development. In this case they develop from dP3–6 domains in a Shh-independent manner. At birth, ventrally and dorsally derived OPCs are supposedly mixed in the spinal cord, and to date it is unclear what the relative contributions are and whether these cells represent a heterogenic population or are indistinguishable (reviewed by Ligon et al. [2]).

Adding to this developmental heterogeneity of OPCs, there might be additional functional heterogeneity within the OPC population. It has recently been shown that there exist two different populations of OPCs in the rat CNS white matter [3]. One type expresses voltage-gated sodium and potassium channels, can generate action potentials, and can receive synaptic input from axons, whereas the other OPC type lacks action potential and synaptic input. The role of these excitable OPCs and their non-excitable counterparts as well as the contribution of these two distinct OPC types to remyelination remains to be addressed.

The development of OPCs continues beyond birth. Extensive in vitro comparisons of perinatal OPCs with adult OPCs, both isolated from rat optic nerve, demonstrate that the adult OPCs are fundamentally different from their perinatal counterparts [4–6]. Perinatal OPCs have a very limited lifespan, and their properties are perfectly suited to the needs of a developing organism. They give then rise to adult OPCs, which persist throughout adulthood and which have properties are adapted to the needs of the adult CNS. In particular, perinatal OPCs are rapidly dividing, and differentiation into oligodendrocytes usually occurs synchronously in all cells of a clone. Thus the perinatal OPCs can generate a large numbers of oligodendrocytes in a short time-span. They are also highly migratory cells.

In contrast, adult OPCs divide, migrate, and differentiate much more slowly than their perinatal counterparts. While perinatal OPCs proliferate and then differentiate synchronously within a clone, adult OPCs have been to shown to be able to generate daughter cells that will subsequently undergo a different fate than the mother cell [6]. Whether this is due to asymmetrical cell division based on the segregation of cell fate determinants remains unclear. Adult OPCs are generated by a subset of perinatal OPCs that mature into adult OPCs. Moreover, this maturation program has been demonstrated to be an intrinsic process that occurs independently from any environmental cues, as it can be replicated in vitro [7]. During this maturation process, the OPCs also change some of their antigenic properties [4]. Due to their stem-cell-like self-renewing properties, they appear not to require another stem cell in the adult CNS to generate adult OPCs de novo, but are a self-maintaining population.

In vivo, adult OPCs are widespread throughout the CNS and make up around 5–8% of the glial cell population of the CNS [8]. Their role in the normal undisturbed CNS remains largely elusive. As their processes are found to be in contiguity with the nodes

of Ranvier (the spaces between two adjacent myelin sheaths) and synapses, a regulatory role has been proposed at these structures. They are very slowly dividing and quiescent in normal white matter, exhibiting stem-cell-like properties [9–11]. However, upon CNS demyelination these cells form a reactive population that proliferates very quickly and can proceed to replace lost oligodendrocytes [12]. Transcription factors like Nkx2.2 and Olig2 have been shown to identify reactive OPCs [13], but it still remains largely unknown what regulates the transition of OPCs from a quiescent state to an active phenotype that is responsive to mediators of repair, and what exactly characterizes the reactive OPC. It is likely though that the inflammatory response that is associated with demyelination plays an important role in activating the transient-amplifying population of OPCs.

For a long time OPCs have generally been regarded as lineage-restricted precursor cells that can give rise in vitro to different types of glial cells – oligodendrocytes and type II astrocytes [1]. Although in normal development their differentiation is largely restricted to oligodendrocyte differentiation, evidence is emerging that the OPC may possess a much wider differentiation potential than previously assumed. Under appropriate conditions, they have been shown to generate neurons in vitro [14–16]. This suggests that the OPC is multipotent, but is restricted by its environment to only differentiate along a certain lineage in vivo. The boundary between neural stem cells and OPCs hence becomes more blurred, and one can consider the OPC to be a multipotential adult stem cell that contributes to tissue homeostasis and repair. Adult OPCs also have been shown to have high levels of telomerase activity, allowing them to undergo many rounds of proliferation without senescence, which is another typical characteristic for stem cells [17].

Oligodendrocyte precursor cells and remyelination

Upon demyelination, OPCs can engage in a spontaneous repair process called remyelination that restores the myelin sheaths on demyelinated axons. Different experimental models have shown that remyelination is a robustly occurring phenomenon in the adult CNS [18, 19]. On a cellular level, remyelination can be divided into several key phases. The first phase involves the activation of a population of OPCs, which then rapidly proliferate and repopulate an area of demyelination [20–22]. After the recruitment of the OPCs to the lesion, the repair proceeds towards the second phase, in which the recruited cells differentiate into oligodendrocytes, which can then generate new myelin sheaths and engage the demyelinated axons in order to complete remyelination.

Even though OPCs are considered to be the key players in this process, there are other cell types that play crucial roles in setting the stage for remyelination and helping to create an environment in the demyelinated lesion that is conducive to the recruitment and differentiation of OPCs. Astrocytes generally become activated after CNS injury and contribute to the signaling environment [23, 24], and demyelination forms no exception to this rule [25, 26]. The role of microglia that become activated after demyelination is equally important. There is a long-standing debate whether the inflammatory response associated with demyelination is detrimental or beneficial to the repair process. While it is clear that certain aspects of inflammation are effectors of the pathological autoimmune response to myelin, evidence emerges that at least in a toxin-induced model of demyelination, the inflammatory response is in fact beneficial to repair. Macrophages, which originate from a quiescent pool of microglia present in the CNS as well as from monocytes from the blood stream that invade the CNS, have received special attention in this context: they have been shown to be not only a key source of growth factors during early phases of remyelination and thereby contribute to the orchestration of the process [26], but also to help with the clearance of myelin debris which is imperative for successful remyelination [27], as myelin debris has been shown to inhibit OPC differentiation [28].

Furthermore, inflammation has been shown to stimulate myelination by transplanted OPCs [29, 30], adding more and direct evidence to the hypothesis that inflammation can have beneficial effects on remyelination. This has important implications for immunomodulatory therapies used in the treatment of multiple sclerosis (MS).

Indirect evidence for the remyelination potential of OPCs comes from various transplantation experiments. Transplantation of rodent OPCs effectively repairs experimental demyelination [26, 31, 32] and rescues myelination in animal models of congenital demyelinating diseases [33, 34], and therefore provides proof of principle that transplantation of OPCs could be used as a remyelination-enhancing repair strategy in various demyelinating disorders.

The human OPC

How do human OPCs compare to rodent OPCs?

Evidence for a human OPC has come early on from studies of MS lesions. Cells expressing PDGFαR/NG2 were found to be present in normal white matter as well as enriched in MS lesions. A wealth of histopathological data on the presumptive human OPC accumulated. However, the characterization of the human OPC in tissue sections based only on antigen expression did not allow characterization of its lineage potential, and could therefore not unambiguously prove the existence of a human OPC. In vitro characterization of the human OPC lagged behind that of the rodent cell because of the difficulty in extracting this cell from human CNS tissue. Early in vitro studies on fresh human white matter dissociates obtained from temporal lobe resections indeed confirmed the presence of immature oligodendroglia [35], which can give rise to oligodendrocytes in vitro, but not to type II astrocytes. The isolated immature oligodendroglia were not proliferating, and exposure to the known mitogens of rodent OPCs revealed that these human cells respond differently to humoral growth factors than their rodent counterparts. When exposed to FGF, PDGF, or IGF-1 or to combinations of these factors – each of which is a mitogen on its own for rodent OPCs – cells do not enter mitosis. Furthermore, they prove mitotically unresponsive to astrocyte-conditioned medium [35–37]. Due to the postmitotic state of these cells, these first studies called the cells pre-oligodendrocytes, rather than progenitor or precursor cells. These pre-oligodendrocytes have a similar antigenic phenotype to rodent adult OPCs, $O4^+/vimentin^-/GalC^-$ [35]. Cells with the same antigenic properties were identified in vivo using tissue prints. Further studies on human brain tissue revealed also that an estimate of 2% of the total oligodendrocyte lineage express PDGFαR as well as MyT1, both recognized OPC markers, and we can thus conclude that the human brain harbors a small pool of OPCs [36].

Later studies however identified a proliferative human OPC in cultures from human white matter, and this cell proves to be identical to the rodent progenitor with respect to its morphology, antigenic properties, and bipotential capacity for differentiation in vitro [38]. Culturing of human OPCs on an astrocyte monolayer was sufficient to induce proliferation in the human OPCs, similar to rodent OPCs. The rodent and human OPCs thus share many features; this indicates that the substantial body of knowledge about the rodent OPC may be directly relevant to human neurobiology. However, some interspecies differences are apparent, e.g., proliferation could not be induced by soluble growth factors, including human conditioned-astrocyte medium. It may be that human OPCs depend more closely on contact with astrocytes for proliferation than rodent cells. But also other salient differences have been described in the responsiveness of OPCs in adult rats and humans [39]. Furthermore, differences between OPCs from different species in response to various growth factors have been reported.

Despite these studies of the human OPC in mixed glial cultures, purification of human OPCs had remained an elusive goal for a long time. Several studies have therefore explored methods to purify or generate human OPCs in sufficient quantity and purity for further characterization of this cell as well as for transplantation-based therapy. It has been demonstrated that OPCs can be generated from neural spheres derived from human embryos, which not only allows the study of oligodendrocyte development in humans and identification of factors that influence it, but also provides an in vitro system that allows expansion of human neural precursors for several passages without losing the ability to generate different CNS cell types [40]. However, the generation of OPCs from human embryonic neurospheres did not solve the problem of how to purify the adult human OPC to characterize it and analyze its remyelination potential. This was achieved with the development of a fluorescence-activated cell sorting (FACS) strategy of human white matter dissociates [41]. With the identification of appropriate markers for human OPCs it was possible to label OPCs in human white matter dissociates, by transfecting the dissociated cells with a green fluorescent protein (GFP) construct under a CNP2 promotor, which is active in the early oligodendrocyte lineage. A population of the cultured and transfected cells began to express GFP after a couple of days. The GFP-positive cells could then be extracted by FACS in sufficient quantity and purity

to characterize them better in vitro and in vivo. These purified cells yielded a distinct pool of bipolar, A2B5-positive progenitors, half of which were mitotically active. They gave rise primarily but not exclusively to oligodendrocytes in vitro, and their abundance in vivo was estimated to be 4% of the total cells in the human adult subcortical white matter, which is slightly more abundant than what had been reported previously using PDGFαR as a marker [36]. Because all the isolated cells were A2B5-positive, it has later been shown that the A2B5 immunoreactivity of the adult human OPCs can be used as a surrogate marker in the FACS strategy, which avoids the transfection step necessary for the promotor-based FACS labeling strategy [42]. Adult human OPCs have been compared in their phenotypic and functional properties to their fetal counterparts, with similar results to the studies comparing perinatal to adult OPCs in rodents. Adult human OPCs are intrinsically different from fetal human OPCs: they divide at a reduced rate, are phenotypically more committed to the oligodendroglial lineage than the fetal OPCs, and show reduced survival and process outgrowth in vitro [43]. However, consistent with previous studies, amongst the cells that did survive the transplantation a higher proportion contributes to myelination of the dysmyelinated mouse mutants. This raises important issues regarding the remyelination potential of adult OPCs that have not been resolved to date. Interestingly, a head-to-head comparison of the myelinogenic potential of purified fetal and adult OPCs transplanted into shiverer mice showed that adult OPCs differed substantially from their fetal counterparts in their myelinating efficacy, as the adult cells myelinated the shiverer brain much more rapidly than fetal OPCs [44]. Transcriptional profiling of adult human OPCs has revealed several interesting signaling pathways that appear to characterize the interaction of OPCs with the white matter in which they reside [45]. The OPCs differentially express several receptors that allow them to interact and respond to their environment, such as the PDGFαR, type 3 FGF receptor (FGFR3), receptor tyrosine phosphatase-ζ (RTPZ), notch, and syndecan.

What is the lineage potential of the human precursor cells? Like their rodent counterparts, the human adult OPCs might not be strictly committed to oligodendrocytic differentiation, but also be pluripotent progenitors that generate a certain lineage depending on the environment to which they are exposed. As mentioned before, OPCs purified by FACS give rise largely to oligodendrocytes, but generate occasional neurons in low-density cultures [41]. It has been demonstrated that human adult OPCs can indeed generate both types of glial cells – oligodendrocytes and astrocytes – as well as neurons in vitro and also in vivo upon xenograft into fetal rat brain [15]. Together with our knowledge about the pluripotency of rodent OPCs, this finding leads to the view that the OPC may indeed be a type of neural stem cell that is restricted in vivo to the oligodendrocyte lineage by its environment. This view is also supported by findings from several groups that non-white-matter neural stem cells become similarly restricted to the oligodendrocyte lineage when presented to adult white matter. An example of this phenomenon is the study in which murine epidermal growth factor (EGF)-expanded neural stem cells were transplanted in shiverer mice, and have been shown to differentiate as oligodendrocytes and achieve widespread myelination [46].

Human OPCs in demyelination/remyelination

The fact that human OPCs are strongly enriched in remyelinating MS lesions suggests that these cells contribute to remyelination. In MS, substantial areas of remyelination can be found in the so-called shadow plaques [47–49], and the extent of remyelination has been shown to be very variable between different patients [50]. Therefore, it seems likely that OPCs contribute to myelin repair in MS. Even though there is no direct clinical evidence to date that could positively correlate the amount of remyelination and functional improvement in MS patients, a wealth of data, mostly from rodent models, suggests that enhancing remyelination, which fails for unknown reasons in MS, could be beneficial to MS patients. The development of strategies to achieve such an enhancement of remyelination in acquired demyelination – either by manipulating endogenous OPCs or by supplying exogenous OPCs – has been the focus of intense research for quite some time.

Many studies have been carried out assessing the myelination potential of rodent as well as human OPCs in congenital dysmyelinated models, and widespread myelination can be achieved. However, much less is known about the behavior of the human OPC in a repair situation rather than a developmental one. Direct evidence for the remyelination potential of human OPCs comes from a study in which human OPCs purified by FACS were transplanted into experimentally demyelinated focal lesions in the rat brain [42]. Human OPCs have been shown to migrate rapidly throughout the lesion and differentiate into oligodendrocytes that express various myelin markers. In contrast to the demyelinated lesions, normal adult white matter is non-permissive to OPC migration. Despite their rapid population of the lesions, the engrafted OPCs rarely extended into normal white matter. The fact that OPCs which are grafted into normal white matter tracts remain localized at the site of injection suggests that this is due to an absolute non-permissive state of the white matter to progenitor migration rather than a relative preference of the human OPCs for the demyelinated lesion over the normally myelinated tracts [42]. The signals that restrict progenitor migration have yet to be identified.

Some of the properties of human OPCs that have been discussed are encouraging for transplantation approaches for cell-based therapy of demyelinating diseases like MS, but others present obstacles. The apparent pluripotency of OPCs is an important issue that has to be considered in a therapeutic strategy that would involve transplantation of these cells. Remaining immature cells could ectopically differentiate; the consequences of this can be variable but should not be left unconsidered. Also, the normal white matter that presents itself non-permissive to migration of OPCs is a serious obstacle for transplantation approaches, as engrafted cells, unless they are transplanted right into the lesion environment, might not be able to reach their target. Targeted cell transplantation into each lesion is not feasible in MS patients with multiple lesions.

In conclusion, even though remyelination-enhancing approaches might harbor great potential for clinical benefit in demyelinating diseases, we are only beginning to understand the biology of the human OPCs, but before it can be efficiently and safely used in cell-based therapies several obstacles are yet to be overcome. Similarly, for an endogenous approach to enhance remyelination, the signals and mechanisms that control the self-renewal, activation, and differentiation of the human OPC in a repair situation need to be much better characterized before we can manipulate them in our favor.

References

1. Raff M C, Miller R H, Noble M. A glial progenitor cell that develops in vitro into an astrocyte or an oligodendrocyte depending on culture medium. *Nature* 1983;**303**:390–6

2. Ligon K L, Fancy S P, Franklin R J M, Rowitch D H. Olig gene function in CNS development and disease. *Glia* 2006;**54**:1–10

3. Karadottir R, Hamilton N B, Bakiri Y, Attwell D. Spiking and nonspiking classes of oligodendrocyte precursor glia in CNS white matter. *Nat Neurosci* 2008;**11**:450–6

4. Wolswijk G, Noble M. Identification of an adult-specific glial progenitor cell. *Development* 1989;**105**:387–400

5. Noble M, Wren D, Wolswijk G. The O-2A(adult) progenitor cell: a glial stem cell of the adult central nervous system. *Semin Cell Biol* 1992;**3**:413–22

6. Wren D, Wolswijk G, Noble M. In vitro analysis of the origin and maintenance of O-2A adult progenitor cells. *J Cell Biol* 1992;**116**:167–76

7. Tang D G, Tokumoto Y M, Raff M C. Long-term culture of purified postnatal oligodendrocyte precursor cells: evidence for an intrinsic maturation program that plays out over months. *J Cell Biol* 2000;**148**:971–84

8. Levine J M, Reynolds R, Fawcett J W. The oligodendrocyte precursor cell in health and disease. *Trends Neurosci* 2001;**24**:39–47

9. Chang A, Nishiyama A, Peterson J, Prineas J, Trapp B D. NG2-positive oligodendrocyte progenitor cells in adult human brain and multiple sclerosis lesions. *J Neurosci* 2000;**20**:6404–12

10. Horner P J, Power A E, Kempermann G, *et al.* Proliferation and differentiation of progenitor cells throughout the intact adult rat spinal cord. *J Neurosci* 2000;**20**:2218–28

11. Dawson M R, Polito A, Levine J M, Reynolds R. NG2-expressing glial progenitor cells: an abundant and widespread population of cycling cells in the adult rat CNS. *Mol Cell Neurosci* 2003;**24**:476–88

12. Franklin R J M. Why does remyelination fail in multiple sclerosis? *Nat Rev Neurosci* 2002;**3**:705–14

13. Fancy S P, Zhao C, Franklin R J M. Increased expression of Nkx2.2 and Olig2 identifies reactive oligodendrocyte progenitor cells responding to demyelination in the adult CNS. *Mol Cell Neurosci* 2004;**27**:247–54

14. Kondo T, Raff M. Oligodendrocyte precursor cells reprogrammed to become multipotential CNS stem cells. *Science* 2000;**289**:1754–7

15. Nunes M C, Roy N S, Keyoung H M, *et al.* Identification and isolation of multipotential neural progenitor cells from the subcortical white matter of the adult human brain. *Nat Med* 2003;**9**:439–47

16. Rivers L E, Young K M, Rizzi M, *et al.* PDGFRA/NG2 glia generate myelinating oligodendrocytes and piriform projection neurons in adult mice. *Nat Neurosci* 2008;**11**:1392–401

17. Tang D G, Tokumoto Y M, Apperly J A, Lloyd A C, Raff M C. Lack of replicative senescence in cultured rat oligodendrocyte precursor cells. *Science* 2001;**291**:868–71

18. Bunge M B, Bunge R P, Ris H. Ultrastructural study of remyelination in an experimental lesion in adult cat spinal cord. *J Biophys Biochem Cytol* 1961;**10**:67–94

19. Miller D J, Asakura K, Rodriguez M. Central nervous system remyelination: clinical application of basic neuroscience principles. *Brain Pathol* 1996;**6**:331–44

20. Carroll W M, Jennings A R. Early recruitment of oligodendrocyte precursors in CNS demyelination. *Brain* 1994;**117**(*3*):563–78

21. Franklin R J M, Gilson J M, Blakemore W F. Local recruitment of remyelinating cells in the repair of demyelination in the central nervous system. *J Neurosci Res* 1997;**50**:337–44

22. Sim F J, Zhao C, Penderis J, Franklin R J M. The age-related decrease in CNS remyelination efficiency is attributable to an impairment of both oligodendrocyte progenitor recruitment and differentiation. *J Neurosci* 2002;**22**:2451–9

23. Eddleston M, Mucke L. Molecular profile of reactive astrocytes: implications for their role in neurologic disease. *Neuroscience* 1993;**54**:15–36

24. Pekny M, Nilsson M. Astrocyte activation and reactive gliosis. *Glia* 2005;**50**:427–34

25. Komoly S, Hudson L D, Webster H D, Bondy C A. Insulin-like growth factor I gene expression is induced in astrocytes during experimental demyelination. *Proc Natl Acad Sci USA* 1992;**89**:1894–8

26. Hinks G L, Franklin R J M. Distinctive patterns of PDGF-A, FGF-2, IGF-I, and TGF-beta1 gene expression during remyelination of experimentally-induced spinal cord demyelination. *Mol Cell Neurosci* 1999;**14**:153–68

27. Kotter M R, Setzu A, Sim F J, Van Rooijen N, Franklin R J M. Macrophage depletion impairs oligodendrocyte remyelination following lysolecithin-induced demyelination. *Glia* 2001;**35**:204–12

28. Kotter M R, Li W W, Zhao C, Franklin R J M. Myelin impairs CNS remyelination by inhibiting oligodendrocyte precursor cell differentiation. *J Neurosci* 2006;**26**:328–32

29. Foote A K, Blakemore W F. Inflammation stimulates remyelination in areas of chronic demyelination. *Brain* 2005;**128**:528–39

30. Setzu A, Lathia J D, Zhao C, *et al*. Inflammation stimulates myelination by transplanted oligodendrocyte precursor cells. *Glia* 2006; **54**:297–303

31. Groves A K, Barnett S C, Franklin R J M, *et al*. Repair of demyelinated lesions by transplantation of purified O-2A progenitor cells. *Nature* 1993;**362**:453–5

32. Franklin R J M. Remyelination of the demyelinated CNS: the case for and against transplantation of central, peripheral and olfactory glia. *Brain Res Bull* 2002;**57**:827–32

33. Duncan I D, Milward E A. Glial cell transplants: experimental therapies of myelin diseases. *Brain Pathol* 1995;**5**:301–10

34. Nistor G I, Totoiu M O, Haque N, Carpenter M K, Keirstead H S. Human embryonic stem cells differentiate into oligodendrocytes in high purity and myelinate after spinal cord transplantation. *Glia* 2005;**49**:385–96

35. Armstrong R C, Dorn H H, Kufta C V, Friedman E, Dubois-Dalcq M E. Pre-oligodendrocytes from adult human CNS. *J Neurosci* 1992;**12**:1538–47

36. Gogate N, Verma L, Zhou J M, *et al*. Plasticity in the adult human oligodendrocyte lineage. *J Neurosci* 1994; **14**:4571–87

37. Prabhakar S, D'Souza S, Antel J P, *et al*. Phenotypic and cell cycle properties of human oligodendrocytes in vitro. *Brain Res* 1995;**672**:159–69

38. Scolding N J, Rayner P J, Sussman J, Shaw C, Compston D A. A proliferative adult human oligodendrocyte progenitor. *Neuroreport* 1995; **6**:441–5

39. Scolding N. Glial precursor cells in the adult human brain. *Neuroscientist* 1998;**4**:264–227

40. Murray K, Dubois-Dalcq M. Emergence of oligodendrocytes from human neural spheres. *J Neurosci Res* 1997;**50**:146–56

41. Roy N S, Wang S, Harrison-Restelli C, *et al*. Identification, isolation, and promoter-defined separation of mitotic oligodendrocyte progenitor cells from the adult human subcortical white matter. *J Neurosci* 1999;**19**:9986–95

42. Windrem M S, Roy N S, Wang J, *et al*. Progenitor cells derived from the adult human subcortical white matter disperse and differentiate as oligodendrocytes within demyelinated lesions of the rat brain. *J Neurosci Res* 2002;**69**:966–75

43. Ruffini F, Arbour N, Blain M, Olivier A, Antel J P. Distinctive properties of human adult brain-derived myelin progenitor cells. *Am J Pathol* 2004;**165**: 2167–75

44. Windrem M S, Nunes M C, Rashbaum W K, *et al*. Fetal and adult human oligodendrocyte progenitor cell isolates myelinate the congenitally dysmyelinated brain. *Nat Med* 2004;**10**:93–7

45. Sim F J, Lang J K, Waldau B, *et al*. Complementary patterns of gene expression by human oligodendrocyte progenitors and their environment predict determinants of progenitor maintenance and differentiation. *Ann Neurol* 2006;**59**:763–79

46. Mitome M, Low H P, van den Pol A, *et al*. Towards the reconstruction of central nervous system white matter using neural precursor cells. *Brain* 2001;**124**:2147–61

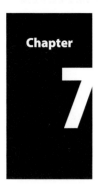

Tissue regeneration and repair in multiple sclerosis: the role of neural stem cells

Stefano Pluchino, Roberto Furlan, Luca Muzio, and Gianvito Martino

The brain repair system

Regeneration is a fundamental part of life. While physiological (spontaneous) regeneration naturally occurs upon cell attrition, injury-reactive (reparative) regeneration occurs as a consequence of tissue damage and greatly differs among different animals and tissues. After the first observation of reparative regeneration in a limb – via blastema formation in the crayfish – made in 1712 by René-Antoine Ferchault de Réaumur, the scientific community had to await Francisco Tello's work, in the early twentieth century, to have preliminary evidence that also the central nervous system (CNS) has the ability to regenerate after an injury [1].

The potential value of this observation was first recognized by Ramón y Cajal who described as "curious and significant" the experiment carried out by Tello: "When a piece of the distal stump of a sectioned nerve is introduced in a cerebral wound of a rabbit a regenerative capacity appears in the apathetic [axons] of the white substance. This demonstrates that the impotence of the central [axons] to restore the peripheral stump is neither fatal nor irremediable" [2]. The seminal work of Tello has been recently rejuvenated by detailed in vitro and in vivo mechanistic evidence supporting the existence of an innate self-maintenance program, "the brain repair system," sustaining brain homeostasis and repair upon injury.

Several molecular and cellular events sustaining intrinsic brain repair mechanisms have been described so far. They can be divided into three distinct, although strictly interrelated, categories: inflammation-driven processes, CNS plasticity, and neuro(glio)genesis (for review see Martino [3]). On the one hand, humoral and cellular inflammatory components shift sense (function) over time from a tissue-damaging mode to

a mode promoting tissue repair (e.g., neurotrophic support from inflammatory cells) (for review see Martino *et al.* [4]). On the other hand, the recruitment of alternative "non-damaged" functioning neuronal pathways (cortical maps), occurring mainly via axonal branching and synaptogenesis, takes place as a consequence of brain damage. Whether or not (and to what extent) the recapitulation of precise developmental pathways underlies the whole brain plasticity is still matter of investigation. Finally, endogenous neural stem/precursor cells (NPCs) – the self-renewing and multipotent cells of the CNS capable of driving neurogenesis and gliogenesis in adult life – may adapt targeted migration into damaged areas and promote repair via several mechanisms of action (e.g., neuro- and gliogenesis, immunomodulation, neuroprotection) [5]. It is still a matter of investigation whether (or not) equally robust brain repair/protection can occur following the recruitment within the CNS of transdifferentiating stem cells of a different embryonic origin (e.g., developmental plasticity vs. cell fusion).

Central nervous system regeneration in multiple sclerosis

Multiple sclerosis (MS) is an inflammatory (auto) immune-mediated disease of the CNS characterized by multifocal white matter plaques of demyelination leading to irreversible axonal loss and degeneration [6]. Spontaneous repair (i.e., remyelination) occurs in MS lesions although its extent is variable among cases [7]. In a correlative radiological–pathological study in postmortem human MS brains, remyelinated areas were found in 42% of the lesions studied; partial remyelination was observed in 19% of the lesions, while 23% of the lesions were completely remyelinated "shadow" plaques [8]. In a more recent study

Multiple Sclerosis: Recovery of Function and Neurorehabilitation, eds. J. Kesselring, G. Comi, and A. J. Thompson.
Published by Cambridge University Press. © Cambridge University Press 2010.

performed on 51 autopsies of MS patients with different clinical courses and disease durations, the extent of remyelination was variable between cases. In 20% of patients – both relapsing and progressive patients – the extent of remyelination was extensive with 60–96% of the global lesion area remyelinated [9].

Despite plenty of evidence indicating that remyelination occurs in MS, there is also evidence that this phenomenon is transient, often incomplete, and limited. Although it is still unknown what is the ultimate reason why spontaneous remyelination fails over time in MS, some explanations can be put forward. The most likely causes of remyelination failure in MS (for review see Franklin [10]) can be summarized as follows: (1) quantitative reduction of oligodendrocyte precursor cells (OPCs) as well as scarce ability of these cells to differentiate into myelinating oligodendrocytes; (2) failure of OPCs to "respond" to demyelination; (3) selective depletion of myelinating cells around demyelinating areas over years; (4) inhibition of remyelination as result of a "critical" balance between pro-inflammatory and pro-remyelinating effects of cytokines; (5) limitation of endogenous OPC migration to sites of injury by reactive astrocytic scar formation; and (6) acute and/or chronic loss of axons. Recently accumulated evidence shows that an inflammatory CNS microenvironment may alter the self-renewal, proliferation, differentiation, and migration capacities of NPCs so to impair their "physiological" capacity to promote CNS homeostasis and repair [5]. This can be an additional important cause of remyelination failure in MS, which has to be taken into consideration.

Neural stem/precursor cells (NPCs)

In the adult CNS, proliferating neural cells represent an heterogeneous population of mitotically active, self-renewing, and multipotent cells showing complex patterns of gene expression that vary in space and time [11]. The category NPCs is used as a generic term encompassing both stem and progenitor cells and includes bona fide CNS stem cells, (intermediate stage) multipotent neural progenitors, and lineage-oriented neural precursors. Stem cells in the CNS display cardinal features such as (virtually) unlimited capacity for self-renewal and ability to proliferate in response to mitogens, and multipotency for the different neuro-ectodermal lineages of the CNS (astrocytes, oligodendrocytes, and neurons). Multipotent progenitors

are proliferative cells with only limited self-renewal that can differentiate into at least two different cell lineages [12], while lineage-oriented precursors are cells with restriction to one distinct neural lineage.

Self-renewal and differentiation of NPCs are regulated by specialized microenvironment(s) – referred to as CNS germinal niche(s) – in which these cells reside. Both environmental cues and intrinsic genetic programs are required to maintain stem cell properties and to direct/regulate proliferation and differentiation within CNS niches [13]. The subventricular zone (SVZ) of the lateral ventricles and the subgranular zone (SGZ) of the dentate gyrus (DG) of the hippocampus are the two most-studied brain germinal regions in which CNS stem cells reside and sustain neurogenesis and gliogenesis throughout adult life [14]. Cells with structural and molecular characteristics of astrocytes (e.g., expression of glial fibrillary acidic protein [GFAP]) are the neurogenic units (putative stem cells or type B cells) in the germinal regions of both the SVZ and SGZ [15].

In the SVZ, GFAP$^+$ astrocytes (type B cells) are in intimate contact with all other SVZ cell types, including the rapidly dividing transit amplifying cells (type C cells) and the lineage-committed (postmitotic) migratory neuroblasts (type A cells). Interestingly enough, some type B cells and a small subpopulation of type C cells express the oligodendrocyte lineage transcription factor 2 (Olig2), thus suggesting that oligodendrocyte differentiation in the SVZ begins early in the lineage [16]. Further, type B cells generate a small number of non-myelinating NG2$^+$ OPCs and mature myelinating oligodendrocytes [16]. The cell lineage differentiation pathway in the SVZ goes from type B, through type C to type A cells, with type B cells believed to be the self-renewing primary precursors [15].

In the SGZ, GFAP$^+$ astrocytes function as putative (type B) stem cells, and undergo self-renewal, proliferation, and differentiation into transit amplifying (type D) cells, which then differentiate into lineage-committed (type G) migratory granule neurons [17, 18].

The maintenance and differentiation of NPCs in CNS germinal niches very likely relies on their physical contact with the basal lamina which, acting as a scaffold, sequesters and/or modulates cytokines and growth factors derived from local cells (such as fibroblasts, macrophages, and pericytes) [19]. Type B cells in the SVZ are in close contact (interdigitated) with both the basal lamina and the blood vessels, while in the SGZ, bursts of endothelial cell division are spatially and temporally related to clusters of neurogenesis [17].

Adult NPCs, inflammation, and demyelination

Neural precursor cells contributing to the endogenous CNS stem cell compartment within brain germinal niches might assist in tissue repair owing to their ability to support neurogenesis and gliogenesis during adulthood [14]. Nevertheless, self-renewal, proliferation, differentiation, and migration of endogenous NPCs may vary, depending on the molecular composition of the local microenvironment characterizing the different types of CNS injuries (e.g., acute vs. chronic, focal vs. multifocal) (Fig. 7.1) [5].

Increased numbers of nestin-expressing proliferating as well as doublecortin-reactive NPCs are detected at the boundaries of the injury site as early as 1 week after experimental acute focal inflammatory CNS disorders, such as spinal cord injury (SCI) and stroke [20–23]. Experimental acute stroke in rodents triggers neurogenesis and migration of newborn neurons from their sites of origin into ischemic brain regions [24]. The transient occlusion of the middle cerebral artery in the rat increases the incorporation of BrdU (marker of proliferating cells) into neural cells in the SGZ, the effect correlating with activation

of the cAMP-response-element-binding protein (CREB) [25]. Neural cells labeled with BrdU co-express the immature neuronal markers doublecortin and proliferating cell nuclear antigen (PCNA), while they do not express the more mature cell markers neuronal nuclear (NeuN) and Hu, thus suggesting that they are nascent neurons [26]. The acute stroke is associated with a shortened length of the cell cycle, a decreased G1 phase, and an increased cell cycle length of SVZ-resident neural progenitors [27] regulating a transient increase in both (terminal) symmetric cell division as well as generation of neuronal progenitors migrating through the ischemic striatum towards the damage, closely associated with blood vessels [22, 28]. In patients with stroke, neural cells that express markers associated with newborn neurons are present in the ischemic penumbra surrounding cerebral cortical infarcts and preferentially localize in the vicinity of blood vessels [29]. In mouse SCI, neural progenitors in the ependymal zone (EZ) of the central canal of the spinal cord mobilize and migrate vigorously toward the direction where the contusion injury is generated – the most favorable migration occurring in the adjacent region close to the epicenter of the lesion – and differentiate optimally into NeuN-immunoreactive neurons, while not into astrocytes or oligodendrocytes [30]. After cervical SCI in the adult rhesus monkey, BrdU-based analysis of cell proliferation in vivo reveals an 80-fold

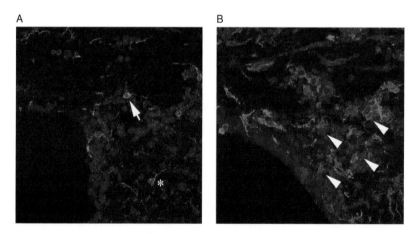

A   B

Fig. 7.1. Inflammation in experimental autoimmune encephalomyelitis (EAE) affects CNS (germinal) areas where neural stem/precursor cells (NPCs) reside. The figure shows infiltrating microglia in the SVZ of EAE and healthy control mice (HC). Coronal sections from brains of HC (panel A) and myelin oligodendrocyte glycoprotein (MOG)35–55-induced EAE (panel B) mice are stained for Iba1 (macrophage/microglia marker, red staining) and DAPI (nuclear marker, blue staining). In HC mice, few ramified Iba1+ cells are located within the dorsolateral SVZ (arrow in panel A) while resting Iba1+ ramified cells are sparse throughout the CNS parenchyma (asterisk in panel A). In EAE mice 20 days post-immunization, many Iba1+ cells are found within the dorsolateral SVZ (arrowheads in panel B) and appear more hyperthophic than those found in HC. (See also color plate.)

Knowledge Spa
Royal Cornwall Hospital
Treliske
Truro. TR1 3HD

Chapter 7: Tissue regeneration and repair

increase in the number of newly divided cells in the spinal cord. By 7 months after injury, 15% of these newly generated neural cells express markers of mature oligodendrocytes while 12% express astrocytic markers. These newly born oligodendrocytes are present in zones of injury-induced demyelination and appear to ensheath or remyelinate host axons [31]. In experimental models of chronic multifocal inflammatory demyelinating disorders such as experimental autoimmune encephalomyelitis (EAE), the animal model of MS, mitotically active neural progenitor cells, which reside either in the SVZ of the brain or in the EZ, subvert their physiological destiny – the rostral migration to the olfactory bulb or the radial migration to the lateral columns of the spinal cord – and migrate into areas of demyelination where they differentiate into glial cells [32, 33]. SVZ-resident type B "putative" stem cells appearing as GFAP$^+$/Olig2$^+$/polysialylated neural cell adhesion molecule (PSA-NCAM)$^+$/platelet-derived growth factor (PDGF) receptor alpha$^+$/beta-tubulin$^-$ (oligodendrocyte/neuron ratio = 1/30) migrate into the corpus callosum, the striatum, and the fimbria fornix, and differentiate into NG2$^+$ non-myelinating and mature myelinating oligodendrocytes [16]. Interestingly enough, when studied in a mouse model of focal CNS demyelination, a 4.3-fold increase in the number of type B cell-derived OPCs is observed in the corpus callosum of lysolecithin-injected brain hemispheres, as compared with the control (vehicle) hemispheres. These cells concentrate within and around the demyelination site and display morphological features suggestive of both mature and immature oligodendrocytes [16]. Activation (or recapitulation) of (oligodendro)gliogenesis has been very recently described in the SVZ and MS lesions of the human postmortem brain. The SVZ from MS patients showed higher (two- to threefold increase) cell density and enhanced numbers of PSA-NCAM$^+$/GFAP$^+$/Sox9$^+$ neural progenitors, as compared to controls. Interestingly, PSA-NCAM$^+$ neural progenitors expressing the markers of oligodendroglial specification Sox10 and Olig2 were detected in demyelinated MS lesions, thus suggesting that activation of (oligodendro)gliogenesis and mobilization of SVZ-derived early glial progenitors to periventricular demyelinating lesions occurs at certain levels in MS [34].

Though accumulating evidence indicates that endogenous neurogenesis and gliogenesis occur as part of an "intrinsic" self-repair process during inflammatory CNS disorders, such as MS, there are no convincing explanations about the overall incapacity of the endogenous stem cell compartment to promote full and long-lasting CNS repair [35]. Since it has been recently postulated that the dialog between inflammatory components and NPCs might have important consequences for CNS homeostasis and repair [36], it can be hypothesized that certain inflammatory components, such as CNS-infiltrating blood-borne inflammatory mononuclear cells, reactive CNS-resident cells (e.g., astrocytes, brain endothelial cells, and microglia), and humoral mediators (e.g., cytokines and chemokines), might orchestrate over time an inflammatory-driven derangement of the appropriate temporal and spatial relationship between cells residing within the germinal neurogenic niches which might, in turn, contribute to the demyelinating process as well as to the remyelination failure occurring in MS (Fig. 7.1) [5].

Is the mechanism underlying such phenomena attributable, at least in part, to the fact that inflammatory components trigger an "aberrant" recapitulation of developmental morphogens (e.g., stem cell regulators) within demyelinated CNS areas? Several recently published studies support such a conjecture. Activated encephalitogenic lymphocytes and reactive CNS-resident cells from EAE mice, which cause patchy demyelination and co-exist within the same perivascular inflamed CNS areas, secrete the morphogen bone morphogenetic protein BMP4 and its antagonist Noggin — two key factors in regulating self-renewal and differentiation of CNS stem cells within the SVZ [37–40]. Sonic hedgehog (Shh), a key fate determinant for embryonic CNS ventral interneuron progenitors of the neural tube [41], is re-expressed in inflammatory demyelinated lesions in rats with EAE [42]. Notch 1 and Jagged 1, which are crucial for axonal patterning and myelination during embryogenesis [43], are re-expressed at the lesion borders of inflammatory demyelinating lesions in MS patients [44]. However, the expression of both Notch and Jagged by OPCs might be of a limited functional significance for remyelination, as recently challenged in Notch 1-depleted OPCs from proteolipid protein (PLP)-creER Notch1(lox/lox) transgenic mice following administration of the demyelinating compound cuprizone [45]. Furthermore, it has been shown that interleukin (IL)-6 released by lipopolysaccharide (LPS)-activated microglia significantly impairs neurogenesis in the hippocampus in vivo and that such impairment is fully restored when non-steroidal anti-inflammatory drugs (such as indomethacin) are used [46]. In vitro generation of new neurons and oligodendrocytes from NPCs is induced and supported by mouse microglia that have encountered T-cell-associated cytokines (such as interferon-γ and IL-4), but blocked by those that have encountered endotoxins (such as LPS) [36]. Finally, when studied in immune-deficient mice, hippocampal neurogenesis has been found markedly impaired and not enhanced by environmental enrichment, while restored and boosted by T cells recognizing a specific CNS antigen, such as myelin basic protein (MBP) [47].

Whether or not primary CNS inflammatory reactions can affect proliferation and differentiation of NPC, either directly or indirectly via the aberrant (uncoordinated) re-expression of developmental genetic programs that regulate stem cell behavior, is still matter of debate. However, it can be speculated that chronic inflammation may ultimately lead to the exhaustion of the capacity of NPCs to exert their homeostatic and repairing program within the CNS.

Regional tropism of NPC-mediated repair

Can disease progression in MS patients be viewed as the consequence of the dysfunction of the neural stem cell compartment rather than caused by an uncontrolled, and still undiscovered, pathogenic alien(s)? How can we combine the apparently contradicting evidence that inflammation, on one hand, drives NPC-mediated gliogenesis and, on the other hand, inhibits NPC proliferation and differentiation?

Magnetic resonance imaging (MRI) and postmortem histological studies indicate that inflammation, demyelination, and remyelination differ according to the regional location of MS lesions (heterogeneity). Gadolinium (Gd) enhancement (highly suggestive of site-specific inflammation), as well as hyperintense T_2-weighted lesions, are frequently visible within the periventricular region at the MRI of human MS brain. Moreover, lesion accumulation probability maps of hyperintense T_2-weighted and Gd-enhancing T_1 lesion volumes in MS suggests that a substantial proportion of the periventricular T_2 lesion volumes arise from mechanisms other than those associated with early breakdown of the blood–brain barrier leading to T_1 Gd enhancement. This asymmetry of T_1/T_2 lesion distribution includes the possibility that the central white matter might have a greater susceptibility to persistent T_2 hyperintense changes following inflammation [48]. Patrikios and colleagues have recently showed that – although complete remyelination may be present in some periventricular plaques – the global extent of remyelination is lower in these lesions, as compared to subcortical or deep white matter lesions [9]. This is true not only in the global MS sample, but also in cases with a high extent of remyelination, in whom large (hemispheric or double hemispheric) sections were analyzed [9].

All together these data prompt us to speculate that diverse, and possibly alternative, stem/precursor cell-mediated repair programs operate within different CNS areas in MS patients. Multipotent white matter progenitors (i.e., OPCs) – which are described as widely spread within the adult CNS parenchyma – may sustain glio(oligodendro)genesis within MS lesions located outside the periventricular areas (e.g., deep white matter, subcortical, and cortical areas) [49], while SVZ-resident NPCs may promote lesion repair in the periventricular areas by switching from a *default* neurogenic to a *injury-reactive* gliogenic program of differentiation. This scenario would be not only be favorable in terms of energy expenditure – cells should not travel too far in order to accomplish a biological priority such as repair – but would also explain the apparent divergent and contradictory effect of inflammation on NPCs. As a consequence, inflammatory players (both cellular and molecular) might interfere with both the proliferation and the differentiation program(s) sustaining NPC-mediated repair in a regionally oriented manner. Inflammation would impair NPC-mediated periventricular lesion repair owing to the facts that (1) periventricular inflammatory demyelinating lesions in MS – frequently visible through the ventricular lining as elongated gray sleeves – are closed to subependymal veins and are very often associated with a granular ependymitis [50], and (2) cell proliferation and differentiation within CNS germinal niche(s) depend on the physical contact between the different cell types of the niche, the basal lamina, and a brain microvessel [15]. On the other hand, parenchymal multipotent white matter progenitors are likely to be less flexible in their repair program as the inflammatory process in MS tends to become less intense as soon as it gets distant from lateral ventricles.

Conclusions

The involvement of neural stem and/or precursor cells in the process of demyelination and remyelination occurring in experimental and human MS is still far from being elucidated. However, the dissection of molecular and cellular components regulating neural stem/precursor cell proliferation, differentiation, and migration following demyelination and remyelination in MS is of key value. A better understanding of the underlying mechanisms of these phenomena might provide clues for the design of future clinical trials aimed at promoting CNS repair in MS.

References

1. Tello F. La influencia del neurotropismo en la regeneraciòn de los centros nerviosos. *Trab Lab Invest Biol Univ Madr* 1911;**9**:123–59

2. Ramón y Cajal S. Neuronismo o reticularismo? Las pruebas objectivas de la unidad anatòmica de las cèlulas nerviosas. *Arch Neurobiol* 1933; **13**:217–91

3. Martino G. How the brain repairs itself: new therapeutic strategies in inflammatory and degenerative CNS disorders. *Lancet Neurol* 2004;**3**:372–8

4. Martino G, Adorini L, Rieckmann P, *et al.* Inflammation in multiple sclerosis: the good, the bad, and the complex. *Lancet Neurol* 2002;**1**:499–509

5. Martino G, Pluchino S. The therapeutic potential of neural stem cells. *Nat Rev Neurosci* 2006; **7**:395–406

6. Martino G, Hartung H P. Immunopathogenesis of multiple sclerosis: the role of T cells. *Curr Opin Neurol* 1999; **12**:309–21

7. Kieseier B C, Hartung H P. Multiple paradigm shifts in multiple sclerosis. *Curr Opin Neurol* 2003;**16**:247–52

8. Barkhof F, Rocca M, Francis G, *et al.* Validation of diagnostic magnetic resonance imaging criteria for multiple sclerosis and response to interferon beta-1a. *Ann Neurol* 2003;**53**:718–24

9. Patrikios P, Stadelmann C, Kutzelnigg A, *et al.* Remyelination is extensive in a subset of multiple sclerosis patients. *Brain* 2006;**129**:3165–72

10. Franklin R J M. Why does remyelination fail in multiple sclerosis? *Nat Rev Neurosci* 2002;**3**:705–14

11. Ivanova N B, Dimos J T, Schaniel C, *et al.* A stem cell molecular signature. *Science* 2002;**298**:601–4

12. Weiss S, Reynolds B A, Vescovi A L, *et al.* Is there a neural stem cell in the mammalian forebrain? *Trends Neurosci* 1996; **19**:387–93

13. Doetsch F. The glial identity of neural stem cells. *Nat Neurosci* 2003;**6**:1127–34

14. Ming G L, Song H. Adult neurogenesis in the mammalian central nervous system. *Annu Rev Neurosci* 2005;**28**:223–50

15. Doetsch F, Caille I, Lim D A, Garcia-Verdugo J M, Alvarez-Buylla A. Subventricular zone astrocytes are neural stem cells in the adult mammalian brain. *Cell* 1999;**97**:703–16

16. Menn B, Garcia-Verdugo J M, Yaschine C, *et al.* Origin of oligodendrocytes in the subventricular zone of the adult brain. *J Neurosci* 2006; **26**:7907–18

17. Palmer T D, Willhoite A R, Gage F H. Vascular niche for adult hippocampal neurogenesis. *J Comp Neurol* 2000;**425**:479–94

18. Seri B, Garcia-Verdugo J M, McEwen B S, Alvarez-Buylla A. Astrocytes give rise to new neurons in the adult mammalian hippocampus. *J Neurosci* 2001;**21**:7153–60

19. Mercier F, Kitasako J T, Hatton G I. Anatomy of the brain neurogenic zones revisited: fractones and the fibroblast/macrophage network. *J Comp Neurol* 2002;**451**:170–88

20. Yagita Y, Kitagawa K, Ohtsuki T, *et al.* Neurogenesis by progenitor cells in the ischemic adult rat hippocampus. *Stroke* 2001;**32**:1890–6

21. Tureyen K, Vemuganti R, Sailor K A, Bowen K K, Dempsey R J. Transient focal cerebral ischemia-induced neurogenesis in the dentate gyrus of the adult mouse. *J Neurosurg* 2004;**101**:799–805

22. Zhang R, Zhang Z, Zhang C, *et al.* Stroke transiently increases subventricular zone cell division from asymmetric to symmetric and increases neuronal differentiation in the adult rat. *J Neurosci* 2004; **24**:5810–5

23. Carmichael S T. Gene expression changes after focal stroke, traumatic brain and spinal cord injuries. *Curr Opin Neurol* 2003;**16**:699–704

24. Zhang R, Zhang Z, Wang L, *et al.* Activated neural stem cells contribute to stroke-induced neurogenesis and neuroblast migration toward the infarct boundary in adult rats. *J Cereb Blood Flow Metab* 2004;**24**:441–8

25. Zhu D Y, Lau L, Liu S H, Wei J S, Lu Y M. Activation of cAMP-response-element-binding protein (CREB) after focal cerebral ischemia stimulates neurogenesis in the adult dentate gyrus. *Proc Natl Acad Sci USA* 2004;**101**:9453–7

26. Jin K, Minami M, Lan J Q, *et al.* Neurogenesis in dentate subgranular zone and rostral subventricular zone after focal cerebral ischemia in the rat. *Proc Natl Acad Sci USA* 2001; **98**:4710–5

27. Zhang R L, Zhang Z G, Lu M, *et al.* Reduction of the cell cycle length by decreasing G1 phase and cell cycle reentry expand neuronal progenitor cells in the

subventricular zone of adult rat after stroke. *J Cereb Blood Flow Metab* 2006; **26**:857–63

28. Thored P, Wood J, Arvidsson A, *et al.* Long-term neuroblast migration along blood vessels in an area with transient angiogenesis and increased vascularization after stroke. *Stroke* 2007; **38**:3032–9

29. Jin K, Wang X, Lin X, *et al.* Evidence for stroke-induced neurogenesis in the human brain. *Proc Natl Acad Sci USA* 2006; **103**:13198–202

30. Ke Y, Chia L, Xua R, *et al.* Early response of endogenous adult neural progenitor cells to acute spinal cord injury in mice. *Stem Cells* 2006; **24**:1011–19

31. Yang H, Lu P, McKay H, *et al.* Endogenous neurogenesis replaces oligodendrocytes and astrocytes after primate spinal cord injury. *J Neurosci* 2006;**26**:2157–66

32. Brundin L, Brismar H, Danilov A I, Olsson T, Johansson C B. Neural stem cells: a potential source for remyelination in neuroinflammatory disease. *Brain Pathol* 2003;**13**:322–8

33. Picard-Riera N, Decker L, Delarasse C, *et al.* Experimental autoimmune encephalomyelitis mobilizes neural progenitors from the subventricular zone to undergo oligodendrogenesis in adult mice. *Proc Natl Acad Sci USA* 2002;**99**:13–211–16

34. Nait-Oumesmar B, Picard-Riera N, Kerninon C, *et al.* Activation of the subventricular zone in multiple sclerosis: Evidence for early glial progenitors. *Proc Natl Acad Sci USA* 2007; **104**:4694–9

35. Elias B E. Oligodendrocyte development and the natural hystory of mulitple sclerosis. *Arch Neurol* 1987;**44**:1294–9

36. Martino G, Pluchino S. Neural stem cells: guardians of the brain. *Nat Cell Biol* 2007; **9**:1031–4

37. Lim D A, Tramontin A D, Trevejo J M, *et al.* Noggin antagonizes BMP signaling to create a niche for adult neurogenesis. *Neuron* 2000;**28**:713–26

38. Butovsky O, Ziv Y, Schwartz A, *et al.* Microglia activated by IL-4 or IFN-gamma differentially induce neurogenesis and oligodendrogenesis from adult stem/progenitor cells. *Mol Cell Neurosci* 2006;**31**:149–60

39. Vallieres L, Campbell I L, Gage F H, Sawchenko P E. Reduced hippocampal neurogenesis in adult transgenic mice with chronic astrocytic production of interleukin-6. *J Neurosci* 2002;**22**:486–92

40. Pluchino S, Zanotti L, Rossi B, *et al.* Neurosphere-derived multipotent precursors promote neuroprotection by an immunomodulatory mechanism. *Nature* 2005;**436**:266–71

41. Pierani A, Brenner-Morton S, Chiang C, Jessell T M. A sonic hedgehog-independent, retinoid-activated pathway of neurogenesis in the ventral spinal cord. *Cell* 1999;**97**:903–15

42. Seifert T, Bauer J, Weissert R, Fazekas F, Storch M K. Differential expression of sonic hedgehog immunoreactivity during lesion evolution in autoimmune encephalomyelitis. *J Neuropathol Exp Neurol* 2005;**64**:404–11

43. Irvin D K, Nakano I, Paucar A, Kornblum H I. Patterns of Jagged1, Jagged2, Delta-like 1 and Delta-like 3 expression during late embryonic and postnatal brain development suggest multiple functional roles in progenitors and differentiated cells. *J Neurosci Res* 2004;**75**:330–43

44. John G R, Shankar S L, Shafit-Zagardo B, *et al.* Multiple sclerosis: re-expression of a developmental pathway that restricts oligodendrocyte maturation. *Nat Med* 2002; **8**:1115–21

45. Stidworthy M F, Genoud S, Li W-W, *et al.* Notch1 and Jagged1 are expressed after CNS demyelination, but are not a major rate-determining factor during remyelination. *Brain* 2004;**127**:1928–41

46. Monje M L, Toda H, Palmer T D. Inflammatory blockade restores adult hippocampal neurogenesis. *Science* 2003;**302**:1760–5

47. Ziv Y, Ron N, Butovsky O, *et al.* Immune cells contribute to the maintenance of neurogenesis and spatial learning abilities in adulthood. *Nat Neurosci* 2006;**9**:268–75

48. Lee M A, Smith S, Palace J, *et al.* Spatial mapping of T2 and gadolinium-enhancing T1 lesion volumes in multiple sclerosis: evidence for distinct mechanisms of lesion genesis? *Brain* 1999;**122** (7):1261–70

49. Sim F J, Goldman S A. White matter progenitor cells reside in an oligodendrogenic niche. *Ernst Schering Res Found Workshop* 2005;**61**–81

50. Adams C W, Abdulla Y H, Torres E M, Poston R N. Periventricular lesions in multiple sclerosis: their perivenous origin and relationship to granular ependymitis. *Neuropathol Appl Neurobiol* 1987;**13**:141–52

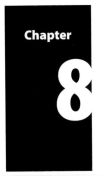
Schwann cells as a potential cell-based therapy for multiple sclerosis

Violetta Zujovic and Anne Baron-Van Evercooren

Introduction

Multiple sclerosis (MS) is an autoimmune disease of the central nervous system (CNS). Successive inflammatory attacks lead to the damage of an essential component of the neuronal circuit: the myelin. The destruction of myelin in demyelinating disorders such as MS leads to severe disabilities due, notably, to the alteration and, possibly, interruption of the saltatory conduction of the nerve influx. Furthermore, since the myelin sheath serves as a physical barrier around axons protecting them from the pathological environment, its loss can, in the long run, cause irreversible axonal damage.

Over the years, several strategies aiming at restoring the loss of myelin were developed, and cell-based therapy emerged as a potential approach to restore myelin. Experimental grafting of myelin-forming cells has proven to be a very efficient way to remyelinate focal demyelinated lesions of the CNS. However, besides remyelinating CNS axons, cells to be grafted have to fulfill several additional criteria, in order to meet the MS pathological hallmarks. Cells should survive the successive inflammatory attacks, and bypass astrogliosis and potential scarring. The widely disseminated lesions throughout the neuraxis require the candidate cells to have great ability to migrate within the CNS. Since cell transplantation is at risk, the accessibility and availability of the cells to be grafted have also to be taken into consideration. Finally, in order to develop a potential therapeutic approach in humans and avoid complex post-grafting treatment, autologous transplantation rather than allografting has to be preferred.

In this review, we will consider the pros and cons of Schwann cells (SC), the myelinating cells of the peripheral nervous system (PNS), as potential candidates for cell therapy, and highlight novel and exciting findings for the field of CNS remyelination.

Myelin-forming cells of the nervous system: Schwann cells and oligodendrocytes

Myelin sheaths are composed of a specific set of proteins and lipids that wrap the axons, allowing the insulation of the covered axonal area. Some parts of the axons remain unwrapped. This specific region, called the node of Ranvier, is present at regular distances along the axon and is highly enriched with voltage-gated ion channels. The nerve influx arising from the cell body bypasses the insulated area and jumps from one node of Ranvier to the other. This so-called saltatory conduction enables rapid and efficient nerve conduction along the axons, which, sometimes, extends over the distance of 1 meter in humans.

Myelin wrapping is completed by two kinds of cells, the oligodendrocytes in the CNS and the SC in the PNS. Both of these cells undergo various transitional phases before becoming mature myelin-forming cells. The SC adopt a one-to-one relationship with axons, while oligodendrocytes, with their numerous processes, myelinate up to 40 axons. Internodes in the PNS are surrounded by a basement membrane, and the PNS nodal regions are covered by SC processes and its basement membrane. Internodes in the CNS are devoid of basal lamina, and nodes are covered by astrocyte end-feet. The composition of PNS and CNS myelin also differs [1], the P-zero myelin protein (P0) being the major constituent of PNS myelin, and the myelin basic protein (MBP) the major component in the CNS. Finally, SC and oligodendrocytes originating from different neural tube compartments are under the

Multiple Sclerosis: Recovery of Function and Neurorehabilitation, eds. J. Kesselring, G. Comi, and A. J. Thompson.
Published by Cambridge University Press. © Cambridge University Press 2010.

influence of different epigenic factors. The morphogens bone morphogenetic proteins (BMPs) and sonic hedgehog (Shh) drive respectively the SC and the oligodendroglial lineage. While axon-derived neuregulins control SC survival, proliferation, and differentiation including their myelin sheath thickness [2], platelet-derived growth factor (PDGF), fibroblast growth factor (FGF), and insulin-like growth factor (IGF) control the various steps of the oligodendrocyte lineage. Finally, SC transcriptional regulation is dominated by Krox 20 [3, 4], while oligodendrocyte development is largely controlled by the Olig1/2 gene family. Yet both these cell types serve the same function: the formation of myelin around axons.

The other main difference between these two cell types is their behavior in pathological conditions. In MS, oligodendrocytes are the main target of the inflammatory attacks, while SC do not seem to be sensitive to the disease. Animal models provided evidence that after demyelination of the CNS both oligodendrocytes and SC participate in the remyelination process. While each cell type forms myelin in its own developmental compartment, SC can invade the CNS and remyelinate central demyelinated axons in pathological conditions. However, the recruitment of oligodendrocytes to the pathological PNS has not been reported so far. While new oligodendrocytes are mainly generated from endogenous oligodendrocyte precursors and neural stem cells [4], there are still uncertainties about the origin of SC and the reason for their presence in the lesioned CNS [5]. Several studies have convincingly demonstrated that myelin repair conducted by recruited SC efficiently re-established axonal conduction [6] with the restoration of well-organized nodes of Ranvier [7], and led in certain circumstances to the restoration of functional deficits [8].

Schwann cell plasticity during PNS development and repair

The therapeutic interest in SC is dictated by their impressive plasticity during development and repair. During development, the migrating neural crest cells give rise to a multitude of neural and non-neural cells including SC. Migrating neural crest cells generate SC precursors, the first transitional phase of SC development. Before birth, SC precursors differentiate into immature SC that associate with axons and encircle

them. After radial sorting of the nerves, immature SC adopt a one-to-one relationship with the axons. From this moment on, the fate of SC is determined by the size of the axon they are associated with. When in contact with a small-caliber axon, they mature in non-myelinating SC and form Remak bundles. When in association with large-caliber axons, SC start to wrap myelin around single axons.

Because of its regenerative properties, the PNS has been widely studied, to try to understand how its axons regenerate after crush injury or axotomy. Although neuronal intrinsic factors and a permissive environment are essential for the regenerative process, the support of SC is essential for nerve regrowth. After nerve transection, first SC phagocytose myelin debris. They revert to a non-myelinating phenotype with features close to immature SC, and after active proliferation, form bands of Bügner, the "rail"-like structures that allow and direct the growth of regenerating axons. During that time, SC express specific neurotrophins supporting growth cone development. Later, SC re-associate with the regenerated axon and redifferentiate into myelin-forming cells. These specific regenerating properties aroused interest very early on, since no such mechanism has been identified in the injured CNS, and led to the transplantation of SC in the CNS.

Grafting committed Schwann cells in the CNS
The advantages

The first efforts in the field of SC-based therapy focused on committed mature or immature SC. When in the late 1920s Ramón y Cajal implanted a fragment of peripheral nerve into the CNS, he made the observation that CNS axons were capable of integrating into the PNS-specific permissive environment, and were surrounded by PNS myelin. These experiments were further confirmed when fragments of peripheral nerves were grafted in the demyelinated spinal cord [9]. Next, SC were harvested from peripheral nerve biopsies. The discovery of specific growth factors, in particular heregulin, allowed the production of highly purified rodent SC in vitro [10, 11]. These purified and expandable neonate or adult SC were grafted in various species using a panel of models of CNS demyelination targeted to the optic disk, cerebellar white matter, or spinal cord. All these experiments provided solid proof of the ability of SC to remyelinate CNS axons very efficiently. The heregulin discovery combined with the recombinant technology provided a means to generate substantial populations of SC from adult human [12, 13] and monkey [14] nerve biopsies. Viral infections that reliably traced the transplanted cells convincingly demonstrated that autologous macaque SC transplantation in the demyelinated spinal cord led to robust remyelination of single acute spinal lesions [15]. New labeling techniques were also developed to follow the fate of grafted cells by magnetic resonance imaging [16].

These technological achievements provided means to assess the repair potential of purified SC in great detail. It was found that SC myelinated successfully when transplanted into toxin-induced areas of demyelination (reviewed in Baron-Van Evercooren and Blakemore [17]). It was even demonstrated that SC implanted in the demyelinated mouse spinal cord sustained stable myelin for up to 5 months after transplantation [18]. Interestingly, the myelin formed by transplanted SC improved markedly the conduction of the demyelinated axons [19]. These observations were correlated with functional recovery in a model of focal demyelination of mouse spinal cord grafted with macaque SC [20]. In all these experiments, the extent of remyelination achieved was related to the number of SC introduced [21], their purity [22], and their age. In fact, SC from neonate and young adult donors achieved more successful repair than cells derived from older donors [23]. While SC neuroregenerative properties have rarely been studied in models of demyelination where minimal axonal injury occurs, numerous studies performed in models of spinal trauma have highlighted the capacity of transplanted SC to promote axonal regeneration across the injured area [24]. This capacity is of great value for demyelinating diseases in which axonal injury or degeneration often occurs as a result of long-standing demyelination.

While the resistance of transplanted SC to inflammation as well as their ability to sustain clinical recovery in large species remain to be addressed, these encouraging data, in addition to the fact that peripheral myelin in MS is spared, have made SC attractive candidates for therapeutic transplantation. However, despite these promising results, successful clinical translation has so far not been achieved.

The limitations

Several issues have raised concern and in particular the interaction of SC with the axons. Indeed, remyelination by transplanted SC depends upon appropriate axonal signals. It occurs only if the previously demyelinated axon is of sufficient size to be myelinated. Consequently injections of SC into areas that are not myelinated by endogenous myelin-forming cells such as the hippocampus or fimbria does not result in remyelination [25]. However, recent data indicate that lentiviral-driven overexpression of NRG1 type III induced SC to myelinate small-diameter axons [26]. The possibility of directing SC remyelination towards specific axons may thus constitute an approach of interest to enhance their contribution to CNS remyelination. Another concern is the restoration by SC of the aggregation of nodal and paranodal components on CNS axons with a pattern similar to that of the PNS. Therefore, the impact of myelin newly formed by SC on axonal integrity and its ability to ensure proper CNS axonal function remains to be addressed. Finally, SC remyelinate only one axon while oligodendrocytes provide up to 40 nodes. One may therefore argue that an excessive quantity of cells would be required to successfully remyelinate CNS lesions when using SC grafts. However, providing large quantities of SC is not a limitation since they can be successfully expanded in vitro prior to transplantation, and experimental transplantation of SC in CNS lesions has not provided evidence for aberrant graft volumes. Moreover, since PNS newly formed internodes are two- to threefold longer than CNS internodes, one can speculate that the quantity of SC would be far less than 40 : 1 to achieve successful remyelination of a lesion.

While these elements do not seem to constitute serious impediments to efficient remyelination of CNS axons by SC, a major limitation has hindered the development of SC-based therapeutic approach. Despite their high motility in vitro, or in the injured peripheral nerve, SC migrate poorly when grafted in the demyelinated or injured CNS. This restriction results most likely from their poor interface with astrocytes [27, 28]. Indeed, transplantation experiments have shown that endogenous or exogenous astrocytes [29, 30] limit SC remyelination of CNS demyelinated axons [27]. Moreover, transplantation of SC remotely from spinal cord lesions showed that their migration potential largely depends upon the environment in which the cells are placed: SC migrate successfully along meninges and blood vessels, but do not do so through white and gray matter [25, 31–33]. Overcoming this limitation is a prerequisite when considering the need to remyelinate extensive and/or dispersed lesions, such as those found in MS patients.

In search of alternative solutions

Modifying Schwann cell intrinsic properties

These obvious limitations resulted in the search for alternative approaches to the use of committed SC. One of these approaches is to enhance their intrinsic capacity of repair, boosting SC expression of neurotrophins. Neurotrophins such as BDNF and NT3 have profound effects on neural protection, plasticity, and regeneration after spinal cord injury in the developing and adult CNS [34–37]. In addition, NT3 enhanced not only oligodendrocyte proliferation, survival, and differentiation [38] but also SC migration in vitro [39]. Forcing expression of brain-derived neurotrophic factor (BDNF) and neurotrophin-3 (NT3) in macaque SC promoted functional motor recovery after their transplantation in the demyelinated mouse spinal cord [20]. Postmortem analysis indicated that this effect resulted from multiple events including enhanced remyelination by endogenous oligodendrocytes and SC, enhanced neuroprotection, and reduced scar formation (astrogliosis, basal membrane). These data highlighted the interest of combining cell therapy and neurotrophin delivery to enhance global repair of demyelinated lesions associated with axonal loss.

As mentioned above, one major inconvenience of SC-based therapy is their poor potential of migration within the CNS. Unlike SC, neural precursors, oligodendrocyte precursors, and olfactory ensheathing cells migrate more efficiently within the CNS environment and interact more efficiently with astrocytes. Interestingly, all of these cells express the polysialylated form of NCAM (PSA-NCAM), a cell adhesion molecule highly expressed during development and involved in CNS plasticity, remodeling, and repair (reviewed in Rutishauser [40]). Since SC express NCAM but not PSA, it has been speculated that forcing NCAM polysialylation in SC would improve their interaction with the CNS environment. Lavdas and colleagues [41] genetically modified SC to express the sialytransferase X (STX), the enzyme responsible for NCAM polysialylation. They showed that ectopic expression of PSA by rodent SC enhanced their

migratory properties without altering their myelination potential in vitro [41]. Moreover, SC grafted in a model of spinal trauma promoted functional recovery and improved SC integration and remyelination associated with an increased sprouting of seretoninergic fibers [42]. Recently, we demonstrated the therapeutic benefit of such a strategy by promoting adult macaque SC migration in the demyelinated CNS [43]. Indeed, ectopic expression of PSA-NCAM in adult SC improved SC interaction with astrocytes, accelerated their migration towards the demyelinated lesion, and promoted their remyelination potential.

Modifying the Schwann cell environment

The poor potential of migration of SC in the CNS is in part due to their inability to mix with astrocytes. Strategies to overcome this difficulty target specific molecular interactions, such as chondroitin sulfate proteoglycans (CSPG) and N-Cadherins, that prevent SC from entering into astrocyte-enriched areas. Reducing levels of CSPG [44, 45] and N-Cadherin–N-Cadherin [46] contact promoted SC–astrocyte interactions in vitro. However, the consequence of SC–astrocyte interaction extends beyond the limitation of migration of SC by astrocytes. In fact, SC contact with astrocytes results in astrocyte hypertrophy, with increased expression of glial fibrillary acidic protein (GFAP) and CSPG, and the formation of boundaries between the two cell types. Since this astrocyte stress response seems to be mediated by SC-derived factors [45], identifying these factors could provide a means to minimize the astrocyte stress response and considerably improve SC–astrocyte interactions.

Alternative sources of Schwann cells

An alternative to facilitate SC migration/integration in the CNS would be the use of earlier stages of the SC lineage, which have greater plasticity. In this last part of the chapter, we will focus on the new somatic sources of SC, whether they are derived from embryonic or from adult stem cell niches.

Embryonic sources

Like all PNS cells, SC are neural crest derivatives. They go through different transitional stages before becoming myelin-competent cells (reviewed into Zujovic et al. [5]). Neural crest cells (NCC) differentiate into SC precursors before becoming immature SC, and a subpopulation of NCC arrests transiently at the PNS–CNS boundary to

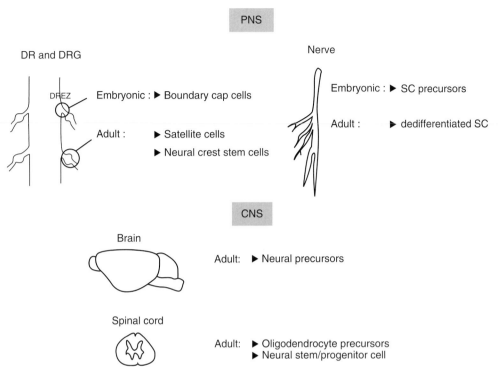

Fig. 8.1. The nervous system, the primary source of SC. The first isolates of SC were obtained with nerve explants, where the capacity of SC to dedifferentiate and proliferate was exploited. In the search for less differentiated cells, intermediate stages of SC development such as SC precursors or boundary cap (BC) cells were isolated at different embryonic stages. Recently, the persistence of neural crest stem cell precursor niches in the adult dorsal root ganglion (DRG) has been suggested. CNS (neural or oligodendrocyte) precursor cells, whether isolated from the brain or the spinal cord, can also generate SC. DREZ, dorsal root entry zone.

form the boundary cap cells (BC). Woodhoo and colleagues tested the repair potential of SC precursor cells isolated from E14 rat embryonic sciatic nerves [47]. They compared the behavior of neonate SC and embryonic SC precursors grafted in the unlesioned or demyelinated spinal cord. While neonate SC survived poorly in normal CNS tissue and did not integrate well in the lesion, SC precursors survived in the normal tissue and invaded massively the lesion where they differentiated into myelin-forming cells.

More recently, BC were identified as potential stem cells [48] and a source of SC of the embryonic mouse spinal roots [49, 50]. Their advantage over SC precursor cells would be the possibility of their unlimited expansion, in view of their self-renewability. When grown in specific culture conditions, BC differentiate into SC, sensory neurons, and smooth muscle cells. However when grafted in the demyelinated sciatic nerve, acute preparations of undifferentiated BC failed to differentiate into myelin-forming SC, unless primed to become committed SC in culture prior to being grafted [50]. Using cell fate mapping technology and

microdissection, we gained evidence that acutely dissociated BC migrate profusely in the demyelinated CNS and compete aggressively with host myelin-forming cells to remyelinate axons of a far-distant spinal cord lesion (Zujovic et al., unpublished data). These data highlight the therapeutic interest of this novel stem cell reservoir. However, despite these promising results, one has to bear in mind the problems that such a therapy may constitute in humans since like any embryonic source, SC precursor or BC will raise ethical concerns about the use of human embryos. This has led to the search for alternative adult stem cell sources.

Adult sources

During development of the neural tube, neural crest cells colonize various embryonic tissues and differentiate into a wide range of cells including neurons and glia in the PNS, pigment cells in the skin, and endocrine cells in the adrenal and thyroid gland (Figs. 8.1 and 8.2). They also contribute to the mesenchymal lineage,

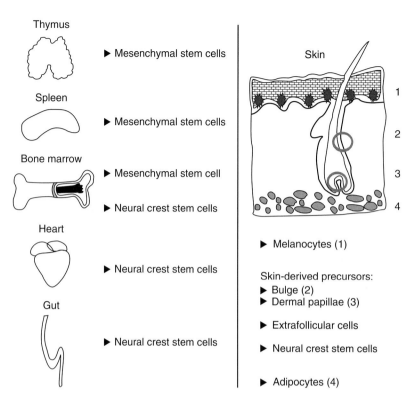

Thymus ▶ Mesenchymal stem cells

Spleen ▶ Mesenchymal stem cells

Bone marrow
▶ Mesenchymal stem cell
▶ Neural crest stem cells

Heart ▶ Neural crest stem cells

Gut ▶ Neural crest stem cells

Skin

▶ Melanocytes (1)

Skin-derived precursors:
▶ Bulge (2)
▶ Dermal papillae (3)

▶ Extrafollicular cells

▶ Neural crest stem cells

▶ Adipocytes (4)

Fig. 8.2. Alternative sources of SC. Although the plasticity of neural crest cells becomes restricted after their migration, several studies have shown that in different organs, neural crest derivatives conserve some differentiation potential. Thus mesenchymal stem cells isolated from the thymus, spleen, and bone marrow can give rise in vitro and in vivo to myelinating SC. The presence of neural-crest-derived stem cells at postnatal stages was evidenced in different organs such as the bone marrow, heart, gut and skin. The skin provided also different sets of cells such as melanocytes, adipocytes, and a subpopulation of skin-derived precursors (isolated from the bulge, the dermal papillae, or extrafollicular cells) that differentiate into SC.

giving rise to cartilage, bone, dermis, adipose tissue from the craniofacial area, and the vascular smooth muscle cells. Neural-crest-derived stem cells (NCSC) were identified in embryonic tissue, such as embryonic sciatic nerve [51] but also in various adult tissues such as gut [52], skin [53, 54], heart [55], dorsal root ganglia (DRG) [56, 57], and bone marrow [58–60] (Figs. 8.1 and 8.2). The persistence of such a stem cell reservoir in adult tissues opens new perspectives for cell therapy.

Dorsal root ganglia satellite cells

In order to gain insights into the mechanisms of regeneration of DRG neurons in response to peripheral nerve injury, Li *et al.* [57] questioned the existence of NCSC in the adult DRG. They isolated a subpopulation of cells emigrating from the DRG with NCSC characteristics and the capacity to give rise to neurons and SC (Fig. 8.1). The existence of such a stem cell reservoir in the adult DRG was further confirmed and better characterized with transgenic mice [61] (see below).

Skin-derived precursors

A number of studies have underlined the multipotency and the self-renewing capacity of skin-derived precursors (SKP) and evidenced their ability to generate cells of both neural and mesenchymal lineage. Of particular interest, is the capacity of SKP to differentiate in vitro into neural-crest-derived cell types such as SC [53]. When rodent and human SKP were cultured with peripheral nerve explants, SKP proliferated and expressed myelin proteins. When transplanted into the injured peripheral nerve or into the dysmyelinated neonatal shiverer mouse brain, the majority of SKP-derived cells generated functional SC that associated with and remyelinated CNS axons [62]. Likewise implanted hair follicle stem cells generated myelinating SC in the injured peripheral nerve [63].

Skin-derived precursors were isolated either from global skin or whisker follicle but skin stem cell niches were identified. Sieber-Blum *et al.* isolated neural-crest-derived stem cells named epidermal neural crest cells from the hair bulge and achieved their differentiation in SC in vitro [64]. Interestingly, these bulge-derived precursors differentiated into neurons and oligodendrocytes when implanted in the contused spinal cord [54, 64]. Finally, the presence of SKP in the human foreskin, a region devoid of hair follicles, also gave evidence of the presence of an extrafollicular niche in the human skin [65].

Skin-derived precursors are of clinical interest since they constitute an accessible source of cells (Fig. 8.2). While these cells can be readily expanded from embryonic and neonatal sources using neuregulins, their expansion from adult tissue has proven to be more problematic. However, a recent study pointed to the possibility of isolating and increasing over 1000-fold dermal papilla-derived precursors in spheres with neuronal and glial potential from a single adult rodent or human hair follicule [66]. Whether adult versus embryonic or neonate cells, and bulge, papilla, or extrafollicular SKP, they have similar repair potential will be of great interest for the therapeutic field.

Mesenchymal stem cells (bone marrow, fat, spleen, thymus)

Mesenchymal stem cells (MSC) are stromal stem cells that can be isolated from various tissues and differentiate into cells of mesodermal (bone, fat, cartilage) and neuroectodermal lineages (neurons, glia). The most commonly studied MSC were isolated from bone marrow [58–60] but also from fat [60, 67], spleen, and thymus [60]. Mesenchymal stem cells originating from these various tissues were able to transdifferentiate into SC-like phenotype in vitro (Fig. 8.2). Adipocyte or bone marrow MSC-derived SC myelinated PC12 neurites in vitro [59, 67] and participated in the axonal regeneration process when implanted into a biogenic muscle graft to bridge a sciatic nerve gap [59].

Intraparenchymal transplantation of the bone marrow CD117+ subpopulation into the neonatal mouse brain resulted in the generation of oligodendrocytes [68]. However, when implanted into X-Eb lesions, freshly isolated rat bone marrow [69] and purified mouse bone marrow stromal cells [70] resulted in SC remyelination. Intravenous injection of rat bone marrow acutely fractionated for mononuclear cells into animals with X-Eb lesions also resulted in SC and possibly oligodendrocyte remyelination [71]. Although MSC may contribute to generating myelin-forming cells, the possibility of their efficacy via an indirect effect on the host environment should not be excluded.

A same neural-crest-derived stem cell?

Several publications by Dupin and Le Douarin have underlined the capacity of neural-crest-derived cells to reverse into a precursor cell stage [72]. It has been found that SC, isolated from quail embryo and exposed to endothelin 3, can transdifferentiate and give rise to a glial melanocytic NC precursor (Fig. 8.3) [73]. On the other hand, endothelin 3 induced the dedifferentiation of pigment cells into NCSC, which in vitro can give rise to SC [74]. SC can also give rise to myofibroblasts in presence of transforming growth factor-$\beta\beta$ (TGF-$\beta\beta$) [75] or after the downregulation of Sox 10 [76]. The capacity to transdifferentiate from one cell type to another might involve a dedifferentiation into a neural-crest-like progenitor/stem cell stage.

Furthermore, the presence of NCSC niches were detected in various tissues such as the gut [52], heart [55], bone marrow [59], the skin (Fig. 8.2), and the DRG (Fig. 8.1). The NCSC isolated from the heart [55] and the gut [52] differentiate both in vitro and in vivo into neurons and glial cells. In a very elegant study, the multipotency of stem cells derived from adult whisker pad, bone marrow, and DRG was tested in parallel. Using lineage tracing with P0 and Wnt1-Cre/Floxed EGFP mice, Nagoshi and colleagues targeted the NCSC niches in the whisker pad, bone marrow, and the DRG. Although these various stem cells share the neural crest origin and all of them give rise to neurons, glia, and myofibroblasts, the DRG-derived stem cells show a higher proportion of tripotent cells, and a greater ability to form secondary spheres [61]. While several tissues can give rise to stem cells sharing the same origin and similar self-renewing and multipotential capacities, it is important to keep in mind that these stem cells have tissue-dependent characteristics.

CNS neural precursors

Until recently, authors did not take into account the possibility that SC could be generated from CNS neural precursors. This possibility was, however, suggested by both in vitro and in vivo studies. In vitro, cloned CNS neural precursors gave rise to both oligodendrocytes and SC (Fig. 8.1) [77]. In vivo experiments using the X-irradiated ethidium bromide lesion demonstrated that transplantation of fibroblast growth factor (FGF)-2 expanded PSA-NCAM glial restricted precursors [78] or myelin oligodendrocyte glycoprotein (MOG)-expressing oligodendrocytes precursors [79] resulted in both SC and oligodendrocyte remyelination. Furthermore, introduction into the same type of lesion of cloned human neural precursors isolated from the adult human brain also resulted in SC remyelination [80].

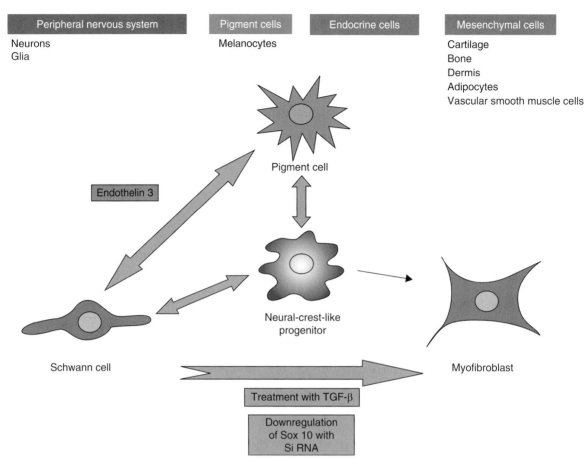

Fig. 8.3. Plasticity of neural-crest-derived cells. The neural crest gives rise to a wide variety of cells from the neurons and the glia of the PNS to endocrine cells, pigment cells, and mesenchymal cells. Several studies have shown the transdifferentiation potential of these cells. Endothelin 3 induces SC and pigment cells to convert into each other in vitro. Furthermore SC in presence of transforming growth factor-β (TGF-β) can differentiate in myofibroblasts. Likewise, Sox 10 downregulation with small interference RNA induces the transdifferentiation of schwannoma cells into myofibroblasts. These transdifferentiation steps might be explained by the capacity of pigment and SC to reverse to a neural crest progenitor stage.

These studies underlined an important role for astrocytes in the fate of CNS precursors. In the presence of astrocytes, CNS precursors that enter areas of demyelination differentiate into oligodendrocytes, while in their absence, they are under the influence of factors that will induce SC differentiation. In this respect, recent data have identified a role for BMP in instructing CNS precursor into the SC fate. In vitro, BMP and FGF-2 were found to cooperate to induce neural-crest-like fate including SC differentiation from fetal and adult neural stem cells [81]. In addition, Talbott *et al.* [82] found that grafted OPCs differentiated preferentially into SC when in the presence of BMP. Mothe & Tator [83] found evidence that, depending on the environment into which they are transplanted, neural stem/progenitor cells derived from the spinal cord give rise to different cells. In the adult shiverer mouse spinal cord, the neural stem/progenitor cells generate oligodendrocytes while in focal demyelinated lesions of the spinal cord they differentiate into both oligodendrocytes and SC. These data suggest that boundaries between CNS and PNS cells are not as clear-cut as expected, and that a common neural progenitor for oligodendrocytes and SC may exist.

Conclusion

Over the years, SC have proven to be eligible candidates for myelin repair due to their great plasticity and manipulability. However, their poor integration in the CNS remains an unresolved issue. This is why the discovery of the NCSC niche in the adult tissue has raised such an interest over the last few years. Indeed, NCSC present all the advantages of stem cells since they are highly proliferative and multipotential. When in presence of axons, NCSC can give rise to mature myelin-forming SC with all the advantages described in this review. The fact that earlier stages of SC development (SC precursors, BC) integrate and migrate more successfully in the CNS than SC leads to the speculation that NCSC share the same capacity. While this hypothesis still remains to be proven, the possibility of isolating stem/precursor cells from hair or skin opens new perspectives for SC-based therapy in myelin disorders. Moreover, understanding the molecular mechanisms involved in their improved CNS integration/migration may foster the development of strategies aimed at promoting endogenous or exogenous CNS remyelination by SC.

Acknowledgments

We would like to thank Cedric Doucerain and Céline Caillava for their artistic contribution, Dr. Nait-Oumesmar for his critical review, and all the past and present members of the Baron's laboratory. This work was supported by several grants from Wings for Life, the NMSS, and the AP-HP contrat d'interface.

References

1. Simons M, Trotter J. Wrapping it up: the cell biology of myelination. *Curr Opin Neurobiol* 2007;**17**(5): 533–40

2. Birchmeier C, Nave K A. Neuregulin-1, a key axonal signal that drives Schwann cell growth and differentiation. *Glia* 2008;**56**(14):1491–7

3. Murphy P, Topilko P, Schneider-Maunoury S, *et al.* The regulation of Krox-20 expression reveals important steps in the control of peripheral glial cell development. *Development* 1996;**122**(9):2847–57

4. Nait-Oumesmar B, Picard-Riera N, Kerninon C, Baron-Van Evercooren A. The role of SVZ-derived neural precursors in demyelinating diseases: from animal models to multiple sclerosis. *J Neurol Sci* 2008;**265** (1–2):26–31

5. Zujovic V, Bachelin C, Baron-Van Evercooren A. Remyelination of the central nervous system: a valuable contribution from the periphery. *Neuroscientist* 2007;**13** (4):383–91

6. Felts P A, Smith K J. Conduction properties of central nerve fibers remyelinated by Schwann cells. *Brain Res* 1992;**574**(1–2):178–92

7. Black J A, Waxman S G, Smith K J. Remyelination of dorsal column axons by endogenous Schwann cells restores the normal pattern of Nav1.6 and Kv1.2 at nodes of Ranvier. *Brain* 2006;**129**(5):1319–29

8. Jasmin L, Janni G, Moallem T M, Lappi D A, Ohara P T. Schwann cells are removed from the spinal cord after effecting recovery from paraplegia. *J Neurosci* 2000;**20** (24):9215–23

9. Blakemore W F. Remyelination of CNS axons by Schwann cells transplanted from the sciatic nerve. *Nature* 1977;**266**(5597):68–9

10. Wood P M. Separation of functional Schwann cells and neurons from normal peripheral nerve tissue. *Brain Res* 1976;**115**(3):361–75

11. Brockes J P, Fields K L, Raff M C. Studies on cultured rat Schwann cells. I. Establishment of purified populations from cultures of peripheral nerve. *Brain Res* 1979;**165**(1):105–18

12. Rutkowski J L, Kirk C J, Lerner M A, Tennekoon G I. Purification and expansion of human Schwann cells in vitro. *Nat Med* 1995;**1**(1):80–3

13. Levi A D. Characterization of the technique involved in isolating Schwann cells from adult human peripheral nerve. *J Neurosci Methods* 1996;**68**(1):21–6

14. Avellana-Adalid V, Bachelin C, Lachapelle F, *et al.* In vitro and in vivo behaviour of NDF-expanded monkey Schwann cells. *Eur J Neurosci* 1998;**10**(1):291–300

15. Bachelin C, Lachapelle F, Girard C, *et al.* Efficient myelin repair in the macaque spinal cord by autologous grafts of Schwann cells. *Brain* 2005;**128**(3):540–9

16. Dunning M D, Kettunen M I, Ffrench Constant C, Franklin R J, Brindle K M. Magnetic resonance imaging of functional Schwann cell transplants labelled with magnetic microspheres. *Neuroimage* 2006;**31**(1):172–80

17. Baron Van-Evecooren A, Blakemore W F. Schwann cell development. In: Lazzarini R A, ed. Myelin biology and disorders. Amsterdam: Elsevier, 2004:143–72

18. Duncan I D, Aguayo A J, Bunge R P, Wood P M. Transplantation of rat Schwann cells grown in tissue culture into the mouse spinal cord. *J Neurol Sci* 1981;**49**(2):241–52

19. Honmou O, Felts P A, Waxman S G, Kocsis J D. Restoration of normal conduction properties in demyelinated spinal cord axons in the adult rat by transplantation of exogenous Schwann cells. *J Neurosci* 1996;**16**(10):3199–208

20. Girard C, Bemelmans A P, Dufour N, *et al.* Grafts of brain-derived neurotrophic factor and neurotrophin 3-transduced primate Schwann cells lead to functional recovery of the demyelinated mouse spinal cord. *J Neurosci* 2005;**25**(35):7924–33

21. Iwashita Y, Blakemore W F. Areas of demyelination do not attract significant numbers of Schwann cells transplanted into normal white matter. *Glia* 2000;**31**(3):232–40

22. Brierley C M, Crang A J, Iwashita Y, *et al.* Remyelination of demyelinated CNS axons by transplanted human Schwann cells: the deleterious effect of contaminating fibroblasts. *Cell Transplant* 2001;**10**(3):305–15

23. Lankford K L, Imaizumi T, Honmou O, Kocsis J D. A quantitative morphometric analysis of rat spinal cord remyelination following transplantation of allogenic Schwann cells. *J Comp Neurol* 2002;**443**(3):259–74

24. Oudega M, Xu X M. Schwann cell transplantation for repair of the adult spinal cord. *J Neurotrauma* 2006;**23**(3–4):453–67

25. Brook G A, Lawrence J M, Raisman G. Morphology and migration of cultured Schwann cells transplanted into the fimbria and hippocampus in adult rats. *Glia* 1993;**9**(4):292–304

26. Taveggia C, Zanazzi G, Petrylak A, *et al.* Neuregulin-1 type III determines the ensheathment fate of axons. *Neuron* 2005;**47**(5):681–94

27. Franklin R J, Crang A J, Blakemore W F. The reconstruction of an astrocytic environment in glia-deficient areas of white matter. *J Neurocytol* 1993;**22**(5):382–96

28. Lakatos A, Barnett S C, Franklin R J. Olfactory ensheathing cells induce less host astrocyte response and chondroitin sulphate proteoglycan expression than Schwann cells following transplantation into adult CNS white matter. *Exp Neurol* 2003;**184**(1):237–46

29. Blakemore W F, Crang A J, Curtis R. The interaction of Schwann cells with CNS axons in regions containing normal astrocytes. *Acta Neuropathol* 1986;**71**(3–4): 295–300

30. Franklin R J, Crang A J, Blakemore W F. Transplanted type-1 astrocytes facilitate repair of demyelinating lesions by host oligodendrocytes in adult rat spinal cord. *J Neurocytol* 1991;**20**(5):420–30

31. Baron-Van Evercooren A, Gansmuller A, Duhamel E, Pascal F, Gumpel M. Repair of a myelin lesion by Schwann cells transplanted in the adult mouse spinal cord. *J Neuroimmunol* 1992;**40**(2–3):235–42

32. Langford L A, Owens G C. Resolution of the pathway taken by implanted Schwann cells to a spinal cord lesion by prior infection with a retrovirus encoding beta-galactosidase. *Acta Neuropathol* 1990;**80**(5):514–20

33. Iwashita Y, Fawcett J W, Crang A J, Franklin R J, Blakemore W F. Schwann cells transplanted into normal and X-irradiated adult white matter do not migrate extensively and show poor long-term survival. *Exp Neurol* 2000;**164**(2):292–302

34. Kromer L F, Cornbrooks C J. Transplants of Schwann cell cultures promote axonal regeneration in the adult mammalian brain. *Proc Natl Acad Sci USA* 1985;**82**(18):6330–4

35. Martin D, Schoenen J, Delree P, Leprince P, Rogister B, Moonen G. Grafts of syngenic cultured, adult dorsal root ganglion-derived Schwann cells to the injured spinal cord of adult rats: preliminary morphological studies. *Neurosci Lett* 1991;**124**(1):44–8

36. Montero-Menei C N, Pouplard-Barthelaix A, Gumpel M, Baron-Van Evercooren A. Pure Schwann cell suspension grafts promote regeneration of the lesioned septo-hippocampal cholinergic pathway. *Brain Res* 1992;**570**(1–2):198–208

37. Levi A D, Bunge R P. Studies of myelin formation after transplantation of human Schwann cells into the severe combined immunodeficient mouse. *Exp Neurol* 1994;**130**(1):41–52

38. McTigue D M, Horner P J, Stokes B T, Gage F H. Neurotrophin-3 and brain-derived neurotrophic factor induce oligodendrocyte proliferation and myelination of regenerating axons in the contused adult rat spinal cord. *J Neurosci* 1998;**18** (14):5354–65

39. Yamauchi J, Miyamoto Y, Tanoue A, Shooter E M, Chan J R. Ras activation of a Rac1 exchange factor, Tiam1, mediates neurotrophin-3-induced Schwann cell migration. *Proc Natl Acad Sci USA* 2005; **102**(41):14 889–94

40. Rutishauser U. Polysialic acid in the plasticity of the developing and adult vertebrate nervous system. *Nat Rev Neurosci* 2008;**9**(1):26–35

41. Lavdas A A, Franceschini I, Dubois-Dalcq M, Matsas R. Schwann cells genetically engineered to express PSA show enhanced migratory potential without impairment of their myelinating ability in vitro. *Glia* 2006;**53**(8):868–78

42. Papastefanaki F, Chen J, Lavdas A A, *et al.* Grafts of Schwann cells engineered to express PSA-NCAM promote functional recovery after spinal cord injury. *Brain* 2007;**130**(8):2159–74

43. Bachelin C, Zujovic V, Buchet D, Maller J, Baron-Van Evercooren A. Ectopic expression of PSA-NCAM in adult macaque Schwann cells promotes their migration and remyelination potential in the CNS *Brain* 2010;**133**(2):406–20

44. Grimpe B, Silver J. A novel DNA enzyme reduces glycosaminoglycan chains in the glial scar and allows microtransplanted dorsal root ganglia axons to regenerate beyond lesions in the spinal cord. *J Neurosci* 2004;**24**(6):1393–7

45. Santos-Silva A, Fairless R, Frame M C, *et al*. FGF/heparin differentially regulates Schwann cell and olfactory ensheathing cell interactions with astrocytes: a role in astrocytosis. *J Neurosci* 2007;**27**(27):7154–67

46. Fairless R, Frame M C, Barnett S C. N-cadherin differentially determines Schwann cell and olfactory ensheathing cell adhesion and migration responses upon contact with astrocytes. *Mol Cell Neurosci* 2005;**28**(2):253–63

47. Woodhoo A, Sahni V, Gilson J, *et al*. Schwann cell precursors: a favourable cell for myelin repair in the central nervous system. *Brain* 2007;**130**(8):2175–85

48. Hjerling-Leffler J, Marmigere F, Heglind M, *et al*. The boundary cap: a source of neural crest stem cells that generate multiple sensory neuron subtypes. *Development* 2005;**132**(11):2623–32

49. Maro G S, Vermeren M, Voiculescu O, *et al*. Neural crest boundary cap cells constitute a source of neuronal and glial cells of the PNS. *Nat Neurosci* 2004;**7**(9):930–8

50. Aquino J B, Hjerling-Leffler J, Koltzenburg M, *et al*. In vitro and in vivo differentiation of boundary cap neural crest stem cells into mature Schwann cells. *Exp Neurol* 2006;**198**(2):438–49

51. Morrison S J, White P M, Zock C, Anderson D J. Prospective identification, isolation by flow cytometry, and in vivo self-renewal of multipotent mammalian neural crest stem cells. *Cell* 1999;**96**(5):737–49

52. Kruger G M, Mosher J T, Bixby S, *et al*. Neural crest stem cells persist in the adult gut but undergo changes in self-renewal, neuronal subtype potential, and factor responsiveness. *Neuron* 2002;**35**(4):657–69

53. Fernandes K J, McKenzie I A, Mill P, *et al*. A dermal niche for multipotent adult skin-derived precursor cells. *Nat Cell Biol* 2004;**6**(11):1082–93

54. Sieber-Blum M, Grim M, Hu Y F, Szeder V. Pluripotent neural crest stem cells in the adult hair follicle. *Dev Dyn* 2004;**231**(2):258–69

55. Tomita Y, Matsumura K, Wakamatsu Y, *et al*. Cardiac neural crest cells contribute to the dormant multipotent stem cell in the mammalian heart. *J Cell Biol* 2005;**170**(7):1135–46

56. Hagedorn L, Suter U, Sommer L. P0 and PMP22 mark a multipotent neural crest-derived cell type that displays community effects in response to TGF-beta family factors. *Development* 1999;**126**(17):3781–94

57. Li H Y, Say E H, Zhou X F. Isolation and characterization of neural crest progenitors from adult dorsal root ganglia. *Stem Cells* 2007;**25**(8):2053–65

58. Dezawa M, Takahashi I, Esaki M, Takano M, Sawada H. Sciatic nerve regeneration in rats induced by transplantation of in vitro differentiated bone-marrow stromal cells. *Eur J Neurosci* 2001;**14**(11):1771–6

59. Keilhoff G, Stang F, Goihl A, Wolf G, Fansa H. Transdifferentiated mesenchymal stem cells as alternative therapy in supporting nerve regeneration and myelination. *Cell Mol Neurobiol* 2006;**26**(7–8):1235–52

60. Krampera M, Marconi S, Pasini A, *et al*. Induction of neural-like differentiation in human mesenchymal stem cells derived from bone marrow, fat, spleen and thymus. *Bone* 2007;**40**(2):382–90

61. Nagoshi N, Shibata S, Kubota Y, *et al*. Ontogeny and multipotency of neural crest-derived stem cells in mouse bone marrow, dorsal root ganglia, and whisker pad. *Cell Stem Cell* 2008;**2**(4):392–403

62. McKenzie I A, Biernaskie J, Toma J G, Midha R, Miller F D. Skin-derived precursors generate myelinating Schwann cells for the injured and dysmyelinated nervous system. *J Neurosci* 2006;**26**(24):6651–60

63. Amoh Y, Li L, Campillo R, *et al*. Implanted hair follicle stem cells form Schwann cells that support repair of severed peripheral nerves. *Proc Natl Acad Sci USA* 2005;**102**(49):17 734–8

64. Sieber-Blum M, Schnell L, Grim M, *et al*. Characterization of epidermal neural crest stem cell (EPI-NCSC) grafts in the lesioned spinal cord. *Mol Cell Neurosci* 2006;**32**(1–2):67–81

65. Toma J G, McKenzie I A, Bagli D, Miller F D. Isolation and characterization of multipotent skin-derived precursors from human skin. *Stem Cells* 2005;**23**(6):727–37

66. Hunt D P, Morris P N, Sterling J, *et al*. A highly enriched niche of precursor cells with neuronal and glial potential within the hair follicle dermal papilla of adult skin. *Stem Cells* 2008;**26**(1):163–72

67. Xu Y, Liu Z, Liu L, *et al*. Neurospheres from rat adipose-derived stem cells could be induced into functional Schwann cell-like cells in vitro. *BMC Neurosci* 2008;**9**:21

68. Bonilla S, Alarcon P, Villaverde R, *et al*. Haematopoietic progenitor cells from adult bone marrow differentiate into cells that express oligodendroglial antigens in the neonatal mouse brain. *Eur J Neurosci* 2002;**15**(3):575–82

69. Sasaki M, Honmou O, Akiyama Y, *et al*. Transplantation of an acutely isolated bone marrow fraction repairs demyelinated adult rat spinal cord axons. *Glia* 2001;**35**(1):26–34

70. Akiyama Y, Radtke C, Kocsis J D. Remyelination of the rat spinal cord by transplantation of identified bone marrow stromal cells. *J Neurosci* 2002;**22**(15):6623–30

71. Akiyama Y, Radtke C, Honmou O, Kocsis J D. Remyelination of the spinal cord following intravenous delivery of bone marrow cells. *Glia* 2002;**39**(3):229–36

72. Dupin E, Calloni G, Real C, Goncalves-Trentin A, Le Douarin N M. Neural crest progenitors and stem cells. *C R Biol* 2007;**330**(6–7):521–9

73. Dupin E, Real C, Glavieux-Pardanaud C, Vaigot P, Le Douarin N M. Reversal of developmental restrictions in neural crest lineages: transition from Schwann cells to glial–melanocytic precursors in vitro. *Proc Natl Acad Sci USA* 2003;**100**(9):5229–33

74. Real C, Glavieux-Pardanaud C, Le Douarin N M, Dupin E. Clonally cultured differentiated pigment cells can dedifferentiate and generate multipotent progenitors with self-renewing potential. *Dev Biol* 2006;**300**(2):656–69

75. Real C, Glavieux-Pardanaud C, Vaigot P, Le-Douarin N, Dupin E. The instability of the neural crest phenotypes: Schwann cells can differentiate into myofibroblasts. *Int J Dev Biol* 2005;**49**(2–3):151–9

76. Roh J, Cho E A, Seong I, *et al.* Down-regulation of Sox10 with specific small interfering RNA promotes transdifferentiation of Schwannoma cells into myofibroblasts. *Differentiation* 2006;**74**(9–10):542–51

77. Mujtaba T, Mayer-Proschel M, Rao M S. A common neural progenitor for the CNS and PNS. *Dev Biol* 1998;**200**(1):1–15

78. Keirstead H S, Ben-Hur T, Rogister B, *et al.* Polysialylated neural cell adhesion molecule-positive CNS precursors generate both oligodendrocytes and Schwann cells to remyelinate the CNS after transplantation. *J Neurosci* 1999;**19**(17):7529–36

79. Crang A J, Gilson J M, Li W W, Blakemore W F. The remyelinating potential and in vitro differentiation of MOG-expressing oligodendrocyte precursors isolated from the adult rat CNS. *Eur J Neurosci* 2004;**20**(6):1445–60

80. Akiyama Y, Honmou O, Kato T, *et al.* Transplantation of clonal neural precursor cells derived from adult human brain establishes functional peripheral myelin in the rat spinal cord. *Exp Neurol* 2001;**167**(1):27–39

81. Sailer M H, Hazel T G, Panchision D M, *et al.* BMP2 and FGF2 cooperate to induce neural-crest-like fates from fetal and adult CNS stem cells. *J Cell Sci* 2005;**118**(24):5849–60

82. Talbott J F, Cao Q, Enzmann G U, *et al.* Schwann cell-like differentiation by adult oligodendrocyte precursor cells following engraftment into the demyelinated spinal cord is BMP-dependent. *Glia* 2006;**54**(3):147–59

83. Mothe A J, Tator C H. Transplanted neural stem/progenitor cells generate myelinating oligodendrocytes and Schwann cells in spinal cord demyelination and dysmyelination. *Exp Neurol* 2008;**213**(1):176–90

9

Magnetic resonance imaging to study white matter damage in multiple sclerosis

Massimo Filippi, Annalisa Pulizzi, and Marco Rovaris

The integrity of white matter (WM) pathways is important for the preservation of brain functioning and the promotion of recovery after structural damage. Multiple sclerosis (MS) is characterized by the presence of both macroscopic (focal) and "occult" (diffuse) WM damage, whose features may range from reversible inflammation and edema to persistent demyelination and loss of axons. In the present chapter, we review the contributions given by magnetic resonance (MR)-based techniques to our understanding of the pathophysiology of WM damage in MS, as well as their possible role as paraclinical markers to monitor the evolution of such a damage over time.

Conventional magnetic resonance imaging

T2-weighted MR images are highly sensitive for the detection of MS WM lesions. Such a sensitivity makes them very useful for diagnosing MS, monitoring its short-term activity, and assessing the overall WM disease burden. Post-contrast (gadolinium – Gd) T1-weighted scans allow one to distinguish active from inactive MS lesions, since Gd enhancement occurs as a result of increased blood–brain barrier (BBB) permeability and corresponds to areas with ongoing inflammation, but does not provide information on tissue damage [1]. Chronically hypointense lesions on T1-weighted images (known as "black holes") represent areas where severe demyelination and axonal loss have occurred [1]. Measurements of brain and cervical cord atrophy can also be obtained from MRI scans to assess the extent of tissue loss in MS. Thanks to the advances in image post-processing, it is now possible to assess the evolution of WM and gray matter (GM) atrophy separately. However, the

pathological basis of MS-related atrophy is still unclear and atrophy can be considered an end-stage phenomenon [2], whose measurement is unable to provide us with any information about the dynamics of progressive WM loss, if any.

Despite the aforementioned limitations, the study of WM damage using conventional MRI (cMRI) remains the main tool for diagnosing MS. As a matter of fact, semiquantitative cMRI features (based on WM lesion number and site) are part of consensus-based criteria for demonstrating the dissemination in space and time of the disease and potentially achieve an earlier and firmer diagnosis than that based upon clinical findings in isolation [3]. Moreover, cMRI can contribute to the diagnostic work-up of MS also by detecting some features of WM damage that are "not suggestive" of MS, thus reducing the likelihood of a false-positive diagnosis, or indicating the need for performance of additional tests.

The relationship between cMRI findings and clinical disability in MS remains suboptimal. This phenomenon is known as the "clinico-radiological paradox" of MS [1]. In patients with established MS, the burden of cMRI-visible lesions explains, at most, about 10–15% of the observed variance of clinical disability [1]. A large-scale cross-sectional study [4] suggested that such a limited correlation may depend upon a plateauing effect of cMRI measurements of disease burden in established MS patients with pronounced locomotor disability, i.e., those with expanded disability status scale (EDSS) scores above 4.5. However, a more recent study showed that the plateauing relationship between T2 lesion volume and disability in MS is not always present and is likely due to the reduced frequency of "inflammatory" events in the most common form of secondary progressive (SP) MS [5].

Conversely, in patients at presentation with clinically isolated syndromes (CIS) suggestive of MS, the burden of brain T2-visible lesions can be a strong predictor of the severity of neurological disability up to 20 years later [6]. Gadolinium-enhanced cMRI is more sensitive than either clinical evaluations or T2-weighted images in detecting MS activity. In established MS, the frequency of enhancing lesions is five to ten times higher than that of clinical relapses, but, once again, the relationship between these lesions and the clinical activity of MS is weak [1]. The harvest of enhancing MS lesions can be markedly increased when administering a triple dose (TD) of Gd. Since those lesions enhancing only after a TD are likely to represent areas with only mildly increased BBB permeability, the simultaneous presence of lesions enhancing at different Gd doses suggests that the severity of cMRI-detectable inflammation is highly variable among WM lesions from the same MS patients [7]. The use of TD-enhanced MRI might be useful in the context of clinical trials to grade the efficacy of treatment on cMRI-detectable inflammation and to reduce the sample sizes and follow-up periods needed to run studies powerful enough to detect a treatment effect [7]. Nevertheless, this approach does not seem to increase the strength of the clinical/cMRI relationship, possibly because of the high inter-patient variability of the resulting findings.

Even though a seminal study showed a significant correlation between the burden of T1-hypointense WM lesions and the severity of clinical disability [8], subsequent studies based on larger samples of patients seemed to deny these findings [1]. The assessment of T1-hypointense lesions has some pitfalls which may explain its limited value for monitoring MS evolution. First, the identification of "black holes" remains operator-, scanner-, and sequence-dependent. Moreover, the assessment of T1-hypointense lesions does not provide information about the pathology of the normal-appearing WM (NAWM) [1].

Recent studies (see Pirko *et al.* [9] for a review) seem to suggest that the measurement of brain atrophy is more rewarding for the assessment of GM than for that of WM damage. Nevertheless, it is well known that a significant reduction of WM volume can be seen in established MS [10], which correlates with patients' locomotor disability [10] and cognitive impairment [11] at a greater magnitude than T2 lesion burden. The reduction of WM volume in MS mainly depends upon the loss of myelin and

axons, which, on turn, is, at least partially, correlated with the burden of focal lesions [12]. Thanks to recent advances in image post-processing techniques the measurement of atrophy in selected pathways, such as the corpus callosum (CC) and the corticospinal tracts (CST) [13], may also represent a novel strategy to improve the in vivo monitoring of MS damage in clinically eloquent WM regions.

Structural magnetic resonance-based techniques

Structural MR-based techniques have the potential to improve our understanding of the features and evolution of MS-related WM damage. Among these techniques, magnetization transfer imaging (MTI), diffusion tensor imaging (DTI) and proton MR spectroscopy (^{1}H-MRS) have, at least, two advantages over cMRI in the study of WM damage. First, they may provide quantitative information with increased specificity for the heterogeneous substrates of MS pathology. Second, they enable us to quantify the damage occurring in the NAWM outside T2-visible lesions [1].

The technique of MTI is based on the interactions between protons in a relatively free environment and those where motion is restricted. Off-resonance irradiation is applied, which saturates the magnetization of the less mobile protons, but this is transferred to the mobile protons, thus reducing the signal intensity from the observable magnetization. Thus, low MT ratio (MTR) indicates a reduced capacity of the macromolecules in the central nervous system to exchange magnetization with the surrounding water molecules, reflecting damage to myelin or to the axonal membrane. The most compelling among the many lines of evidence indicating that markedly decreased MTR values correspond to areas where severe tissue loss has occurred is the strong correlation of MTR values from MS lesions and NAWM with the percentage of residual axons and the degree of demyelination found in postmortem studies of patients with MS [14].

Diffusion is the microscopic random translational motion of molecules. Water molecular diffusion can be measured in vivo using DTI, in terms of an apparent diffusion coefficient (ADC) [15]. Although diffusion is inherently a three-dimensional process, in some tissues with an oriented microstructure, such as brain WM, the molecular mobility is not the same in all directions. This property is called anisotropy, and results in a variation of the measured diffusivity with tissue measurement direction. Fiber tracts in the WM consist of aligned myelinated axons and, therefore, hindrance of water diffusion is much greater across rather than along the major axis of axonal fibers. Under these conditions, a full characterization of diffusion can only be found in terms of a tensor, a matrix where the on-diagonal elements represent the diffusion coefficients along the axes of the reference frame, while the off-diagonal elements account for the correlations between molecular displacement along orthogonal directions. From the tensor, it is possible to derive some scalar indices. These include the mean diffusivity (MD), which is affected by cellular size and integrity, and the fractional anisotropy (FA), which reflects the degree of alignment of cellular structures within fiber tracts, as well as their structural integrity. The main postmortem correlates of diffusivity changes in MS are demyelination and axonal loss [16]. This seems to be more evident for anisotropy indexes than for ADC.

Water-suppressed, proton MR spectra of the human brain at long echo times reveal four major resonances: one from choline-containing phospholipids (Cho), one from creatine and phosphocreatine (Cr), one from N-acetylaspartate (NAA), and one from the methyl resonance of lactate (Lac). Of these, NAA is a marker of axonal integrity, whereas Cho and Lac are considered as chemical correlates of acute inflammatory or demyelinating changes [17]. Studies using ^{1}H-MRS with shorter echo times can detect additional metabolites, such as lipids and myoinositol (mI), which are also regarded as markers of ongoing myelin damage.

Magnetization transfer imaging studies

A reduction of MTR values is already detectable in the NAWM prior to T2-visible lesion appearance [18, 19], in NAWM areas adjacent to focal T2-weighted lesions, particularly in progressive MS patients [20], and in patients with MS and no cMRI-visible WM abnormalities [21]. This indicates that MTI is sensitive to NAWM damage in MS and can reflect the presence of an increased amount of unbound water due to edema, perivascular inflammation, demyelination, and axonal loss before these features may cause T2-visible MR signal abnormalities. To investigate these aspects of WM damage, macroscopic lesions segmented on T2-weighted images can be superimposed

onto the co-registered MTR maps of the brain and the areas corresponding to the segmented lesions can be masked out, thus obtaining MTR maps of normal-appearing brain tissue (NABT), including the NAWM [22], and a histogram-based analysis can then be applied. Using such an approach, it has been shown that NABT MTR histogram-derived measures are different and evolve at a different pace in the major MS clinical phenotypes [22, 23]. When a multivariate analysis of several cMRI- and MTI-derived variables was run, it was found that average NABT MTR can be more strongly associated with cognitive impairment in MS patients than the extent of T2-visible lesions and their intrinsic tissue damage [24]. Reduced NABT MTR has also been found in asymptomatic relatives of patients with MS and in patients who present with CIS [25]. Although not confirmed by other studies, the extent of NABT changes in patients presenting with CIS has been found to be an independent predictor of subsequent evolution to clinically definite MS (25). A significant prognostic value of NAWM MTR abnormalities for the medium-term evolution of disability in patients with established MS has also been independently reported by different longitudinal studies [26, 27]. In recent studies, voxel-based analysis has been applied to brain MTR maps to better assess the severity of tissue damage in specific WM regions [28, 29]. Patients with CIS suggestive of MS showed significantly lower MTR values than healthy controls in multiple WM regions including the CC, the occipito-frontal fascicles, the external capsule, and the optic radiations [28, 29]. Significant correlations between regional MTR values and the Multiple Sclerosis Functional Composite (MSFC) scores were found for the right superior longitudinal fasciculus, the right frontal WM, the splenium, and the genu of the CC; MTR values in the right superior longitudinal fasciculus and in the splenium of the CC were also correlated with the patients' performance at the Paced Auditory Serial Addition Task (PASAT) test [29]. These results suggest a potential role for voxel-based analysis of brain MTR data to achieve a better understanding of the relationship between the location of NAWM damage and its functional impact in patients with MS.

Diffusion tensor imaging studies

Similarly to what was found using MTI, numerous DTI studies have consistently shown the presence of diffusion abnormalities in the NAWM of patients with MS, which can even precede the development of T2-visible lesions by several weeks (see Rovaris *et al.* [30] for a review). Studies with DTI assessing changes in different brain regions showed that NAWM abnormalities in MS are widespread, but tend to be more severe in sites where MRI-visible lesions are usually located and in peri-plaque regions. A recent study, using histogram-based analysis of segmented diffusion maps of the brain, reported a significant increase of MD and decrease of FA values in CIS patients with paraclinical evidence of disease dissemination in space, although the changes did not predict the short-term occurrence of cMRI disease activity [31]. Seminal cross-sectional studies did not find significant correlations between the average NAWM diffusivity or anisotropy values and the severity of MS neurological disability, as assessed by the EDSS score, nor significant differences between MS clinical phenotypes as regards the severity of overall DTI changes in the NAWM (see Rovaris *et al.* [30] for a review). However, when the DTI characteristics of clinically eloquent NAWM regions were studied, a significant relationship with patients' EDSS was found for the CC and internal capsule FA [32] and for cerebral peduncle MD and FA [33]. In addition, in a preliminary DTI study of cognitive impairment in patients with relapsing–remitting (RR) MS [34] moderate correlations were found between several NAWM histogram-derived DTI quantities and neuropsychological test scores. The application of voxel-based analysis techniques to diffusivity maps of the brain may represent a rewarding strategy to highlight the correlations between WM damage and clinical features of MS. In a seminal DTI study using a 3T magnet, Ceccarelli *et al.* [35] were able to demonstrate a different spatial distribution of NAWM damage between patients with benign (B) MS and those with RRMS, which was in apparent contrast with the between-group similarity of the overall extent of WM structural changes.

Studies using ^{1}H-MRS

Regional increases in the concentrations of Cho and mobile lipids, as well as decreases in NAA concentrations, can precede the appearance of cMRI-visible WM lesions by several months [17]. Studies using ^{1}H-MRS reveal that Cho and Lac increase and Cr decreases in the early phases following the acute onset

of WM lesions [17]. Changes in the resonance intensity of Cho reflect membrane turnover, while raised Lac concentrations can be explained by the metabolism of inflammatory cells. At short echo times ^{1}H-MRS may also better detect temporary increases in lipids that are released during myelin disruption, as well as revealing raised mI levels. For several months after the acute stage of WM lesions, the signal intensity of NAA may remain decreased or just show a partial recovery. In patients with BMS, chronic lesions have higher NAA signal intensities than those in SPMS patients, indicating a more efficient tissue integrity recovery in patients with less severe disability [17]. Decreases in NAA concentrations are also well known to occur in the NAWM of MS patients [36]. De Stefano *et al.* [37] demonstrated reversible changes in NAA concentration in the NAWM of the hemisphere contralateral to large, acute demyelinating lesions, suggesting that part of these diffuse changes in the NAWM may be related to a sublethal damage of axons passing through inflammatory lesions. In the NAWM of patients with CIS [38] and established MS [39] an increase of mI levels has also been detected, confirming the hypothesis that increased glial cell activity is an important feature of "occult" WM damage together with axonal damage. A significant correlation of ^{1}H-MRS findings with neurological disability or selective motor impairment has been shown by several studies [16], but these findings have not been confirmed by others [39]. In a recent study [40], patients' EDSS was found to correlate with mI and glutamate–glutamine concentrations in the NAWM, suggesting that ^{1}H-MRS markers of NAWM pathological features other than axonal damage may also have a functional relevance in MS.

Novel magnetic resonance-based strategies: tractography and perfusion imaging

The examination of diffusion tensor (DT) eigenvectors, which represent the diffusion coefficients along the axes of the diffusion ellipsoid, may provide a signature of Wallerian degeneration in the NAWM of MS patients. These DT tractography methods can also be used to segment clinically eloquent WM pathways in MS patients, such as the CST and the CC. Thanks to DT tractography, probing functional pathways with DT MRI measures may enable us to achieve a better reflection of the NAWM disease burden and also allow the strength of the correlations between clinical and MRI findings to be improved. Wilson et al. [41] produced maps of CST from DTI scans of 25 patients with RRMS and measured the relative anisotropy along these pathways. Significant correlations were found between the latter parameter and patients' EDSS and pyramidal functional system scores, whereas T2 lesion burden and diffusion histogram parameters did not correlate with clinical findings. Similarly, Lin et al. [42] performed DT fiber tracking in a group of 29 patients with RRMS and 13 normal controls matched for age and gender, to map the CST and the CC, and correlated the ADC values in these regions with clinical evaluations, such as patients' scores of the pyramidal functional system and PASAT. The mean ADC in the CST correlated with pyramidal functional system scores, and the mean ADC of the CC with the performance at PASAT. In addition, DT tractography has been used to build a probability map of the CST from healthy volunteers, which can then be applied to patients, to overcome some of the expected difficulties for fiber tracking in the MS brain [43]. In a study of CIS patients [43], the CST increase of transverse diffusion eigenvalues was correlated with the presence of motor impairment. Vaithianathar et al. [44] mapped the CST of 25 patients with RRMS and sampled T1 relaxation time values along the corresponding trajectories on co-registered whole-brain T1 maps. Values of CST T1, but not global WM T1 values, correlated significantly with the severity of patients' neurological disability. Beyond DT tractography, newer acquisition schemes for DTI, such as high b-value images [45], may also increase the sensitivity of "conventional," low b-value DTI in the detection of NAWM abnormalities and, therefore, provide a more accurate picture of the severity of MS damage.

Cerebral perfusion is defined as the volume of blood flowing through a definite volume of tissue per unit of time; this phenomenon can be described by MRI in terms of cerebral blood flow (CBF), cerebral blood volume (CBV), and mean transit time (MTT). Perfusion MRI still suffers from some technical limitations, such as poor spatial resolution and limited brain coverage. Moreover, in MS patients the presence of BBB disruption may cause leakage artefacts that can lead to wrong estimates of the CBV. However, thanks to the use of high field scanners, perfusion MRI is receiving increasing attention in the study of NAWM

damage in the MS brain. Some studies [46, 47] have suggested the presence of perfusion abnormalities both in T2-visible lesions and in the NAWM. A longitudinal MRI study of RRMS patients, who underwent monthly scans, has revealed that changes in NAWM perfusion may precede T2-visible lesion formation, before any evidence of BBB breakdown and ADC increases [48]. A recent 3T study of patients with primary progressive (PP) MS and RRMS investigated the correlation between perfusion abnormalities and clinical disability [49]. Compared to controls, CBF and CBV were significantly lower in all NAWM regions from both PPMS and RRMS patients; compared to RRMS patients, those with PPMS showed significantly lower CBF in the periventricular NAWM and lower CBV in the periventricular and frontal NAWM. Patients' EDSS was significantly correlated with periventricular CBF and with the periventricular and frontal CBV. These findings indicate that the severity of perfusion abnormalities in the NAWM may have some impact on the clinical status of patients with MS. On the other hand, however, another recent 3T study investigating the relationship between regional perfusion changes and cognitive dysfunctions in RRMS and PPMS patients [50] found that the only significant correlations were those between deep GM CBF/CBV values and some neuropsychological test scores.

Conclusions

The high sensitivity of cMRI for the detection of focal WM lesions makes this technique a sort of paraclinical "gold standard" for diagnosing MS and monitoring its evolution. On the other hand, cMRI has a limited value for improving our understanding of the pathophysiology of WM damage, since it provides limited information about its heterogeneous features and does not account for the presence and severity of NAWM pathology. Numerous studies have consistently shown that quantitative MR-based techniques may overcome some of the aforementioned limitations of cMRI, but their application to the work-up of individual MS patients in a clinical setting is still premature. Several pieces of evidence seem also to indicate that none of these techniques taken in isolation is able to provide a complete picture of the complexity of the MS process in the WM and this should call for the definition of aggregates of MR quantities, thought to reflect different aspects of MS pathology, to improve our ability to monitor the evolution of the disease.

References

1. Filippi M, Grossman R I. MRI techniques to monitor MS evolution: the present and the future. *Neurology* 2002;**58**:1147–53

2. Miller D H, Barkhof F, Frank J A, Parker G J, Thompson A J. Measurement of atrophy in multiple sclerosis: pathological basis, methodological aspects and clinical relevance. *Brain* 2002;**125**:1676–95

3. Polman C H, Reingold S C, Edan G, *et al.* Diagnostic criteria for multiple sclerosis: 2005 revisions to the "McDonald Criteria." *Ann Neurol* 2005;**58**:840–6

4. Li D K B, Held U, Petkau J, *et al.* MRI T2 lesion burden in multiple sclerosis: a plateauing relationship with clinical disability. *Neurology* 2006;**66**:1884–8

5. Sormani M P, Rovaris M, Comi G, Filippi M. A reassessment of the plateauing relationship between T2 lesion load and disability in MS. *Neurology* 2009;**73**:1538–42

6. Fisniku L K, Brex P A, Altmann D R, *et al.* Disability and T2 MRI lesions: a 20-year follow-up of patients with relapse onset of multiple sclerosis. *Brain* 2008;**131**:808–17

7. Filippi M, Rovaris M, Capra R, *et al.* A multi-centre longitudinal study comparing the sensitivity of monthly MRI after standard and triple dose gadolinium-DTPA for monitoring disease activity in multiple sclerosis: implications for phase II clinical trials. *Brain* 1998;**121**:2011–20

8. Truyen L, van Waesberghe J H, van Walderveen M A, *et al.* Accumulation of hypointense lesions ("black holes") on T1 spin-echo MRI correlates with disease progression in multiple sclerosis. *Neurology* 1996;**47**:1469–76

9. Pirko I, Lucchinetti C F, Sriram S, Bakshi R. Gray matter involvement in multiple sclerosis. *Neurology* 2007;**68**:634–42

10. Tedeschi G, Lavorgna L, Russo P, *et al.* Brain atrophy and lesion load in a large population of patients with multiple sclerosis. *Neurology* 2005;**65**:280–5

11. Sanfilipo M P, Benedict R H, Weinstock-Guttman B, Bakshi R. Gray and white matter brain atrophy and neuropsychological impairment in multiple sclerosis. *Neurology* 2006;**66**:685–95

12. Evangelou N, Konz D, Esiri M M, *et al.* Regional axonal loss in the corpus callosum correlates with cerebral white matter lesion volume and distribution in multiple sclerosis. *Brain* 2000;**123**:1845–9

13. Audoin B, Ibarrola D, Malikova I, *et al.* Onset and underpinnings of white matter atrophy at the very early stage of multiple sclerosis: a two-year longitudinal MRI/MRSI study of corpus callosum. *Mult Scler* 2007;**13**:41–51

14. Schmierer K, Scaravilli F, Altmann D R, Barker G J, Miller D H. Magnetization transfer ratio and myelin in postmortem multiple sclerosis brain. *Ann Neurol* 2004;**56**:407–15

15. Pierpaoli C, Jezzard P, Basser P J, Barnett A, Di Chiro G. Diffusion tensor MR imaging of the human brain. *Radiology* 1996;**201**:637–48

16. Schmierer K, Wheeler-Kingshott C A M, Boulby P A, *et al.* Diffusion tensor imaging of postmortem multiple sclerosis brain. *NeuroImage* 2007;**35**:467–77

17. Filippi M, Arnold D L, Comi G (eds). *Magnetic Resonance Spectroscopy in Multiple Sclerosis.* Milan: Springer-Verlag, 2001

18. Filippi M, Rocca M A, Martino G, Horsfield M A, Comi G. Magnetization transfer changes in the normal appearing white matter precede the appearance of enhancing lesions in patients with multiple sclerosis. *Ann Neurol* 1998;**43**:809–14

19. Laule C, Vavasour I M, Whittall K P, *et al.* Evolution of focal and diffuse magnetisation transfer abnormalities in multiple sclerosis. *J Neurol* 2003;**250**:924–31

20. Filippi M, Campi A, Dousset V, *et al.* A magnetization transfer imaging study of normal-appearing white matter in multiple sclerosis. *Neurology* 1995;**45**: 478–82

21. Filippi M, Rocca M A, Minicucci L, *et al.* Magnetization transfer imaging of patients with definite MS and negative conventional MRI. *Neurology* 1999;**52**:845–8

22. Tortorella C, Viti B, Bozzali M, *et al.* A magnetization transfer histogram study of normal appearing brain tissue in multiple sclerosis. *Neurology* 2000;**54**:186–93

23. Filippi M, Inglese M, Rovaris M, *et al.* Magnetization transfer imaging to monitor the evolution of MS: a 1-year follow-up study. *Neurology* 2000;**55**:940–6

24. Filippi M, Tortorella C, Rovaris M, *et al.* Changes in the normal appearing brain tissue and cognitive impairment in multiple sclerosis. *J Neurol Neurosurg Psychiatry* 2000;**68**:157–61

25. Miller D, Barkhof F, Montalban X, Thompson A, Filippi M. Clinically isolated syndromes suggestive of multiple sclerosis. 2: Non-conventional MRI, recovery processes, and management. *Lancet Neurol* 2005;**4**:341–8

26. Santos C A, Narayanan S, De Stefano N, *et al.* Magnetization transfer can predict clinical evolution in patients with multiple sclerosis. *J Neurol* 2002; **249**:662–8

27. Khaleeli Z, Sastre-Garrga J, Ciccarelli O, Miller D H, Thompson A J. Magnetization transfer ratio in the normal appearing white matter predicts progression of disability over 1 year in early primary progressive

multiple sclerosis. *J Neurol Neurosurg Psychiatry* 2007;**78**:1076–82

28. Audoin B, Ranjeva J P, Au Duong M V, *et al.* Voxel-based analysis of MTR images: a method to locate gray matter abnormalities in patients at the earliest stage of multiple sclerosis. *J Magn Reson Imaging* 2004;**20**:765–71

29. Ranjeva J P, Audoin B, Au Duong M V, *et al.* Local tissue damage assessed with statistical mapping analysis of brain magnetization transfer ratio: relationship with functional status of patients in the earliest stage of multiple sclerosis. *Am J Neuroradiol* 2005;**26**:119–27

30. Rovaris M, Gass A, Bammer R, *et al.* Diffusion MRI in multiple sclerosis. *Neurology* 2005;**65**:1526–32

31. Gallo A, Rovaris M, Riva R, *et al.* Diffusion tensor MRI detects normal-appearing white matter damage unrelated to short-term disease activity in patients at the earliest clinical stage of multiple sclerosis. *Arch Neurol* 2005;**62**:803–8

32. Filippi M, Cercignani M, Inglese M, Horsfield M A, Comi G. Diffusion tensor magnetic resonance imaging in multiple sclerosis. *Neurology* 2001;**56**:304–11

33. Ciccarelli O, Werring D J, Wheeler-Kingshott C A, *et al.* Investigation of MS normal-appearing brain using diffusion tensor MRI with clinical correlations. *Neurology* 2001;**56**:926–33

34. Rovaris M, Iannucci G, Falautano M, *et al.* Cognitive dysfunction in patients with mildly disabling relapsing–remitting multiple sclerosis: an exploratory study with diffusion tensor MR imaging. *J Neurol Sci* 2002;**195**:103–9

35. Ceccarelli A, Rocca M A, Pagani E, *et al.* The topographical distribution of tissue injury in benign MS: a 3T multiparametric MRI study. *NeuroImage* 2008;**39**:1499–509

36. Caramanos Z, Narayanan S, Arnold D L. ^{1}H-MRS quantification of tNA and tCr in patients with multiple sclerosis: a meta-analytic review. *Brain* 2005;**128**:2483–506

37. De Stefano N, Narayanan S, Matthews P M, *et al.* In vivo evidence for axonal dysfunction remote from focal cerebral demyelination of the type seen in multiple sclerosis. *Brain* 1999;**122**:1933–9

38. Fernando K T, McLean M A, Chard D T, *et al.* Elevated white matter myo-inositol in clinically isolated syndromes suggestive of multiple sclerosis. *Brain* 2004;**127**:1361–9

39. Vrenken H, Barkhof F, Uitdehaag B M, *et al.* MR spectroscopic evidence for glial increase but not for neuro-axonal damage in MS normal-appearing white matter. *Magn Reson Med* 2005;**53**:256–66

40. Sastre-Garriga J, Ingle G T, Chard D T, *et al.* Metabolite changes in normal-appearing gray and white matter are linked with disability in early primary progressive multiple sclerosis. *Arch Neurol* 2005;**62**:569–73

41. Wilson M, Tench C R, Morgan P S, Blumhardt L D. Pyramidal tract mapping by diffusion tensor magnetic resonance imaging in multiple sclerosis: improving correlations with disability. *J Neurol Neurosurg Psychiatry* 2003;**74**:203–7

42. Lin X, Tench C R, Morgan P S, Niepel G, Constantinescu C S. "Importance sampling" in MS: use of diffusion tensor tractography to quantify pathology related to specific impairment. *J Neurol Sci* 2005;**237**:13–19

43. Pagani E, Filippi M, Rocca M A, Horsfield M A. A method for obtaining tract-specific diffusion tensor MRI measurements in the presence of disease: application to patients with clinically isolated syndromes suggestive of multiple sclerosis. *NeuroImage* 2005;**26**:258–65

44. Vaithianathar L, Tench C R, Morgan P S, Wilson M, Blumhardt L D. T1 relaxation time mapping of white matter tracts in multiple sclerosis defined by diffusion tensor imaging. *J Neurol* 2002;**249**:1272–8

45. Assaf Y, Ben-Bashat D, Chapman J, *et al.* High *b*-value *q*-space analyzed diffusion-weighted MRI: application to multiple sclerosis. *Magn Reson Med* 2002;**47**:115–26

46. Law M, Saindane A M, Ge Y, *et al.* Microvascular abnormality in relapsing–remitting multiple sclerosis: perfusion MRI imaging findings in normal-appearing white matter. *Radiology* 2004;**231**:645–52

47. Ge Y, Law M, Johnson G, *et al.* Dynamic susceptibility contrast perfusion MR imaging of multiple sclerosis lesions: characterizing hemodynamic impairment and inflammatory activity. *Am J Neuroradiol* 2005;**26**:1539–47

48. Wuerfel J, Bellman-Strobl J, Bruneker P, *et al.* Changes in cerebral perfusion precede plaque formation in multiple sclerosis: a longitudinal perfusion MRI study. *Brain* 2004;**127**:111–19

49. Adhya S, Johnson G, Herbert J, *et al.* Pattern of hemodynamic impairment in multiple sclerosis: dynamic susceptibility contrast perfusion MR imaging at 3.0 T. *NeuroImage* 2006;**33**:1029–35

50. Inglese M, Adhya S, Johnson G, *et al.* Perfusion magnetic resonance imaging correlates of neuropsychological impairment in multiple sclerosis. *J Cereb Blood Flow Metab* 2008;**28**:164–71

Chapter 1

Magnetic resonance imaging to assess gray matter damage in multiple sclerosis

Massimo Filippi, Federica Agosta, and Maria A. Rocca

Introduction

Although multiple sclerosis (MS) has been classically regarded as a white matter (WM) disease of the central nervous system (CNS), pathological studies have shown the presence of MS-related damage in the gray matter (GM) of MS patients [1–4]. Cortical GM lesions have been distinguished in mixed WM–GM lesions (type I), and purely intracortical lesions (types II, III, and IV) [5]. In addition to the neocortex, demyelination can also be found in the GM of the thalamus [6], basal ganglia [6], hypothalamus [7], hippocampus [8], cerebellum [9], and spinal cord [10]. A recent study suggested that meningeal inflammation may be a cause for subpial demyelination [11]. MS-related GM pathology is associated with neuronal injury, including neuritic swelling, as well as dendritic and axonal transections [3, 6].

Consistently with pathological studies, recent magnetic resonance imaging (MRI) studies have shown the involvement of the GM in MS, in terms of focal lesion, "diffuse" tissue abnormalities, and irreversible tissue loss (i.e., atrophy) [12]. These studies have also shown that GM damage affects the cortex and deep nuclei in the brain as well as the spinal cord, is present from the earliest clinical stage of the disease, and is at least partially independent of the WM burden of the disease [12].

This chapter summarizes the main results obtained from the use of conventional and modern quantitative MR-based techniques – namely, magnetization transfer (MT) MRI, diffusion-weighted (DW) MRI, and proton MR spectroscopy (^{1}H-MRS) – for the assessment of GM pathology in patients with MS.

Imaging gray matter lesions

Despite the technique's overall high sensitivity for MS abnormalities [13], conventional T2-weighted MRI sequences are unable to reveal the actual burden of GM lesions, because these lesions are small and have longer relaxation times than those of normal WM, which in turn results in poor contrast resolution between them and surrounding normal GM, and, in the case of cortical lesions, because of partial volume effects from the cerebrospinal fluid (CSF) [13]. Fast fluid-attenuated inversion recovery (fast-FLAIR) sequences and post-gadolinium (Gd) T1-weighted sequences have been the first strategies used to increase detection of GM lesions in MS. Due to CSF signal suppression, fast-FLAIR sequences allow the detection of more cortical and juxtacortical lesions than conventional T2-weighted sequences [2, 14–16]. The sharp contrast between enhancing lesions and surrounding tissue also results in an increased harvest of new cortical lesions, which may go undetected on unenhanced scans [2]. More recently, a multi-slab three-dimensional (3D) double-inversion recovery (DIR – i.e., two inversion times are used to suppress the signal from both WM and CSF) sequence has been developed to improve further the detection of GM lesions in MS [17]. As a result of the increased contrast between GM and WM, DIR images were able to detect more intracortical lesions than standard MRI techniques, showing gains of 538% and 152% compared with conventional T2-weighted and FLAIR, respectively [17]. Higher contrast between the lesion and its surroundings also resulted in an improved distinction between juxtacortical and mixed WM–GM lesions on DIR images [17]. In a large cohort of MS patients, intracortical lesions were

Multiple Sclerosis: Recovery of Function and Neurorehabilitation, eds. J. Kesselring, G. Comi, and A. J. Thompson.
Published by Cambridge University Press. © Cambridge University Press 2010.

detected in 58% of cases: 36% of patients with clinically isolated syndromes (CIS) suggestive of MS, 64% of patients with relapsing–remitting (RR) MS, and 73% of patients with secondary progressive (SP) MS [18]. The number of GM lesions was higher in patients with SPMS than in CIS or RRMS patients [18]. Pathological studies reported that the number of intracortical lesions may even amount to 59% of the total lesion count [2]. However, 3D DIR images showed a mean of 4.6% of the total number of lesions to be intracortical [18]. It is likely that many of the intracortical lesions still can not be visualized with 3D DIR imaging. Reliable detection and classification of intracortical lesions in MS have been shown to be greatly improved by the combination of 3D DIR with phase-sensitive inversion recovery (PSIR) images [19].

Although lesional involvement of deep GM in MS patients has not been studied as extensively as that of cortical GM, T2-hyperintense lesions in the basal ganglia have been detected in 25% of patients with MS [20]. T2 hypointensities, probably reflecting iron deposition, have also been described in the deep GM of MS patients [21]. More recently, hippocampal lesions have been visualized with 3D DIR sequences [22].

An additional gain in detection of GM lesions is likely to be achieved in the near future thanks to the increased availability of high-field MRI scanners (3.0 Tesla or more) [23]. Kangarlu *et al.* [23] compared MR images of brain samples from newly deceased MS patients obtained at 8.0 and 1.5 T, and showed that cortical lesions invisible on MRI scans at 1.5 T are clearly seen at 8.0 T.

Although a more precise quantification of focal GM damage in MS patients is expected to increase the strength of the correlation between clinical and MRI findings, especially when considering cognitive impairment and fatigue, heterogeneous results have been obtained so far [16, 18, 24–26]. This, however, does not come as a surprise, since other aspects of MS-related GM involvement have not been considered in these studies (i.e., "diffuse" tissue changes, and irreversible tissue loss).

Imaging "diffuse" gray matter damage

It is likely that GM damage in MS is not limited to focal lesions, but might also cause "diffuse" tissue changes, for instance through retrograde and transsynaptic degeneration. Modern quantitative MR-based techniques have the potential to provide accurate

estimates of "overall" (focal and "diffuse") GM abnormalities, and might, therefore, contribute to a more complete picture of GM damage associated with MS.

With MT MRI it is possible to calculate the MT ratios (MTR) of the CNS tissues [27]. Low MTR values, which indicate a reduced capacity of the protons bound to the brain tissue matrix to exchange magnetization with the surrounding "free" water, provide an accurate estimate of the extent of tissue disruption due to MS pathology [27]. Several studies have demonstrated reduced MTR values in the brain GM (which had been considered to be normal on conventional MR scans) from patients with different MS phenotypes [28–30], including those at the earliest clinical stage of MS [31–33]. Abnormalities in the GM increase with disease duration, since they have been found to be more pronounced in patients with primary progressive (PP) or SPMS [34]. In a recent, large, multi-center study of PPMS patients greater MT MRI-detectable GM damage was found in patients who required walking aids than in those who did not [35]. The distribution of MTR abnormalities in the various brain GM structures still needs to be defined. In a voxel-based MTR study [36], a regional pattern of brain MTR decrease, more evident in the basal ganglia, was found in patients with early MS. By contrast, in another study [37], which assessed thalamic MTR in early RRMS patients, no significant difference was observed at baseline between patients and controls. After 1 and 2 years, however, the mean thalamic MTR became significantly lower in patients [37].

Changes in GM MTR have been found to correlate with clinical disability [29, 30, 33, 38] and cognitive impairment [24, 39], whereas no correlation with fatigue emerged [40]. A voxel-based MTR study [39] showed that regional MTR values of several cortical areas are correlated significantly with the Multiple Sclerosis Functional Composite (MSFC) and the Paced Auditory Serial Addition Task (PASAT) scores. Values of GM MTR were also found to be an independent predictor of subsequent accumulation of disability in patients with MS followed up for 8 years [41].

The DW MRI technique enables the random diffusional motion of water molecules to be measured, thus providing metrics such as mean diffusivity (MD) and fractional anisotropy (FA) that allow the size and geometry of water-filled spaces to be quantified [42]. In line with MT MRI findings, DW MRI confirmed the presence of GM damage in MS [28, 43–46] and showed that the extent of such damage differs among the various disease phenotypes, being more severe in patients with SPMS [28, 43, 46]. An increased diffusivity in the thalami of MS patients has also been found, which was again more pronounced in SPMS than in RRMS patients [47]. More intriguingly, DW MRI has been shown to be sensitive to the evolution of MS damage over short periods of time. Longitudinal studies [44, 45, 48, 49] have demonstrated a worsening of GM damage over time in patients with RRMS [45], SPMS, and PPMS [44, 49]. Several studies have suggested that DW MRI might be more sensitive to the accrual of GM damage than to that of normal-appearing WM [45, 48]. A moderate correlation between MD of the GM and the degree of cognitive impairment has been detected in mildly disabled RRMS patients [50]. Furthermore, GM diffusivity was found to predict accumulation of disability over a 5-year period in patients with PPMS [49].

Studies with ^{1}H-MRS can complement structural MRI in the assessment of patients with MS by simultaneously defining several chemical correlates of the pathological changes occurring in the brain [51]. Using this technique, several studies have found metabolite abnormalities, including reduced concentrations of N-acetylaspartate (NAA) and choline (Cho), and increased concentrations of myoinositol, in the cortical GM [52–54] and subcortical tissue [55–57] from MS patients. This was shown to occur also in early RRMS [52], and in patients with CIS suggestive of MS [58]. This disagrees, at least partially, with the results of another study [59], where significant decreases of Cho, creatine, and NAA concentrations were found in the GM of patients with the progressive forms of the disease, but not in the GM of those with RRMS. Reduction in NAA has also been demonstrated in the thalamus of SPMS [55] and RRMS patients [56, 57, 60]. In addition to an NAA decrease, a reduced concentration of glutamate–glutamine in the cortical GM of patients with PPMS has also been measured [61], which was significantly correlated with the expanded disability status scale (EDSS) score.

Imaging gray matter atrophy

Pathology of the GM is likely to contribute significantly to the development of progressive brain atrophy in MS [62]. High-resolution MRI scans coupled with automated segmentation techniques have allowed us to achieve an accurate quantification of

GM tissue volume and to improve our understanding of the dynamics of GM tissue loss in MS.

Through the assessment of the so-called GM fraction (GMF), which is calculated as the ratio between GM volume and the total intracranial volume, Dalton et al. [63] showed significant GM loss (but not WM fraction [WMF] reduction) in patients presenting with CIS who developed definite MS in the subsequent 3 years. A significant reduction over time of GMF has been observed in patients with early RRMS [64, 65]. A longitudinal study of 117 RRMS patients found a significant decrease of normalized GM volumes on monthly scans over 9 months, whereas WM volumes remained relatively stable [66]. The same trend of GM tissue loss was detected in patients with early PPMS followed up for a 1-year period [67]. In a large-scale study of 597 MS patients (427 with RRMS, 140 with SPMS, and 30 with PPMS), significantly reduced WMF and GMF were found in all phenotypes, the most severe tissue loss being shown in SPMS [68]. Atrophy of GM is associated with clinical disability [68, 69]. Normalized neocortical volumes (NCV) have also been shown to be decreased in RRMS and PPMS patients [70]. Furthermore, the specific contribution of the neocortical pathology to cognitive impairment has been assessed by selectively measuring neocortical volumes in RRMS patients [71, 72]. In these studies, neocortical volume loss was found in patients with even mild cognitive disturbances and was absent in patients with preserved cognition. In addition, only cognitively impaired MS patients seem to show a close relationship between measures of neocortical atrophy and those expressing a degree of cognitive impairment. In a longitudinal study, Chen et al. [73] measured cortical thickness from patients with stable disease and those with progressing disability, showing an increased rate of cortical thickness loss in the latter group.

Regional GM changes have also been assessed. A reduction of the mean cortical thickness in MS patients compared to controls has been described [74]. Regional analysis of these data showed a more pronounced focal cortical thinning in the frontal and temporal regions, also in patients with short disease durations and low disability scores. Interestingly, patients with long-standing disease or severe disability had additional focal thinning of the primary sensorimotor cortex. These observations have been confirmed and extended by other investigators [75–79]. Pagani et al. [76] showed that cortical atrophy is more severe in patients with the progressive forms of MS than in those with RRMS. Prinster *et al.* [77] demonstrated that cortical GM reduction in RRMS patients preferentially affects the fronto-temporal lobes. Morgen *et al.* [78] showed that, compared to controls, RRMS patients had reduced left temporal and prefrontal cortex volumes, and that overall GM volume as well as GM volumes of regions associated with working memory and executive function performance were correlated with the results obtained on several cognitive tasks. In patients with RRMS and SPMS, Benedict *et al.* [75] also found an association between left temporal lobe atrophy and auditory/verbal memory, as well as between both left and right temporal lobe atrophy and visual/spatial memory performance. Compared to controls, benign (B) MS patients had a reduced GM volume in the subcortical and frontoparietal regions and, in comparison with BMS patients, those with SPMS had a significant GM loss in the cerebellum [79], thus suggesting that atrophy of the cerebellar GM is a major determinant of irreversible locomotor disability in MS. In contrast to what happens in adult-onset MS, a recent voxel-based morphometry (VBM) study showed that patients with pediatric MS experience GM atrophy in the thalamus only, with sparing of the cortex and other deep GM nuclei [80].

Imaging gray matter in the spinal cord

Pathological studies have demonstrated that extensive demyelination can occur in the spinal cord GM of MS patients [10, 81], while a recent postmortem study showed that spinal cord atrophy in MS is almost exclusively secondary to WM volume loss [82]. Imaging the spinal cord in vivo is challenging for several reasons, including the small size of this structure and the presence of motion artefacts (due to cardiac pulsation and respiration). Furthermore, the cross-sectional area of the cord is only about 1 cm^2 in size and, as a consequence, submillimeter spatial resolution is necessary to distinguish with relative accuracy GM from WM. Lesions in the spinal cord do not usually spare central GM [83]. Consistently with pathological data, ^{1}H-MRS studies have recently described a reduction of NAA in the cervical cord of MS patients [84–85]. Moreover, patients with RRMS demonstrated lower cervical cord GM average MTR compared to healthy controls [86]. Interestingly, GM average MTR also correlated with the degree of

disability, thus suggesting that cervical cord GM is not spared by MS pathology, and that such damage is an additional factor contributing to the disability of these patients [86].

Conclusions

The application of quantitative MR-based techniques has consistently shown that GM is not spared by MS. These studies have also clearly demonstrated that GM damage, albeit with different patterns of regional distribution, is present in all MS phenotypes, since the earliest clinical stage of the disease affects various GM compartments (i.e., neocortex, deep nuclei GM, and cord GM), and is associated with the main clinical manifestations of MS (i.e., locomotor disability and cognitive impairment). Several factors contribute to overall GM damage, including focal macroscopic lesions, intrinsic "diffuse" changes, and irreversible tissue loss. All of these increase over time and are only partially associated to the extent of WM pathology. Measuring GM MR variables might be a rewarding exercise both to improve our understanding of MS pathobiology and to ameliorate clinical/MR correlations. In this context, an accurate estimate of GM damage might not only be important per se, but also because of its potential influence on the functional capacity of the cortex to readapt after MS-related tissue injury (for details see Chapter 11).

References

1. Brownell B, Hughes J T. The distribution of plaques in the cerebrum in multiple sclerosis. *J Neurol Neurosurg Psychiatry* 1962;**25**:315–20

2. Kidd D, Barkhof F, McConnell R, *et al.* Cortical lesions in multiple sclerosis. *Brain* 1999;**122**:17–26

3. Peterson J W, Bö L, Mork S, Chang A, Trapp B D. Transected neurites, apoptotic neurons, and reduced inflammation in cortical multiple sclerosis lesions. *Ann Neurol* 2001;**50**:389–400

4. Lumsden G E. The neuropathology of multiple sclerosis. In: Vinken P J, Bruny G W, eds. *Handbook of Clinical Neurology.* Amsterdam: North-Holland, 1970:217–309

5. Bo L, Vedeler C A, Nyland H I, Trapp B D, Mork S J. Subpial demyelination in the cerebral cortex of multiple sclerosis patients. *J Neuropath Exp Neurol* 2003;**62**:723–32

6. Vercellino M, Plano F, Votta B, *et al.* Grey matter pathology in multiple sclerosis. *J Neuropathol Exp Neurol* 2005;**64**:1101–7

7. Huitinga I, De Groot C J, Van der Valk P, *et al.* Hypothalamic lesions in multiple sclerosis. *J Neuropathol Exp Neurol* 2001;**60**:1208–18

8. Geurts J J, Bö L, Roosendaal S D, *et al.* Extensive hippocampal demyelination in multiple sclerosis. *J Neuropathol Exp Neurol* 2007;**66**:819–27

9. Kutzelnigg A, Faber-Rod J C, Bauer J, *et al.* Widespread demyelination in the cerebellar cortex in multiple sclerosis. *Brain Pathol* 2007;**17**:38–44

10. Gilmore C P, Bo L, Owens T, *et al.* Spinal cord gray matter demyelination in multiple sclerosis: a novel pattern of residual plaque morphology. *Brain Pathol* 2006;**16**:202–8

11. Magliozzi R, Howell O, Vora A, *et al.* Meningeal B-cell follicles in secondary progressive multiple sclerosis associate with early onset of disease and severe cortical pathology. *Brain* 2007;**130**:1089–104

12. Filippi M, Valsasina P, Rocca M A. Magnetic resonance imaging of grey matter damage in people with MS. *Int MS J* 2007;**14**:12–21

13. Filippi M, Rocca M A. Conventional MRI in multiple sclerosis. *J Neuroimag* 2007;**17** (Suppl 1):3S–9S

14. Filippi M, Yousry T A, Baratti C, *et al.* Quantitative assessment of MRI lesion load in multiple sclerosis: a comparison of conventional spin-echo with fast fluid-attenuated inversion recovery. *Brain* 1996;**119**:1349–55

15. Tubridy N, Barker G J, MacManus D G, Moseley I F, Miller D H. Three-dimensional fast fluid attenuated inversion recovery (3D fast FLAIR): a new MRI sequence which increases the detectable cerebral lesion load in multiple sclerosis. *Br J Radiol* 1998;**71**:840–5

16. Bakshi R, Ariyaratana S, Benedict R H, Jacobs L. Fluid-attenuated inversion recovery magnetic resonance imaging detects cortical and juxtacortical multiple sclerosis lesions. *Arch Neurol* 2001;**58**:742–8

17. Geurts J J, Pouwels P J, Uitdehaag B M, *et al.* Intracortical lesions in multiple sclerosis: improved detection with 3D double inversion-recovery MR imaging. *Radiology* 2005;**236**:254–60

18. Calabrese M, De Stefano N, Atzori M, *et al.* Detection of cortical inflammatory lesions by double inversion recovery magnetic resonance imaging in patients with multiple sclerosis. *Arch Neurol* 2007;**64**:1416–22

19. Nelson F, Poonawalla A H, Hou P, *et al.* Improved identification of intracortical lesions in multiple sclerosis with phase-sensitive inversion recovery in combination with fast double inversion recovery MR imaging. *Am J Neuroradiol* 2007;**28**:1645–9

20. Ormerod I E, Miller D H, McDonald W I, *et al.* The role of NMR imaging in the assessment of multiple sclerosis and isolated neurological lesions: a quantitative study. *Brain* 1987;**110**:1579–616

21. Bakshi R, Benedict R H, Bermel R A, *et al.* T2 hypointensity in the deep gray matter of patients with multiple sclerosis: a quantitative magnetic resonance imaging study. *Arch Neurol* 2002;**59**:62–8

22. Roosendaal S D, Moraal B, Vrenken H, *et al.* In vivo MR imaging of hippocampal lesions in multiple sclerosis. *J Magn Reson Imaging* 2008; **27**:726–31

23. Kangarlu A, Bourekas E C, Ray-Chaudhury A, Rammohan K W. Cerebral cortical lesions in multiple sclerosis detected by MR imaging at 8 Tesla. *Am J Neuroradiol* 2007;**28**:262–6

24. Rovaris M, Filippi M, Minicucci L, *et al.* Cortical/subcortical disease burden and cognitive impairment in patients with multiple sclerosis. *Am J Neuroradiol* 2000;**21**:402–8

25. Moriarty D M, Blackshaw A J, Talbot P R, *et al.* Memory dysfunction in multiple sclerosis corresponds to juxtacortical lesion load on fast fluid-attenuated inversion recovery MR images. *Am J Neuroradiol* 1999;**20**:1956–62

26. Catalaa I, Fulton J C, Zhang X, *et al.* MR imaging quantitation of grey matter involvement in multiple sclerosis and its correlation with disability measures and neurocognitive testing. *Am J Neuroradiol* 1999;**20**:1613–18

27. Filippi M, Agosta F. Magnetization transfer MRI in multiple sclerosis. *J Neuroimaging* 2007;**17** (Suppl 1):22S–26S

28. Cercignani M, Bozzali M, Iannucci G, Comi G, Filippi M. Magnetization transfer ratio and mean diffusivity of normal-appearing white and gray matter from patients with multiple sclerosis. *J Neurol Neurosurg Psychiatry* 2001;**70**:311–17

29. Ge Y, Grossman R I, Udupa J K, *et al.* Magnetization transfer ratio histogram analysis of gray matter in relapsing–remitting multiple sclerosis. *Am J Neuroradiol* 2001;**22**:470–5

30. Dehmeshki J, Chard D T, Leary S M, *et al.* The normal appearing gray matter in primary progressive multiple sclerosis: a magnetization transfer imaging study. *J Neurol* 2003;**250**:67–74

31. Fernando K T, Tozer D J, Miszkiel K A, *et al.* Magnetization transfer histograms in clinically isolated syndromes suggestive of multiple sclerosis. *Brain* 2005;**128**:2911–25

32. Davies G R, Altmann D R, Hadjiprocopis A, *et al.* Increasing normal-appearing gray and white matter magnetization transfer ratio abnormality in early relapsing–remitting multiple sclerosis. *J Neurol* 2005;**252**:1037–44

33. Ramio-Torrenta L, Sastre-Garriga J, Ingle G T, *et al.* Abnormalities in normal appearing tissues in early

primary progressive multiple sclerosis and their relation to disability: a tissue specific magnetisation transfer study. *J Neurol Neurosurg Psychiatry* 2006;**77**:40–5

34. Rovaris M, Bozzali M, Santuccio G, *et al.* In vivo assessment of the brain and cervical cord pathology of patients with primary progressive multiple sclerosis. *Brain* 2001;**124**:2540–9

35. Rovaris M, Judica E, Sastre-Garriga J, *et al.* Large-scale, multicentre, quantitative MRI study of brain and cord damage in primary progressive multiple sclerosis. *Mult Scler* 2008;**14**:455–64

36. Audoin B, Ranjeva J P, Au Duong M V, *et al.* Voxel-based analysis of MTR images: a method to locate grey matter abnormalities in patients at the earliest stage of multiple sclerosis. *J Magn Reson Imaging* 2005;**20**:765–71

37. Davies G R, Altmann D R, Rashid W, *et al.* Emergence of thalamic magnetization transfer ratio abnormality in early relapsing–remitting multiple sclerosis. *Mult Scler* 2005;**11**:276–81

38. Oreja-Guevara C, Charil A, Caputo D, *et al.* MT MRI reflects clinical changes over 18 months in relapsing–remitting MS patients. *Arch Neurol* 2006;**63**:736–40

39. Ranjeva J P, Audoin B, Au Duong M V, *et al.* Local tissue damage assessed with statistical mapping analysis of brain magnetization transfer ratio: relationship with functional status of patients in the earliest stage of multiple sclerosis. *Am J Neuroradiol* 2005;**26**:119–27

40. Codella M, Rocca M A, Colombo B, *et al.* A preliminary study of magnetization transfer and diffusion tensor MRI of multiple sclerosis patients with fatigue. *J Neurol* 2002;**249**:535–7

41. Agosta F, Rovaris M, Pagani E, *et al.* Magnetization transfer MRI metrics predict the accumulation of disability 8 years later in patients with multiple sclerosis. *Brain* 2006;**129**:2620–7

42. Rovaris M, Gass A, Bammer R, *et al.* Diffusion MRI in multiple sclerosis. *Neurology* 2005;**65**:1526–32

43. Bozzali M, Cercignani M, Sormani M P, Comi G, Filippi M. Quantification of brain grey matter damage in different MS phenotypes by use of diffusion tensor MR imaging. *Am J Neuroradiol* 2002;**23**:985–8

44. Rovaris M, Bozzali M, Iannucci G, *et al.* Assessment of normal-appearing white and grey matter in patients with primary progressive multiple sclerosis. *Arch Neurol* 2002;**59**:1406–12

45. Oreja-Guevara C, Rovaris M, Iannucci G, *et al.* Progressive grey matter damage in patients with relapsing–remitting multiple sclerosis: a longitudinal diffusion tensor magnetic resonance imaging study. *Arch Neurol* 2005;**62**:578–84

46. Pulizzi A, Rovaris M, Judica E, *et al.* Determinants of disability in multiple sclerosis at various disease stages: a multiparametric magnetic resonance study. *Arch Neurol* 2007;**64**:1163–8

47. Fabiano A J, Sharma J, Weinstock-Guttman B, *et al.* Thalamic involvement in multiple sclerosis: a diffusion-weighted magnetic resonance imaging study. *J Neuroimag* 2003;**13**:307–14

48. Rovaris M, Gallo A, Valsasina P, *et al.* Short-term accrual of gray matter pathology in patients with progressive multiple sclerosis: an in vivo study using diffusion tensor MRI. *NeuroImage* 2005;**24**:1139–46

49. Rovaris M, Judica E, Gallo A, *et al.* Grey matter damage predicts the evolution of primary progressive multiple sclerosis at 5 years. *Brain* 2006;**129**:2628–34

50. Rovaris M, Iannucci G, Falautano M, *et al.* Cognitive dysfunction in patients with mildly disabling relapsing–remitting multiple sclerosis: an exploratory study with diffusion tensor MR imaging. *J Neurol Sci* 2002;**195**:103–9

51. De Stefano N, Filippi M, Miller D, *et al.* Guidelines for using proton MR spectroscopy in multicenter clinical MS studies. *Neurology* 2007;**69**:1942–52

52. Sharma R, Narayana P A, Wolinsky J S. Grey matter abnormalities in multiple sclerosis: proton magnetic resonance spectroscopic imaging. *Mult Scler* 2001;**7**:221–6

53. Chard D T, Griffin C M, McLean M A, *et al.* Brain metabolite changes in cortical gray and normal-appearing white matter in clinically early relapsing–remitting multiple sclerosis. *Brain* 2002;**125**:2342–52

54. Sarchielli P, Presciutti O, Tarducci R, *et al.* Localized ^{1}H magnetic resonance spectroscopy in mainly cortical gray matter of patients with multiple sclerosis. *J Neurol* 2002;**249**:902–10

55. Adalsteinsson E, Langer-Gould A, Homer R J, *et al.* Gray matter *N*-acetyl aspartate deficits in secondary progressive but not relapsing–remitting multiple sclerosis. *Am J Neuroradiol* 2003;**24**:1941–5

56. Cifelli A, Arridge M, Jezzard P, *et al.* Thalamic neurodegeneration in multiple sclerosis. *Ann Neurol* 2002;**52**:650–3

57. Inglese M, Liu S, Babb J S, *et al.* Three-dimensional proton spectroscopy of deep gray matter nuclei in relapsing–remitting MS. *Neurology* 2004;**63**:170–2

58. Kapeller P, Brex P A, Chard D T, *et al.* Quantitative ^{1}H MRS imaging 14 years after presenting with a clinically isolated syndrome suggestive of multiple sclerosis. *Mult Scler* 2002;**8**:207–10

59. Sijens P E, Mostert J P, Oudkerk M, De Keyser J. ^{1}H MR spectroscopy of the brain in multiple sclerosis subtypes with analysis of the metabolite concentrations

in gray and white matter: initial findings. *Eur Radiol* 2006;**16**:489–95

60. Wylezinska M, Cifelli A, Jezzard P, *et al.* Thalamic neurodegeneration in relapsing–remitting multiple sclerosis. *Neurology* 2003;**60**:1949–54

61. Sastre-Garriga J, Ingle G T, Chard D T, *et al.* Metabolite changes in normal-appearing gray and white matter are linked with disability in early primary progressive multiple sclerosis. *Arch Neurol* 2005;**62**:569–73

62. Miller D H, Barkhof F, Frank J A, Parker G J, Thompson A J. Measurement of atrophy in multiple sclerosis: pathological basis, methodological aspects and clinical relevance. *Brain* 2002;**125**:1676–95

63. Dalton C M, Chard D T, Davies G R, *et al.* Early development of multiple sclerosis is associated with progressive gray matter atrophy in patients presenting with clinically isolated syndromes. *Brain* 2004; **127**:1101–7

64. Chard D T, Griffin C M, Parker G J, *et al.* Brain atrophy in clinically early relapsing–remitting multiple sclerosis. *Brain* 2002;**125**:327–37

65. Tiberio M, Chard D T, Altmann D R, *et al.* Grey and white matter volume changes in early RRMS: a 2-year longitudinal study. *Neurology* 2005;**64**:1001–7

66. Valsasina P, Benedetti B, Rovaris M, *et al.* Evidence for progressive grey matter loss in patients with relapsing–remitting MS. *Neurology* 2005;**65**:1126–8

67. Sastre-Garriga J, Ingle G T, Chard D T, *et al.* Gray and white matter volume changes in early primary progressive multiple sclerosis: a longitudinal study. *Brain* 2005;**128**:1454–60

68. Tedeschi G, Lavorgna L, Russo P, *et al.* Brain atrophy and lesion load in a large population of patients with multiple sclerosis. *Neurology* 2005;**65**:280–5

69. Sanfilipo M P, Benedict R H, Sharma J, Weinstock-Guttman B, Bakshi R. The relationship between whole brain volume and disability in multiple sclerosis: a comparison of normalized gray vs. white matter with misclassification correction. *NeuroImage* 2005;**26**:1068–77

70. De Stefano N, Matthews P M, Filippi M, *et al.* Evidence of early cortical atrophy in MS: relevance to white matter changes and disability. *Neurology* 2003;**60**:1157–62

71. Amato M P, Bartolozzi M L, Zipoli V, *et al.* Neocortical volume decrease in relapsing–remitting MS patients with mild cognitive impairment. *Neurology* 2004;**63**:89–93

72. Benedict R H, Bruce J M, Dwyer M G, *et al.* Neocortical atrophy, third ventricular width, and cognitive dysfunction in multiple sclerosis. *Arch Neurol* 2006;**63**:1301–6

73. Chen J T, Narayanan S, Collins D L, *et al.* Relating neocortical pathology to disability progression in multiple sclerosis using MRI. *NeuroImage* 2004;**23**:1168–75

74. Sailer M, Fischl B, Salat D, *et al.* Focal thinning of the cerebral cortex in multiple sclerosis. *Brain* 2003;**126**:1734–44

75. Benedict R H, Zivadinov R, Carone D A, *et al.* Regional lobar atrophy predicts memory impairment in multiple sclerosis. *Am J Neuroradiol* 2005;**26**: 1824–31

76. Pagani E, Rocca M A, Gallo A, *et al.* Regional brain atrophy evolves differently in patients with multiple sclerosis according to clinical phenotype. *Am J Neuroradiol* 2005;**26**:341–6

77. Prinster A, Quarantelli M, Orefice G, *et al.* Grey matter loss in relapsing–remitting multiple sclerosis: a voxel-based morphometry study. *NeuroImage* 2006;**29**:859–67

78. Morgen K, Sammer G, Courtney S M, *et al.* Evidence for a direct association between cortical atrophy and cognitive impairment in relapsing–remitting MS. *NeuroImage* 2006;**30**:891–8

79. Mesaros S, Rovaris M, Pagani E, *et al.* A magnetic resonance imaging voxel-based morphometry study of regional gray matter atrophy in patients with benign multiple sclerosis. *Arch Neurol* 2008;**65**:1223–30

80. Mesaros S, Rocca M A, Absinta M, *et al.* Evidence of thalamic gray matter loss in pediatric multiple sclerosis. *Neurology* 2008;**70**:1107–12

81. Lycklama à Nijeholt G J, Bergers E, Kamphorst W, *et al.* Postmortem high-resolution MRI of the spinal cord in multiple sclerosis: a correlative study with conventional MRI, histopathology and clinical phenotype. *Brain* 2001;**124**:154–66

82. Gilmore C P, DeLuca G C, Bo L, *et al.* Spinal cord atrophy in multiple sclerosis caused by white matter volume loss. *Arch Neurol* 2005;**62**:1859–62

83. Lycklama à Nijeholt G J, Thompson A, Filippi M, *et al.* Spinal-cord MRI in multiple sclerosis. *Lancet Neurol* 2003;**2**:555–62

84. Kendi A T, Tan F U, Kendi M, *et al.* MR spectroscopy of cervical spinal cord in patients with multiple sclerosis. *Neuroradiology* 2004;**46**:764–9

85. Ciccarelli O, Wheeler-Kingshott C A, McLean M A, *et al.* Spinal cord spectroscopy and diffusion-based tractography to assess acute disability in multiple sclerosis. *Brain* 2007;**130**:2220–31

86. Agosta F, Pagani E, Caputo D, Filippi M. Associations between cervical cord gray matter damage and disability in patients with multiple sclerosis. *Arch Neurol* 2007;**64**:1302–5

Application of functional magnetic resonance imaging in multiple sclerosis

Massimo Filippi and Maria A. Rocca

Introduction

Over the past decade, conventional and modern structural magnetic resonance imaging (MRI) techniques have been extensively used to study patients with multiple sclerosis (MS) to increase the understanding of the mechanisms responsible for the accumulation of irreversible disability [1, 2]. In detail, the application of these techniques has provided important insights into the pathobiology of the disease, by showing that: (1) MS-related damage is not restricted to T2-visible lesions, but it involves diffusely the normal-appearing white matter (NAWM) and gray matter (GM); (2) the neurodegenerative component of the disease is not a late phenomenon and it is not completely driven by inflammatory demyelination; and (3) axonal damage makes an important contribution to the clinical manifestations of the disease. Despite this, however, the magnitude of the correlation between MRI and clinical findings remained suboptimal.

Among the reasons for such a discrepancy, the variable effectiveness of reparative and recovery mechanisms following MS-related tissue damage has been suggested to have a role. Among these, brain plasticity is a well-known feature of the human brain, which is likely to have several different substrates (including increased axonal expression of sodium channels, synaptic changes, increased recruitment of parallel existing pathways or "latent" connections, and reorganization of distant sites), and which might have a major adaptive role in limiting the functional consequences of axonal loss in MS.

The signal changes seen during functional MRI (fMRI) studies depend on the blood oxygenation level dependent (BOLD) mechanism, which, in turn, involves changes of the transverse magnetization relaxation time – either T2* in a gradient echo sequence, or T2 in spin echo sequence [3]. Local increases in neuronal activity result in a rise of blood flow and oxygen consumption. The increase of blood flow is greater than the oxygen consumption, thus determining an increased ratio between oxygenated and deoxygenated hemoglobin, which enhances the MRI signal [3].

This chapter summarizes the main contributions to the understanding of MS pathobiology gained by the use of fMRI with different paradigms of stimulation.

General considerations

The main problem in the interpretation of fMRI studies in diseased people is that the observed changes might be biased by differences in task performance between patients and controls. Clearly, this is a major issue in MS, which typically causes impairment of various functional systems. Therefore, despite providing several important pieces of information, the value of the earliest fMRI studies of patients with MS has to be weighted against this background [4]. For this reason, the most recent fMRI studies in MS have been based on larger and more selected patients' groups than the seminal studies. These studies have investigated the brain patterns of cortical activations during the performance of a number of motor, visual, and cognitive tasks in patients with all the major clinical phenotypes of the disease. One of the most solid conclusions that can be drawn from fMRI studies of MS is that cortical reorganization does occur in patients affected by this condition. The correlation between various measures of structural MS damage and the extent of cortical activation also suggests an adaptive role of such cortical changes in contributing to clinical recovery and maintaining a normal level of

Multiple Sclerosis: Recovery of Function and Neurorehabilitation, eds. J. Kesselring, G. Comi, and A. J. Thompson. Published by Cambridge University Press. © Cambridge University Press 2010.

functioning in patients with MS, despite the presence of irreversible axonal/neuronal loss.

The visual system

The method usually applied to investigate the visual system consists of the application of an 8-Hz photic stimulation to one or both eyes. Using this stimulation, compared to healthy controls, patients who had recovered from a single episode of acute unilateral optic neuritis had an extensive activation of the visual network, including the claustrum, lateral temporal and posterior parietal cortices, and thalamus, in addition to the primary visual cortex, when the clinically affected eye was studied [5]. Conversely, when the unaffected eye was stimulated, only activation of the visual cortex and the right insula/claustrum was observed. In these patients, the volume of the extra-occipital activation was strongly correlated with the visual evoked potential (VEP) P100 latency, suggesting that the functional reorganization of the cortex might represent an adaptive response to a persistently abnormal visual input [5]. Toosy et al. [6] replicated the previous study [5], using a longer photic stimulation epoch. Their results confirmed the original findings of a phase-dependent increase of the BOLD signal in the extra-occipital regions during the baseline condition. By combining fMRI and VEP to monitor the functional recovery after an acute unilateral optic neuritis, Russ et al. [7] found a strong relationship between fMRI and VEP latencies, suggesting that fMRI might contribute to the assessment of the temporal evolution of the visual deficits during MS recovery. The role of non-primary visual processing areas in recovery of function has been addressed by more recent studies. Levin et al. [8] showed reduced activation of the primary visual cortex and increased activation of the lateral occipital complex (LOC), an object-related area, in eight subjects with clinical recovery from an episode of optic neuritis, but who still had prolonged VEP latencies in comparison with healthy controls. In a 1-year follow-up study, Toosy et al. [9] demonstrated, early after optic neuritis, a potential adaptive role of reorganization within the extrastriate visual areas, which are regions involved in higher-order visual processing. In this study, an increased optic nerve gadolinium-enhanced lesion length at baseline was associated with a reduced functional activation within the visual cortex and poorer vision. At 3 months, more severe optic

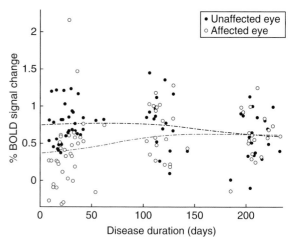

Fig. 11.1. Mean lateral geniculate nucleus (LGN) activation during stimulation of the affected and unaffected eye over time. The dash-dotted lines indicate weighted moving averages for the affected eye (●) and unaffected eye (O). During recovery there is a significant increase in LGN blood oxygenated level dependent (BOLD) signal from stimulation of the affected eye. The LGN BOLD signal from stimulation of the unaffected eye decreases over time in a stepwise fashion. Post hoc analysis showed this decrease to be significant. The BOLD signal changes for the affected and unaffected eye level off at a similar positive value as time increases. (Reproduced from Korsholm et al. [10] Recovery from optic neuritis: an ROI-based analysis of LGN and visual cortical areas. *Brain* 2007;**130**:1244–53, by permission of Oxford University Press and the Guarantors of *Brain*.)

nerve damage was associated with an increased fMRI response in the temporal cortices, whereas at 1 year, the right temporal cortex correlation reversed. These results illustrate how the same regions may play different roles at different times during recovery, reflecting the complexity of brain plasticity and the MS process. This notion has been supported by a recent region-of-interest longitudinal study [10] which demonstrated dynamic changes in the fMRI response following visual stimulation not only in V1, V2, and the LOC, but also in the lateral geniculate nucleus (LGN) in patients with isolated acute optic neuritis (Fig. 11.1).

In patients with established MS and a relapsing–remitting (RR) course with a unilateral optic neuritis a reduced recruitment of the visual cortex has been found after stimulation of the affected and the unaffected eyes [11]. On average, patients with optimal clinical recovery showed increased visual cortex activation compared to those with poor or no recovery, although the extent of the activation remained reduced compared with controls [11].

The motor system

The investigation of the motor system in patients with MS has mainly focused on the analysis of the performance of simple motor tasks with the dominant right upper limbs [4]. Such tasks were either self-paced or paced by a metronome. A few studies assessed the performance of simple motor tasks with the dominant right lower limbs [12–14], while even fewer studies have investigated the performance of more complex tasks, including phasic movements of dominant hand and foot [12, 14], object manipulation [4], and visuo-motor integration tasks [15].

An altered brain pattern of movement-associated cortical activations, characterized by an increased recruitment of the contralateral primary sensorimotor cortex (SMC) during the performance of simple tasks [12, 16] and by the recruitment of additional "classical" and "higher-order" sensorimotor areas during the performance of more complex tasks [12] has been demonstrated in patients with clinically isolated syndrome (CIS) suggestive of MS. Clinical and conventional MRI follow-up of these patients has shown that, at disease onset, CIS patients with a subsequent evolution to clinically definite MS tend to recruit a more widespread sensorimotor network than those without short-term disease evolution [17].

An increased recruitment of several sensorimotor areas, mainly located in the cerebral hemisphere ipsilateral to the limb which performed the task, has also been demonstrated in patients with early RRMS and a previous episode of hemiparesis [18]. In patients with similar characteristics, but who presented with an episode of optic neuritis, this increased recruitment involved sensorimotor areas that were mainly located in the contralateral cerebral hemisphere [19].

In patients with established MS and a RR course, functional cortical changes, mainly characterized by an increased recruitment of "classical" motor areas, including the primary SMC, the supplementary motor area (SMA), and the secondary sensorimotor cortex (SII), have been shown during the performance of simple motor [4, 20] and visuo-motor integration tasks [15]. Movement-associated cortical changes, characterized by the activation of highly specialized cortical areas, have also been described in patients with secondary progressive (SP) MS [13] and in patients with primary progressive (PP) MS [4, 14, 21].

The concept that movement-associated cortical reorganization varies across patients at different stages of the disease has been confirmed by an fMRI study of patients with different disease phenotypes [22], which suggested that early in the course of the disease more areas typically devoted to motor tasks (such as the primary SMC) are recruited, then a bilateral activation of these regions is seen, and late in the course of the disease, areas that healthy people recruit to perform novel or complex tasks are activated [22], perhaps in an attempt to limit the functional consequences of accumulating tissue damage.

The cognitive system

Recent fMRI studies have suggested that functional cortical changes might have an adaptive role also in limiting MS-related cognitive impairment [4, 23–31]. Several cognitive domains have been investigated in MS patients with fMRI [4]. Working memory has been the most extensively studied by means of the Paced Auditory Serial Addition Test (PASAT) or the Paced Visual Serial Addition Task (PVSAT) (which both involve sustained attention, information processing speed, and simple calculation), the n-back task, or a task adapted from the Sternberg paradigm. Additional cognitive domains including attention and planning have been interrogated, too.

In CIS patients, an altered pattern of cortical activations has been described during the performance of the PASAT [23, 24]. During the performance of the PVSAT, RRMS patients with intact task performance had increased activation of several regions located in the frontal and parietal lobes, bilaterally, compared to healthy volunteers, suggesting the presence of functional compensatory mechanisms [25]. Increased recruitment of several cortical areas during the performance of a simple cognitive task has also been shown in patients with RRMS and mild clinical disability [26]. Increased activation of regions exclusively located in the right cerebral hemisphere (mainly in the frontal and temporal lobes) has also been found in MS patients when testing rehearsal within working memory [27]. The degree of right hemisphere recruitment was strongly related to patient neuropsychological performance [27]. In patients with RRMS and no cognitive deficits, during an n-back task, reduced activation of the "core" areas of the working memory circuitry (including prefrontal and parietal regions) and increased activation of other regions within and beyond the typical working memory circuitry (including areas in the frontal, parietal, temporal, and occipital lobes)

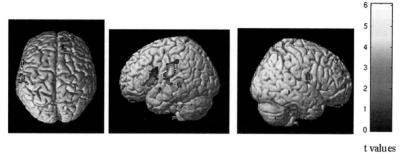

t values

Fig. 11.2. Areas showing increased activations in patients with BMS in comparison with healthy controls during the analysis of the Stroop facilitation condition (random effect interaction analysis, ANOVA, $p < 0.05$ corrected for multiple comparisons). The BMS patients had increased activations of several areas located in the frontal and parietal lobes, bilaterally, including the anterior cingulate cortex, the superior frontal sulcus, the inferior frontal gyrus, the precuneus, the secondary sensorimotor cortex, the bilateral visual cortex, and the cerebellum, bilaterally. Note that the color-encoded activations have been superimposed on a rendered brain and normalized into standard Statistical Parametric Mapping (SPM) space (neurological convention). (See also color plate.)

have been found [28]. This shift of activation was most prominent with increased working memory demands. These findings suggest that, as shown for motor and visual tasks, dynamic cognitive-associated changes of brain activation patterns can occur in RRMS patients. Other studies [4], which also investigated working memory performance in MS patients, demonstrated: (1) increased recruitment of regions related to sensori-motor functions and anterior attentional/executive components of the working memory system in patients compared to healthy controls, and (2) reduced recruitment of several regions in the right cerebellar hemisphere in patients compared with healthy individuals [29], thus suggesting that the cerebellum might play a role in the working memory impairment of MS.

Recently, a study in RRMS patients [30] investigated working memory with an n-back task and functional connectivity analysis. Compared to controls, patients had relatively reduced activation of the superior frontal and anterior cingulate gyri. Patients also showed a variable, but substantially smaller increase of activation than healthy controls with greater task complexity, suggesting a reduced functional reserve for cognition relevant to memory in MS patients. The functional connectivity analysis revealed increased correlations between right dorsolateral prefrontal and superior frontal/anterior cingulate activation in controls, and increased correlation between activation in the right and left prefrontal cortices in patients, indicating that altered inter-hemispheric interactions between dorsal and lateral prefrontal regions may yet be an additional adaptive mechanism distinct from recruitment of novel processing regions [30].

More significant activations of several areas of the cognitive network involved in the performance of the Stroop test have also been demonstrated in a group of 15 cognitively preserved patients with benign MS (BMS) when compared to 19 healthy controls (Fig. 11.2) [31]. The BMS patients also showed an increased connectivity of several cortical areas of the sensorimotor network with the right inferior frontal gyrus and the right cerebellum, as well as a decreased connectivity between some areas and the anterior cingulate cortex. These results suggest an altered inter-hemispheric balance in favor of the right hemisphere in BMS patients in comparison with healthy controls, when performing cognitive tasks.

Functional magnetic resonance imaging of changes of the spinal cord

Recently fMRI has been applied to the assessment of functional changes in the spinal cord in MS. Among the reasons for the paucity of fMRI investigations in the human spinal cord is the significant technical challenge associated with the detection and measurement of activation changes in such a small structure, subjected to periodic movements. Although BOLD fMRI of the spinal cord has provided reliable results in healthy subjects [32], several studies [32] put forward the concept that the exploitation of the so-called signal enhancement by extravascular protons (SEEP) effect rather than the "classical" BOLD [3] effect might be more suitable for the assessment of spinal cord activity. While the BOLD effect depends on the local MR signal change due to variation in blood

C5 C5/C6 C6 C6/C7 C7 C7/C8 C8

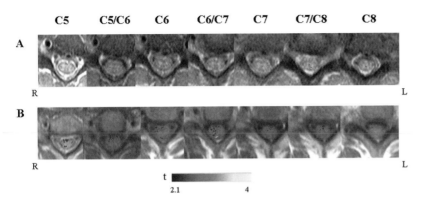

A

R   L

B

R   L

t
2.1   4

Fig. 11.3. Illustrative activation maps (color coded for t values) of cervical cord on axial proton density-weighted spin-echo images from C5 to C8, from a healthy control (A) and a patient with MS (B) during a tactile stimulation of the palm of the right hand. Right (R) and left (L). (See also color plate.)

oxygenation [3], the SEEP effect is proposed to arise from a local change in fluid balance which may result from changes in perfusion pressure, production of extracellular fluid, cellular swelling, and maintenance of ion and neurotransmitter concentrations at sites of neuronal activity [32]. Following tactile stimulation of the palm of the right hand, significant task-related mean signal change in the entire cervical cord has been detected in 12 right-handed healthy subjects [33]. In this study, cord activity was higher in the right than in the left cervical cord and a significant heterogeneity in frequency of fMRI activity between cord levels was also observed, with the highest frequencies of fMRI activity detected at C6 and C7.

Two studies have interrogated cervical cord neuronal activity during a proprioceptive [34] and a tactile [35] (Fig. 11.3) stimulation of the right upper limb in patients with relapsing MS. In the first study [34], MS patients had an higher average fMRI signal change of the overall cord, as well as higher average fMRI signal changes in the anterior section of the right cord at C5 and left cord at C5–C6 in comparison to controls. In MS patients, overall cord average signal change correlated significantly with quantitative MRI measures of cord and brain tissue damage, suggesting an adaptive role of such an abnormal recruitment. In the second study [35], 25 MS patients and 12 matched healthy controls were scanned during a tactile stimulation of the palm of the right hand. The MS patients had a 20% higher cord fMRI signal change than healthy controls. In addition, MS patients also showed a different topographical distribution of fMRI signal changes at the level of the different portions of the cervical cord in comparison with controls, mainly characterized by activation of regions located in the anterior and the left portions of the cord. Such an over-recruitment of the ipsilateral posterior cervical cord associated with a reduced functional lateralization suggests an abnormal function of the spinal relay interneurons in MS patients.

Correlation between the extent of functional cortical reorganization and structural MR damage in MS

The majority of the previous studies described a variable relationship between the extent of fMRI activation and several measures of tissue damage [4, 11–22, 24, 26].

Increased recruitment of several brain areas with increasing T2 lesion load has been shown in patients with RRMS [4, 24, 26] and PPMS [14]. The severity of intrinsic T2-visible lesion damage, measured using T1-weighted images [19], magnetization transfer (MT) and diffusion tensor (DT) MRI [20], has been found to modulate the activity of some cortical areas in these patients. The severity of normal-appearing brain tissue (NABT) injury, measured using proton MR spectroscopy [4, 16], MT MRI [20, 21, 24], and DT MRI [16, 21] is another important factor associated with an increased recruitment of motor- and cognitive-related brain regions, as shown by studies of patients at presentation with CIS suggestive of MS, patients with RRMS and variable degrees of clinical disability, patients with PPMS, and those with SPMS. Finally, subtle GM damage, which goes undetected when using conventional MRI, may also influence functional cortical recruitment, as demonstrated, for the motor system, in patients with RRMS [15] and SPMS [13] and in patients with clinically definite MS and non-specific (less than three focal WM lesions) conventional MRI findings [4]. In cognitively intact MS patients, increased activation of a left prefrontal region during the counting Stroop task has been correlated with normalized brain parenchymal volume [36].

Seminal studies have shown that damage to "strategic" WM pathways connecting functionally relevant areas, such as the corticospinal tract (CST) [19, 37] and the corpus callosum (CC) [38, 39] in case of a motor task, modifies the observed brain patterns of cortical activations in MS patients.

The recent development of diffusion-based tractography methods which allow to define with precision the pathways connecting different central nervous system (CNS) structures and their application to MS patients resulted in an improvement of the correlation between structural and functional abnormalities. Recent works combined measures of abnormal functional connectivity with DT MR measures of damage within selected WM fiber bundles in patients with RRMS [40] and BMS [31]. In patients with RRMS and no clinical disability [40], measures of abnormal connectivity inside the motor network were correlated with structural MRI metrics of tissue damage of the CST and the dentatorubrothalamic tracts, while no correlation was found with measures of damage within "not-motor" WM fiber bundles. These findings suggest an adaptive role of functional connectivity changes in limiting the clinical consequences of structural damage to selected WM pathways in RRMS patients [40]. In patients with BMS, measures of abnormal connectivities inside the cognitive network were moderately correlated with structural MRI metrics of tissue damage within intra- and inter-hemispheric cognitive-related WM fiber bundles, while no correlations were found with the remaining fiber bundles studied, suggesting that functional cortical changes in patients with BMS might represent an adaptive response driven by damage to specific WM structures [31].

In patients with PPMS, a relationship has been demonstrated between the severity of spinal cord pathology, measured using MT MRI, and the extent of movement-associated cortical activations [21].

Role of functional cortical reorganization in MS

The correlations found in the majority of the studies [4] between fMRI measures of abnormal activations and quantitative MRI metrics of structural brain and

cord injury suggest that, at least in some phases of the disease, increased recruitment of the cortical network might contribute in limiting the functional impact of MS-related damage.

The results of a recent experiment highlight the notion that an increased recruitment of areas that are usually activated by healthy individuals when performing complex motor tasks might be one of the mechanisms playing a role in limiting the consequences of MS tissue damage [41]. In detail, this study demonstrated that during the performance of a simple motor task MS patients recruit regions that are part of the mirror-neuron system, a frontoparietal observation–execution matching network activated in humans during action observation, motor learning, and imitation of action. However, several studies have suggested that increased cortical recruitment might not always be beneficial for patients with MS. In patients with PPMS, the recruitment of multimodal integration areas has been observed during the performance of active simple and complex motor tasks [14, 21], as well as during the performance of a passive task with the right lower limb [42]. These results suggest that the lack or exhaustion of the "classical" adaptive mechanisms may lead to widespread brain recruitment, which in turn might be among the factors responsible for an unfavorable clinical evolution. Similar findings have led to similar conclusions in patients with cognitive decline [43], in whom a "reallocation" of neuronal resources and the inefficiency of neuronal processes have been associated with the extent and severity of structural tissue damage.

Finally, comparison of the movement-associated brain patterns of cortical activations between RRMS patients complaining of reversible fatigue after interferon beta-1a administration and those without such a symptom, has demonstrated an association between the presence of fatigue and increased recruitment of several areas of the motor network, including the thalamus, the cingulum, and several regions located in the frontal lobes, such as the SMA and the primary SMC bilaterally [44]. These results suggest that the over-recruitment of brain networks in MS might, at least to some degree, have a detrimental effect.

Use of fMRI to assess longitudinal changes of cortical reorganization

Dynamic functional changes have been described in an MS patient following an acute relapse [45]. These

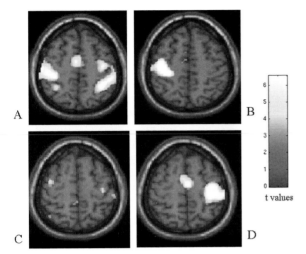

Fig. 11.4. Longitudinal evolution of cortical activations in the primary sensorimotor cortex (SMC), bilaterally, during task performance with impaired hand compared to unimpaired hand in one patient with good clinical recovery during follow-up (A and B), and in one patient with poor/absent clinical recovery (C and D). Scans obtained during a left-hand motor task have been flipped in order to keep the left hemisphere contralateral to movement. At baseline, both patients showed increased activation of the primary SMC of the unaffected (ipsilateral) hemisphere (A and C). During follow-up, the patient with good clinical recovery showed an increased recruitment of the primary SMC of the affected hemisphere (B), while the patient with poor/absent clinical recovery continued to show an increased recruitment of the primary SMC of the unaffected hemisphere (D). Note that the activations are color-coded according to their t values. (See also color plate.)

results have been confirmed and extended by a recent study which assessed the early cortical changes following acute motor relapses secondary to pseudo-tumoral lesions in 12 MS patients and the evolution over time of cortical reorganization in a subgroup of these patients [46]. In this study, short-term cortical changes were mainly characterized by the recruitment of pathways in the unaffected hemisphere. A recovery of function of the primary SMC of the affected hemisphere was found in patients with clinical improvement, while in patients without clinical recovery, there was persistent recruitment of the primary SMC of the unaffected hemisphere, suggesting that the restoration of function of motor areas of the affected hemisphere might be a critical factor for a favorable recovery (Fig. 11.4).

A longitudinal (time interval of 15–26 months) fMRI study of the motor system has been conducted in a group of patients with early RRMS [47]. Patients exhibited greater bilateral activation than controls in both fMRI studies. While no significant differences between the two fMRI scans were observed in controls, a reduction of the functional activity of the ipsilateral SMC and the contralateral cerebellum was seen in patients at follow-up. Moreover, activation changes in ipsilateral motor areas correlated inversely with age, extent, and progression of T1 lesion load,

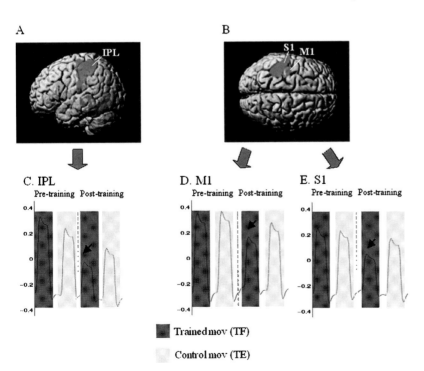

Fig. 11.5. Three-dimensional rendering (A and B) of task-specific reductions of activations in contralateral inferior parietal lobule (IPL) (BA 40; A and C), primary motor cortex (M1) (B and D), and primary somatosensory cortex (S1) (B and E) in healthy volunteers after training. Panels C, D, and E illustrate average signal intensities in voxels representing cluster maxima in IPL (BA 40), M1, and S1 for 30-s blocks of thumb flexion (trained movement, gray bars), extension (control movement, blue bars), and rest. Note that training led to a decrease in signal intensity predominantly for the trained movement (black arrows). Images are in neurological convention. (Reproduced from Morgen *et al.* [49] Training-dependent plasticity in patients with multiple sclerosis. *Brain* 2004; **127**:2506–17, by permission of Oxford University Press and the Guarantors of *Brain*.) (See also color plate.)

and occurrence of a new relapse, suggesting that younger patients with less structural brain damage and a favorable clinical course demonstrate brain plasticity that follows a more lateralized pattern of brain activations [47].

A few studies have used fMRI to monitor the effect of treatments in MS [36, 48, 49]. A preliminary study tested the effects of acute administration of rivastigmine, a central cholinesterase inhibitor, on the patterns of brain activations during the performance of the Stroop task [36]. After treatment administration, a relative normalization of the abnormal Stroop-associated brain activation was observed in patients, while no change in the pattern of brain activation was found in any of the four healthy controls studied. In MS patients, increased activation in the ipsilateral primary SMC and SMA has been observed after a single dose of 3,4-diaminopyridine (a potassium channel blocker), suggesting that this treatment may modulate brain motor activity in patients with MS, probably by enhancing excitatory synaptic transmission [48]. A recent study analyzed how the motor network responds to motor training in MS patients with mild motor impairment of the right upper extremity [49]. Before training, MS patients had a more prominent activation of the contralateral dorsal premotor cortex during thumb movements when compared to controls. After training, unlike the control group, MS patients did not exhibit task-specific reductions in activation of the contralateral primary SMC and adjacent parietal association cortices (Fig. 11.5). The absence of training-dependent reductions in activation supports the notion that MS patients have a decreased capacity to optimize recruitment of the motor network with practice.

Conclusions

Functional fMRI holds promise to improve our understanding of the factors associated with the accumulation of irreversible disability in MS. Although the role of cortical reorganization in limiting the functional impact of structural damage is still not definitively proved, the available data support the notion that cortical adaptive responses may have an important role in compensating for irreversible tissue injury, and that the rate of accumulation of disability in MS might be a function not only of tissue loss, but also of the progressive failure of the adaptive capacity of the MS brain with increasing tissue damage.

References

1. Filippi M, Rocca M A. Magnetization transfer magnetic resonance imaging in the assessment of neurological diseases. (Review.) *J Neuroimag* 2004;**14**:303–13

2. Filippi M, Rocca M A, Comi G. The use of quantitative magnetic-resonance-based techniques to monitor the evolution of multiple sclerosis. *Lancet Neurol* 2003;**2**:337–46

3. Ogawa S, Menon R S, Tank D W, *et al.* Functional brain mapping by blood oxygenation level-dependent contrast magnetic resonance imaging: a comparison of signal characteristics with a biophysical model. *Biophys J* 1993;**64**:803–12

4. Rocca M, Filippi M. Functional MRI in multiple sclerosis. (Review.) *J Neuroimag* 2007;**17**:36S–41S

5. Werring D J, Bullmore E T, Toosy A T, *et al.* Recovery from optic neuritis is associated with a change in the distribution of cerebral response to visual stimulation: a functional magnetic resonance imaging study. *J Neurol Neurosurg Psychiatry* 2000;**68**:441–9

6. Toosy A T, Werring D J, Bullmore E T, *et al.* Functional magnetic resonance imaging of the cortical response to photic stimulation in humans following optic neuritis recovery. *Neurosci Lett* 2002;**330**:255–9

7. Russ M O, Cleff U, Lanfermann H, *et al.* Functional magnetic resonance imaging in acute unilateral optic neuritis. *J Neuroimag* 2002;**12**:339–50

8. Levin N, Orlov T, Dotan S, *et al.* Normal and abnormal fMRI activation patterns in the visual cortex after recovery from optic neuritis. *NeuroImage* 2006;**33**:1161–8

9. Toosy A T, Hickman S J, Miszkiel K, *et al.* Adaptive cortical plasticity in higher visual areas after acute optic neuritis. *Ann Neurol* 2005;**57**:622–33

10. Korsholm K, Madsen K H, Frederiksen J L, *et al.* Recovery from optic neuritis: an ROI-based analysis of LGN and visual cortical areas. *Brain* 2007;**130**:1244–53

11. Rombouts S, Lazeron R H, Scheltens P, *et al.* Visual activation patterns in patients with optic neuritis: an fMRI pilot study. *Neurology* 1998;**50**:1896–9

12. Filippi M, Rocca M, Mezzapesa D M, *et al.* Simple and complex movement-associated functional MRI changes in patients at presentation with clinically isolated syndromes suggestive of MS. *Hum Brain Mapp* 2004;**21**:108–17

13. Rocca M A, Gavazzi C, Mezzapesa D M, *et al.* A functional magnetic resonance imaging study of patients with secondary progressive multiple sclerosis. *NeuroImage* 2003;**19**:1770–7

14. Rocca M A, Matthews P M, Caputo D, *et al.* Evidence for widespread movement-associated functional MRI changes in patients with PPMS. *Neurology* 2002;**58**:866–72

15. Cerasa A, Fera F, Gioia M C, *et al*. Adaptive cortical changes and the functional correlates of visuo-motor integration in relapsing–remitting multiple sclerosis. *Brain Res Bull* 2006;**69**:597–605

16. Rocca M, Mezzapesa D M, Falini A, *et al*. Evidence for axonal pathology and adaptive cortical reorganization in patients at presentation with clinically isolated syndromes suggestive of MS. *NeuroImage* 2003; **18**:847–55

17. Rocca M, Mezzapesa D M, Ghezzi A, *et al*. A widespread pattern of cortical activations in patients at presentation with clinically isolated symptoms is associated with evolution to definite multiple sclerosis. *Am J Neuroradiol* 2005;**26**:1136–9

18. Pantano P, Iannetti G D, Caramia F, *et al*. Cortical motor reorganization after a single clinical attack of multiple sclerosis. *Brain* 2002;**125**:1607–15

19. Pantano P, Mainero C, Iannetti G D, *et al*. Contribution of corticospinal tract damage to cortical motor reorganization after a single clinical attack of multiple sclerosis. *NeuroImage* 2002;**17**:1837–43

20. Rocca M, Falini A, Colombo B, *et al*. Adaptive functional changes in the cerebral cortex of patients with non-disabling MS correlate with the extent of brain structural damage. *Ann Neurol* 2002;**51**:330–9

21. Filippi M, Rocca M, Falini A, *et al*. Correlations between structural CNS damage and functional MRI changes in primary progressive MS. *NeuroImage* 2002;**15**:537–46

22. Rocca M, Colombo B, Falini A, *et al*. Cortical adaptation in patients with MS: a cross-sectional functional MRI study of disease phenotypes. *Lancet Neurol* 2005;**4**:618–26

23. Audoin B, Ibarrola D, Ranjeva J P, *et al*. Compensatory cortical activation observed by fMRI during a cognitive task at the earliest stage of MS. *Hum Brain Mapp* 2003;**20**:51–8

24. Audoin B, Au Duong M V, Ranjeva J P, *et al*. Magnetic resonance study of the influence of tissue damage and cortical reorganization on PASAT performance at the earliest stage of multiple sclerosis. *Hum Brain Mapp* 2005;**24**:216–28

25. Staffen W, Mair A, Zauner H, *et al*. Cognitive function and fMRI in patients with multiple sclerosis: evidence for compensatory cortical activation during an attention task. *Brain* 2002;**125**:1275–82

26. Mainero C, Caramia F, Pozzilli C, *et al*. fMRI evidence of brain reorganization during attention and memory tasks in multiple sclerosis. *NeuroImage* 2004; **21**:858–67

27. Hillary F G, Chiaravalloti N D, Ricker J H, *et al*. An investigation of working memory rehearsal in multiple sclerosis using fMRI. *J Clin Exp Neuropsychol* 2003;**25**:965–78

28. Wishart H A, Saykin A J, McDonald B C, *et al*. Brain activation patterns associated with working memory in relapsing–remitting MS. *Neurology* 2004;**62**:234–8

29. Li Y, Chiaravalloti N D, Hillary F G, *et al*. Differential cerebellar activation on functional magnetic resonance imaging during working memory performance in persons with multiple sclerosis. *Arch Phys Med Rehabil* 2004;**85**:635–9

30. Cader S, Cifelli A, Abu-Omar Y, Palace J, Matthews P M. Reduced brain functional reserve and altered functional connectivity in patients with multiple sclerosis. *Brain* 2006;**129**:527–37

31. Rocca M, Valsasina P, Ceccarelli A, *et al*. Structural and functional MRI correlates of Stroop control in benign MS. *Hum Brain Mapp* 2009; **30**:276–90

32. Stroman P W. Magnetic resonance imaging of neuronal function in the spinal cord: spinal FMRI. (Review.) *Clin. Med Res* 2005;**3**:146–56

33. Agosta F, Valsasina P, Caputo D, Rocca M, Filippi M. Tactile-associated fMRI recruitment of the cervical cord in healthy subjects. *Hum Brain Mapp* 2009; **30**:340–5

34. Agosta F, Valsasina P, Rocca M, *et al*. Evidence for enhanced functional activity of cervical cord in relapsing multiple sclerosis. *Magn Reson Med* 2008; **59**:1035–42

35. Agosta F, Valsasina P, Caputo D, Stroman P W, Filippi M. Tactile-associated recruitment of cervical cord is altered in patients with multiple sclerosis. *NeuroImage* 2008; **39**:1542–8

36. Parry A M, Scott R B, Palace J, Smith S, Matthews P M. Potentially adaptive functional changes in cognitive processing for patients with multiple sclerosis and their acute modulation by rivastigmine. *Brain* 2003;**126**:2750–60

37. Rocca M A, Gallo A, Colombo B, *et al*. Pyramidal tract lesions and movement-associated cortical recruitment in patients with MS. *NeuroImage* 2004;**23**:141–7

38. Lenzi D, Conte A, Mainero C, *et al*. Effect of corpus callosum damage on ipsilateral motor activation in patients with multiple sclerosis: a functional and anatomical study. *Hum Brain Mapp* 2007;**28**: 636–44

39. Manson S C, Palace J, Frank J A, Matthews P M. Loss of interhemispheric inhibition in patients with multiple sclerosis is related to corpus callosum atrophy. *Exp Brain Res* 2006;**174**:728–33

40. Rocca M A, Pagani E, Absinta M, *et al*. Altered functional and structural connectivities in patients with MS: a 3T fMRI study. *Neurology* 2007;**69**:2136–45

41. Rocca M A, Tortorella P, Ceccarelli A, *et al.* The "mirror-neuron system" in MS: a 3 Tesla fMRI study. *Neurology* 2008;**70**:255–62

42. Ciccarelli O, Toosy A T, Marsden J F, *et al.* Functional response to active and passive ankle movements with clinical correlations in patients with primary progressive multiple sclerosis. *J Neurol* 2006;**253**:882–91

43. Morgen K, Sammer G, Courtney S M, *et al.* Distinct mechanisms of altered brain activation in patients with multiple sclerosis. *NeuroImage* 2007;**37**:937–46

44. Rocca M A, Agosta F, Colombo B, *et al.* fMRI changes in relapsing–remitting multiple sclerosis patients complaining of fatigue after IFNβ-1a injection. *Hum Brain Mapp* 2007;**28**:373–82

45. Reddy H, Narayanan S, Matthews P M, *et al.* Relating axonal injury to functional recovery in MS. *Neurology* 2000;**54**:236–9

46. Mezzapesa D M, Rocca M A, Rodegher M A, Comi G, Filippi M. Functional cortical changes of the sensorimotor network are associated with clinical recovery in multiple sclerosis. *Hum Brain Mapp* 2008;**29**:562–73

47. Pantano P, Mainero C, Lenzi D, *et al.* A longitudinal fMRI study on motor activity in patients with multiple sclerosis. *Brain* 2005;**128**:2146–53

48. Mainero C, Inghilleri M, Pantano P, *et al.* Enhanced brain motor activity in patients with MS after a single dose of 3,4-diaminopyridine. *Neurology* 2004;**62**:2044–50

49. Morgen K, Kadom N, Sawaki L, *et al.* Training-dependent plasticity in patients with multiple sclerosis. *Brain* 2004;**127**:2506–17

Functional magnetic resonance imaging in focal CNS damage

Patrizia Pantano and Eytan Raz

Introduction

Functional magnetic resonance imaging (fMRI) provides the opportunity to map brain areas during the performance of specific tasks. It is mainly used in the field of neuroscience to study functional anatomy in healthy subjects and thus define the neural circuits involved in sensorimotor, cognitive, and emotional processes. Within the clinical context, fMRI offers the possibility of investigating differences between patients with neurological or psychiatric disorders and healthy subjects, in order to understand functional changes induced by disease.

Neuroplasticity is a fundamental property of the central nervous system (CNS) – it evolves throughout a person's life and allows the brain to modify the properties of its neural circuits and to adapt to new conditions according to experience, practice, and learning [1, 2]. The electrical, synaptic, and morphological properties of neurons change constantly to optimize behavioral gain.

Adaptive mechanisms of the brain also occur as a response to brain injury. Functional reorganization of adult sensorimotor pathways following injury is now a widely documented phenomenon. A substantial body of information has demonstrated that neuronal properties in sensorimotor circuits can be reorganized in the adult mammalian CNS in response to peripheral or central structure lesions [3, 4]. Following a lesion that impairs the neural pathways subserving a specific function, functional cortical changes may compensate for the lesion, thereby contributing to the maintenance of a normal level of function.

Generally, clinical outcome is the result of a balance between the degree of damage to the CNS and the extent of repair and efficacy of the recovery mechanisms. Mechanisms of recovery include sprouting (new collaterals from undamaged fibers), recruitment of new cortical projection neurons, and formation of detour circuits. These plastic changes are believed to be the basis of the changes in functional activity observed in fMRI studies.

In neurological practice, fMRI may help to predict the extent of recovery after stroke, and to select the appropriate medication and rehabilitation. Longitudinal studies conducted on stroke patients point to increased activation (recruitment) in many cerebral areas, particularly in the intact hemisphere [5], demonstrating a correlation between fMRI changes over time and clinical outcome.

A widely used clinical application of fMRI in neurosurgical practice is the presurgical mapping of motor or language function before focal brain lesions such as tumors and arteriovenous malformations are removed. By identifying important functional regions within the brain, including unpredictable patterns of functional reorganization, fMRI can help in surgical decision-making [6]. Furthermore, fMRI may help to identify epileptic foci and to guide surgery in intractable epilepsy [7].

Unfortunately, as randomized trials or outcome studies designed to assess the benefits provided by fMRI to the final outcome of the patient are lacking, further fMRI studies are warranted to confirm the importance of fMRI as a clinical tool.

Stroke

The World Health Organization (WHO) has developed a method for estimating the incidence and prevalence of stroke in countries without data; using this method, the incidence of stroke in the EU was estimated to be 235 per 100 000, which corresponds to 1 070 000 new strokes per year [8].

Multiple Sclerosis: Recovery of Function and Neurorehabilitation, eds. J. Kesselring, G. Comi, and A. J. Thompson. Published by Cambridge University Press. © Cambridge University Press 2010.

Approximately 800 000 of these are first attacks, while the remaining 300 000 are recurrent attacks. Stroke is the leading cause of disability among adults in the EU, and four out of five families will be affected by a stroke over a lifetime.

Because of the high social impact and economic consequences of stroke [9], researchers have focused on gaining a better understanding of the physiopathological basis of stroke and on potential therapeutic innovations. Within this context, neuroimaging has contributed greatly by shedding light on the mechanisms of recovery following a stroke.

Although the disruption of motor activity and neurological function caused by a stroke may be severe, the clinical recovery is often highly dynamic. Clinical recovery, as demonstrated by both experimental and empirical data, is characterized by a first phase of progressive improvement, which lasts approximately 3 months, followed by a plateau phase; there are, however, data suggesting that recovery lasts many months after stroke [10].

From a physiopathological point of view, clinical recovery is a multifactorial and highly complex event. In the acute phase of stroke, the clinical improvement may be determined by the resolution of cerebral edema, reperfusion of the ischemic penumbra, and hemorrhage reabsorption. In the subsequent phases, recovery depends on the regression of diaschisis and on a complex of neuroplastic events that determine structural and functional reorganization.

Diaschisis is very frequent after stroke, occurring in more than half of patients with an ischemic lesion in the territory of the middle cerebral artery [11]; the underlying mechanism of this phenomenon is decreased excitatory transsynaptic neuronal input into otherwise normal neurological tissue, and the subsequent decrease in the metabolism and blood flow in cerebral areas that are far from the site of the ischemic lesion but are functionally connected to it. For example, diaschisis may manifest itself in the cerebellar hemisphere contralateral to a supratentorial lesion because of the interruption in the corticopontocerebellar pathway (crossed cerebellar diaschisis), or it may manifest itself in the ipsilateral cortex following a subcortical lesion because of the interruption in the thalamocortical pathway [12].

It is a functional and, hence, reversible event; Vallar *et al.* [13] demonstrated that the improvement of some symptoms, such as aphasia or neglect, in patients with subcortical stroke, is related to blood

reperfusion of the cerebral cortex ipsilaterally to the lesion. The clinical symptoms caused by the loss of function of structurally undamaged but disconnected cortex may improve in concomitance with the regression of diaschisis.

Moreover, neuroplasticity exploits neurons that are not normally involved in the damaged circuits and restores pathways that are only partially damaged. Two kinds of neuroplasticity exist: sprouting and redundancy. Sprouting is the generation of new axon collaterals from surviving neurons, while redundancy occurs when the number of neurons available is greater than required and the neurons in excess perform the role of the lost neurons in a vicarious manner.

Plasticity can be improved by extrinsic factors, such as pharmacological agents, electric and magnetic brain stimulation, and environmental stimulation. The key aspect of neuroplasticity is that the changes in the neuronal circuits are use-dependent and that the degree of change is directly proportional to the constraint-induced use of that function.

The study of functional changes observed after a stroke has been rendered possible by two functional imaging techniques, positron emission tomography (PET) and fMRI. The mechanisms involved in motor recovery are those most frequently investigated with these two techniques.

The medical literature contains many experimental studies, conducted on patients who survived a cortical or subcortical stroke, that have used standardized motor tasks with a well-known effect on healthy people. Although hand movement seems at first to be a relatively simple cerebral function, it is actually rather complex. It involves not only the primary motor cortex, but also the premotor cortex, the supplementary motor area, the motor cingulate cortex and the collateral connections with the dorsolateral prefrontal cortex, the parietal cortex, and the insular cortex. The studies published in this field can be divided into cross-sectional studies and longitudinal studies.

Cross-sectional studies

The earliest studies focused on patients who completely recovered after a stroke, on the assumption that the comparison of differences between patients and normal subjects would reveal which adaptation mechanisms had been used.

The very first study used PET during a finger-tapping motor task in six patients who had recovered from a hemiplegic stroke [14]; interestingly, the ipsilateral motor cortex and both cerebellar hemispheres were activated during the movement of the previously affected hand, these activations being interpreted as vicarious mechanisms.

Another PET study, published shortly afterwards by the same scientists, confirmed the activation of both the ipsilateral motor cortex and both sides of the cerebellum, in addition to supplementary sensorimotor areas, the anterior and posterior cingulate cortex, and the prefrontal cortex [15].

Numerous other fMRI studies have been published since [16, 17]. Although there are some discrepancies between the results of these studies, in part due to differences in technical procedures and image post-processing, some conclusions can be drawn: patients with a subcortical infarct displayed the activation of bilateral motor cortex and of the secondary motor and somatosensory cortex, areas that are not normally activated in healthy subjects, and also showed the extension of the hand area in the primary sensorimotor cortex caudally toward the area of the face. In patients with a cortical infarction, the authors observed, along with the bilateral activation pattern, the activation of both the perilesional cortex and the premotor ipsilateral cortex.

Cross-sectional studies have two major limitations: first, they do not provide information on patients in whom the clinical recovery is poor or absent because of the difficulties such patients encounter in executing the motor task during the fMRI examination and, second, the observation of intrinsic differences between patients in the active phase of recovery and those who have already completed their recovery is not possible. The two drawbacks with this kind of studies are thus the inability to study the dynamic processes during recovery and the inability to understand fully the role of the activation changes in order to determine whether such changes are beneficial, detrimental, or merely collateral to the clinical recovery.

Longitudinal studies

Longitudinal studies have focused on patients recovering from stroke so as to allow researchers to assess the dynamic evolution of recovery in the same patient, which is not possible in cross-sectional studies. Although the cerebral pattern of activation in both cerebral hemispheres is the same as that seen in cross-sectional studies, the temporal evolution of activation that emerges is highly interesting.

Marshall et al. [18] examined eight patients using fMRI within a few days of and 3–6 months after stroke: clinical recovery was paralleled by a reduction in bilateral activation and a trend toward the baseline pattern of strongly lateralized activation, similar to that observed in healthy subjects. This phenomenon is known as "focusing." Calautti et al. [19], in a PET study, also observed a delayed activation in other cortical regions, such as the premotor cortex, prefrontal cortex and normal hemisphere putamen.

Feydy et al. [20] demonstrated a marked inter-individual variation, describing three different activation patterns: the first pattern is characterized by early focusing involving above all the sensorimotor cortex contralateral to the plegic limb, as seen in normal subjects; the second is characterized by progressive focusing, from ipsilateral and contralateral cortical activation, towards a gradual return to a normal pattern; the third is characterized by the persistent recruitment of many cortical areas of both cerebral hemispheres. While differences in the activation pattern between patients may be due to the characteristics of the ischemic lesion, there was no significant correlation between variations in cortical function and clinical recovery.

Ward et al. [21], however, investigated a possible correlation: they analyzed the temporal evolution relative to cortical activation, and demonstrated for the first time that there is a linear correlation between the degree of clinical recovery, as measured by clinical evaluation scales, and the extent of the reduction in the cortical activation regions. They also found that in patients with a poorer outcome, some motor areas, such as the ipsilesional premotor cortex, displayed this correlation only in the early post-stroke phase.

These results suggest that there are differences in the cerebral implementation of action in patients with a poor outcome that are dependent on the time lapsed since the stroke. Thus, in those patients with the most to gain from rehabilitation, different therapeutic approaches may be required at different stages after stroke [22].

The effects of neurorehabilitation on the activation motor pattern were studied for the first time by Carey et al. [23] by means of fMRI before and after an intensive motor training program. Such training may induce cerebral plasticity in the absence of a

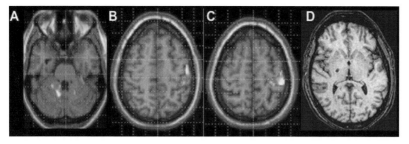

Fig. 12.1. Results obtained in a randomized, cross-over, double-blind study on ten patients with pure motor hemiparesis following a subcortical lacunar infarct. Patients were randomly assigned in two counterbalanced groups and underwent two fMRI examinations a week apart, after donepezil and after placebo. During each fMRI session, patients performed an active motor task consisting of a finger flexion–extension of the paretic hand. A single dose of donepezil induced a significantly reduced activation in sensorimotor areas (sensorimotor cortex of the healthy hemisphere: B and C) and contralateral cerebellum (A) compared to placebo, associated with a significant motor skill improvement of the affected hand. (From Tombari *et al.* [27]). (See also color plate.)

temporal relationship with stroke. Physical exercise tends to restore the cortical activation pattern to a more lateralized pattern, thus accelerating an event already observed in spontaneous recovery [24].

Johansen-Berg *et al.* [25] obtained interesting results by means of transcranial magnetic stimulation (TMS) during rehabilitation. They used TMS to interfere with the function of the primary motor cortex and dorsal premotor cortex of the healthy hemisphere in patients who had survived a stroke. They showed that induced transient inhibition provoked worsened movement capacity, thereby demonstrating the active role of the healthy hemisphere in motor recovery.

Furthermore, some studies have analyzed the effects of pharmacological agents on neuroplasticity. The most important of these is a double-blind placebo-controlled study by Pariente *et al.* [26], who analyzed the effects of a single dose of fluoxetine, a selective serotonin reuptake inhibitor, on motor function and cortical activation after stroke; they showed that fluoxetine induced hyperactivation of the motor cortex in the hemisphere ipsilateral to the stroke and simultaneous reduced activation in other cortical areas, hence determining a strengthening of the focusing process; this fMRI finding was combined with a clinical improvement in motor activity in the plegic side of the body.

A similar experimental study by Tombari *et al.* [27] assessed the efficacy of donepezil, an acetylcholinesterase inhibitor, on motor activity in patients who survived a lacunar subcortical stroke with pure motor hemiparesis. During movement of the previously paretic hand, greater focusing of motor activation and a reduction in cortical activity were

observed in the healthy hemisphere under donepezil than under placebo (Fig. 12.1).

In conclusion, many studies have demonstrated that after stroke there is a phase of metabolic depression, due to diaschisis, followed by a phase of increased activation in several cortical areas, particularly in the healthy hemisphere, and, lastly, by a phase in which normal cortical activity is restored. This has been shown in several neuroimaging studies using PET and fMRI. Clinical recovery seems to be associated with a focusing process that is a return to normal lateralized cortical activity similar to that observed in healthy subjects.

Some more recent studies have investigated whether physical exercise or any drug may accelerate this spontaneous process. In the near future, neuroimaging techniques will be used to understand which patients may benefit most from pharmacological or rehabilitation treatment, and to study the effects of these therapeutic interventions on cortical activity.

Pre-surgical planning

The selection of patients with brain tumor or arteriovenous malformations who are to undergo surgery on the basis of radiological criteria may be insufficient owing to individual variability in the location of eloquent areas, to the distortion of brain functional anatomy by the tumor, and to the fact that function can be at least partially preserved within infiltrated brain tissue. Indeed, the tumor and the associated edema distort the anatomy of the brain, thereby preventing the identification of functional areas using anatomical landmarks (e.g., the central sulcus, the calcarine scissure) on conventional MR images.

Pre-surgical mapping of motor and language function by fMRI is therefore largely used to study the relationship between structure and function in order to optimize the extent of the resection while minimizing permanent morbidity. The main aims of pre-surgical fMRI are to assess the risks of a neurological deficit that follow a surgical procedure and to guide the surgical procedure itself. Some caution is, however, required when basing the surgical procedure on the fMRI findings, as fMRI cannot differentiate between activation in brain areas that are merely correlated with a particular function and activation in brain areas that are truly essential for performing that function.

Although some attempts have be made to identify the minimum distance required between the activation focus and the tumor resection margins to avoid a postoperative neurological deficit [28], there is no standardized rule. Many factors must be taken into account when using fMRI to assess the risk of a neurological deficit that follows a surgical procedure. Indeed, the measurement of the distance between an eloquent area and the lesion margins is influenced by the statistical threshold used in image processing. Moreover, some image processing steps such as realignment, smoothing, and co-registration may reduce the accuracy of fMRI localization. Methods to improve the identification of functional areas have been proposed [29]. Lastly, it should be borne in mind that the brain shifting during the craniotomy may modify the precise location of an eloquent area and its relationship to the lesion.

Functional MRI provides information on gray matter function, though not on the integrity and location of white matter fibers. Diffusion tensor imaging (DTI) is a MR technique that maps white matter bundles [30], which may be distorted and/or disrupted by the tumor. Thus, new pre-surgical mapping methods combine fMRI and DTI to study both gray matter function and white matter connectivity [31]. The DTI technique can be used to identify three patterns of white matter alteration: (1) disruption, (2) displacement, and (3) infiltration [32].

Different stimuli have been used to study functional anatomy in patients with brain tumors and to map the corresponding brain functions, i.e., motor, sensory, visual, auditory, etc. [33]. Motor function and language production and comprehension are the most frequently mapped functions.

Depending on the tumor location, patients can be studied during the performance of movements of the foot, hand, and face. Lehéricy et al. [34] found a close somatotopical structure–function relationship in the primary motor cortex of individual patients by comparing fMRI data with intraoperative electrical stimulation. Depending on the presence and the severity of a motor deficit, patients can be studied during either complex or simple active movements or during passive movements. Finger-tapping is usually used in patients with a normal motor function, hand-clenching in patients with mild to moderate paresis, and passive flexo-extension of the last four fingers in patients with a more severe deficit [35].

Language areas are more difficult to study than motor function on account of the greater variability and complexity of language. A variety of language paradigms (verbal fluency, passive listening, comprehension) have been developed for the study of language processing and its separate components. Activation patterns display interindividual variability [36, 37], which renders the interpretation of data difficult. Language expression is usually tested by word generation tasks such as verbal fluency or verb-to-noun generation, while language comprehension is tested by semantic judgment or sentence listening or reading.

Symptoms in patients with slow-growing tumors develop slowly because the functional network has time to adapt to the lesion. Two main patterns of cortical adaptation may be observed in patients with space-occupying lesions: dislocation and relocation. A dislocation of functional areas may be observed in regions close to, though not involved by, the lesion. Dislocation is due to mass effect and consists of a mechanical shift of functional areas (Fig. 12.2).

Moreover, when neurons deputed to a specific function are destroyed by the tumor, neuroplastic changes lead to the relocation of functional areas. As occurs in stroke patients, reorganization of the cerebral cortex may include activation of previously inactive neuronal pathways (such as the ipsilateral corticospinal tract in the healthy hemisphere) or of neuronal groups that function in a vicarious manner (such as non-primary motor areas in the lesioned hemisphere).

These recovery mechanisms following a CNS lesion depend on the state of maturity of the brain when the damage occurs [38]. Recovery of function is generally greater when brain damage occurs early in life rather than in adulthood since the brain possesses a greater ability to compensate in its immature than

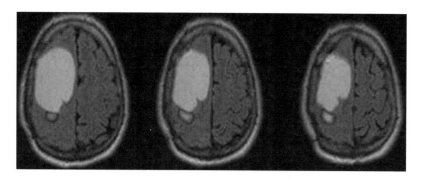

Fig. 12.2. Motor fMRI in a patient with a large neuroepithelial cyst in the right rolandic region in the pre-surgical planning: fMRI during left-hand finger-tapping showed a cortical activation area posteriorly dislocated by the lesion. (See also color plate.)

(A)

(B)

(C)

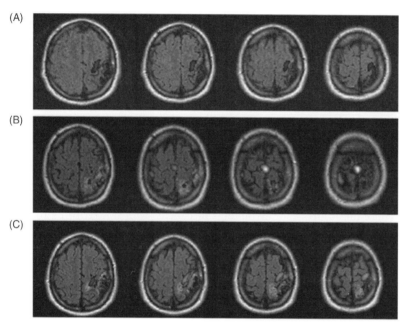

Fig. 12.3. Example of cortical plasticity in a case of arteriovenous malformation (AVM). Motor fMRI in a patient with an AVM located in the left rolandic region during flexo-extension of the last four fingers of the right hand: fMRI was performed at baseline (A), 2 days (B), and 2 months (C) after endovascular embolization. Following embolization, the patient showed a mild motor deficit of the right upper limb which completely recovered in the following weeks. (A) Before embolization: fMRI showed contralateral activation of the sensorimotor cortex located anteriorly to the AVM. (B) 2 days after embolization, in association with the mild right motor deficit: fMRI showed a bilateral activation of sensorimotor cortex and of the supplementary motor area. (C) 2 months after embolization, in association with clinical recovery: fMRI showed the return to a normal activation pattern. (With permission from Raz *et al.* [40]). (See also color plate.)

in its mature state. Relocation is, therefore, to be expected more frequently in patients with lesions that are either congenital or develop early in life, such as arteriovenous malformations [39]. In arteriovenous malformations, fMRI may also allow the documentation of neuroplastic changes after embolization (Fig. 12.3) [40].

Epilepsy

In the field of epilepsy, fMRI is used in two main ways: to assess candidates for surgical treatment of intractable epilepsy and, in conjunction with electroencephalography (EEG), to obtain more information on the physiopathological characteristics of the disease.

Subjects with epilepsy are prone to recurrent seizures; a certain proportion of such subjects do not respond to anti-epileptic medications, and consequently become candidates for neurosurgical treatment. In the pre-surgical assessment, fMRI can be used in conjunction with other methods such as conventional MRI, a neuropsychological assessment, and an electrophysiological examination, so as to spare the functional cortex during resective surgery. In such cases, fMRI reveals when reorganization of function has occurred and shows when abnormal cortex is functionally active, thereby indicating when surgery may not be recommended. Some subjects, in whom the spatial relationship between the epileptogenic focus and functional cortex cannot be defined, require invasive EEG recording, which involves the placement of subdural electrodes on the surface of the brain.

FMRI can therefore be used:

- to help identify brain regions that are associated with ictal or interictal activity and may therefore be targeted for surgical resection;
- to identify critical motor, speech, and language or memory areas during the planning of surgery;
- to investigate the reorganization of brain damage and of seizure activity.

Rendering a patient seizure-free is not the sole criterion for determining the optimum surgical resection in patients with epilepsy; indeed, surgical decision-making must in many cases bear in mind the quality of life, striking a balance between reducing the seizures and maintaining function; an fMRI examination performed in candidates for surgery is likely to help strike the right balance. Moreover, fMRI has the advantage of being non-invasive and can be repeated if necessary; it has also largely replaced the Wada test as a means of determining cerebral dominance for language functions during the pre-surgical epilepsy assessment.

Despite being 75 years old, EEG remains one of the main diagnostic tools in the clinical evaluation of epilepsy; a major reason is that epilepsy is a disease characterized by functional abnormality, while most imaging techniques depict only structure. Yet, the anatomical resolution of EEG is poor and its specificity has clinically significant limitations [7, 41]. As functional abnormalities may propagate through normal tissue, there may be uncertainty as to whether visible discharges arise from the region immediately beneath the electrodes or from another region that is not visible.

Simultaneous EEG and fMRI (SEM) is being investigated as an innovative technique on account of its potential to improve functional imaging in epilepsy [42, 43]. Functional MRI detects regions of activity associated with tasks or stimulation performed during scanning. Indeed, SEM determines the timing of interictal spikes, which may in turn be used to identify the associated blood oxygenation level dependent (BOLD) signal [44].

However, SEM does have some drawbacks: safety, image artefacts, and EEG artefacts. Concerning safety, the EEG recording requires circuits in which both the patient and an electrical amplifier are included. In addition, loops may be formed by overlapping wires when care is not taken to keep all the recording leads parallel from the patient to the amplifier.

Both the circuits and the unintentional loops raise an immediate safety issue, i.e., the induction of an electrical current within a circuit that includes the patient. Another major safety concern linked to the recording apparatus is the heating at the electrode–scalp contact [45, 46].

Regarding image artefacts, the presence of EEG recording electrodes and leads within or near the MRI scanner may affect the image quality, with the magnetic susceptibility artefact being the most straightforward effect. Besides raising a safety concern, the induction of current within the components of the EEG apparatus during scanning also produces artefacts in the EEG recording; moreover, the means of reducing artefacts is different for each of the three MRI features that induce current, i.e., radiofrequency (RF) activity, the static magnetic field, and magnetic gradients. The RF signal is the easiest to filter because its frequency is in the megahertz range, hence far above the EEG frequencies [47, 48].

Once the interictal spikes during continuous fMRI have been identified, the processing of the fMRI data to obtain an image of the discharges is similar to that used in any other fMRI study. Since hemodynamic response function has been defined by sensory stimulation studies, the validity of the hemodynamic response function from such studies should not be assumed for interictal epileptiform discharges. The other significant difference lies in the fact that interictal epileptiform discharges are not predictable events and are not necessarily identical to one another. In standard fMRI experimental designs, the stimulus under study is repeated during scanning to maximize the statistical significance of the imaging results; in SEM, by contrast, the number of interictal spikes cannot be controlled and studies are sometimes based on only a small number of events. More often, the interictal spikes are combined in the analysis to gain more consistent data for image post-processing, though this is not possible when the scalp localization of interictal spikes varies [49–51].

References

1. Karni A, Meyer G, Rey-Hipolito C, *et al.* The acquisition of skilled motor performance: fast and slow experience-driven changes in primary motor cortex. *Proc Natl Acad Sci USA* 1998;**95**:861–8

2. Kleim J A, Barbay S, Nudo R J. Functional reorganization of the rat motor cortex following motor skill learning. *J Neurophysiol* 1998;**80**:3321–5

3. Schady W, Braune S, Watson S, Torebjörk H E, Schmidt R. Responsiveness of the somatosensory system after nerve injury and amputation in the human hand. *Ann Neurol* 1994;**36**:68–75

4. Calautti C, Baron J -C. Functional neuroimaging studies of motor recovery after stroke in adults: a review. *Stroke* 2003;**34**:1553–66

5. Ward N S. The neural substrates of motor recovery after focal damage to the central nervous system. *Arch Phys Med Rehabil* 2006;**87**(12 Suppl 2):S30–5

6. Sunaert S. Presurgical planning for tumor resectioning. *J Magn Reson Imaging* 2006;**23**:887–905

7. Koepp M J, Woermann F G. Imaging structure and function in refractory focal epilepsy. *Lancet Neurol* 2005;**4**:42–53

8. Truelsen T, Piechowski-Jówiak B, Bonita R, *et al*. Stroke incidence and prevalence in Europe: a review of available data. *Eur J Neurol* 2006;**13**:581–98

9. Truelsen T, Ekman M, Boysen G. Cost of stroke in Europe. *Eur J Neurol* 2005;**12**(Suppl 1):78–84

10. Hendricks H T, van Limbeek J, Geurts A C, Zwarts M J. Motor recovery after stroke: a systematic review of the literature. *Arch Phys Med Rehab* 2002;**83**:1629–37

11. Pantano P, Baron J C, Samson Y, *et al*. Crossed cerebellar diaschisis: further studies. *Brain* 1986;**109**:677–94

12. Baron J C, D'Antona R, Pantano P, *et al*. Effects of thalamic stroke on energy metabolism of the cerebral cortex: a positron tomography study in man. *Brain* 1986;**109**:1243–59

13. Vallar G, Perani D, Cappa S F, *et al*. Recovery from aphasia and neglect after subcortical stroke: neuropsychological and cerebral perfusion study. *J Neurol Neurosurg Psychiatry* 1988;**51**:1269–76

14. Chollet F, DiPiero V, Wise R J, *et al*. The functional anatomy of motor recovery after stroke in humans: a study with positron emission tomography. *Ann Neurol* 1991;**29**:63–71

15. Weiller C, Chollet F, Friston K J, Wise R J, Frackowiak R S. Functional reorganization of the brain in recovery from striatocapsular infarction in man. *Ann Neurol* 1992;**31**:463–72

16. Cramer S C, Nelles G, Benson R R, *et al*. A functional MRI study of subjects recovered from hemiparetic stroke. *Stroke* 1997;**28**:2518–27

17. Cao Y, D'Olhaberriague L, Vikingstad E M, Levine S R, Welch K M. Pilot study of functional MRI to assess cerebral activation of motor function after poststroke hemiparesis. *Stroke* 1998;**29**:112–22

18. Marshall R S, Perera G M, Lazar R M, *et al*. Evolution of cortical activation during recovery from corticospinal tract infarction. *Stroke* 2000;**31**:656–61

19. Calautti C, Leroy F, Guincestre J Y, Baron J C. Dynamics of motor network overactivation after striatocapsular stroke: a longitudinal PET study using a fixed-performance paradigm. *Stroke* 2001;**32**:2534–42

20. Feydy A, Carlier R, Roby-Brami A, *et al*. Longitudinal study of motor recovery after stroke: recruitment and focusing of brain activation. *Stroke* 2002;**33**:1610–17

21. Ward N S, Brown M M, Thompson A J, Frackowiak R S J. Neural correlates of motor recovery after stroke: a longitudinal fMRI study. *Brain* 2003;**126**:2476–96

22. Ward N S, Brown M M, Thompson A J, Frackowiak R S J. The influence of time after stroke on brain activations during a motor task. *Ann Neurol* 2004;**55**:829–34

23. Carey J R, Kimberley T J, Lewis S M, *et al*. Analysis of fMRI and finger tracking training in subjects with chronic stroke. *Brain* 2002;**125**:773–88

24. Richards L G, Stewart K C, Woodbury M L, Senesac C, Cauraugh J H. Movement-dependent stroke recovery: a systematic review and meta-analysis of TMS and fMRI evidence. *Neuropsychologia* 2008;**46**:3–11

25. Johansen-Berg H, Rushworth M F S, Bogdanovic M D, *et al*. The role of ipsilateral premotor cortex in hand movement after stroke. *Proc Natl Acad Sci USA* 2002;**99**:14 518–23

26. Pariente J, Loubinoux I, Carel C, *et al*. Fluoxetine modulates motor performance and cerebral activation of patients recovering from stroke. *Ann Neurol* 2001;**50**:718–29

27. Tombari D, Lenzi G, Sirimarco G, *et al*. Modulation of motor cortical activity in chronic stroke patients by a single dose of donepezil. *Cerebrovasc Dis* 2006;**21** (suppl 4) (abstr)

28. Yetkin F Z, Mueller W M, Morris G L, *et al*. Functional MR activation correlated with intraoperative cortical mapping. *Am J Neuroradiol* 1997;**18**:1311–15

29. Hattingen E, Good C, Weidauer S, *et al*. Brain surface reformatted images for fast and easy localization of perirolandic lesions. *J Neurosurg* 2005;**102**:302–10

30. Le Bihan D, Mangin J F, Poupon C, *et al*. Diffusion tensor imaging: concepts and applications. *J Magn Reson Imaging* 2001;**13**:534–46

31. Ramnani N, Behrens T E J, Penny W, Matthews P M. New approaches for exploring anatomical and functional connectivity in the human brain. *Biol Psychiatry* 2004;**56**:613–19

32. Wei C W, Guo G, Mikulis D J. Tumor effects on cerebral white matter as characterized by diffusion tensor tractography. *Can J Neurol Sci* 2007;**34**:62–8

33. Hirsch J, Ruge M I, Kim K H, *et al*. An integrated functional magnetic resonance imaging procedure for preoperative mapping of cortical areas associated with

tactile, motor, language, and visual functions. *Neurosurgery* 2000;**47**:711–21; discussion 721–2

34. Lehéricy S, Duffau H, Cornu P, *et al.* Correspondence between functional magnetic resonance imaging somatotopy and individual brain anatomy of the central region: comparison with intraoperative stimulation in patients with brain tumors. *J Neurosurg* 2000;**92**:589–98

35. Shinoura N, Suzuki Y, Yamada R, *et al.* Restored activation of primary motor area from motor reorganization and improved motor function after brain tumor resection. *Am J Neuroradiol* 2006;**27**:1275–82

36. Roux F -E, Boulanouar K, Lotterie J -A, *et al.* Language functional magnetic resonance imaging in preoperative assessment of language areas: correlation with direct cortical stimulation. *Neurosurgery* 2003;**52**:1335–45; discussion 1345–7

37. Seghier M L, Lazeyras F, Pegna A J, *et al.* Variability of fMRI activation during a phonological and semantic language task in healthy subjects. *Hum Brain Mapp* 2004;**23**:140–55

38. Passingham R E, Perry V H, Wilkinson F. The long-term effects of removal of sensorimotor cortex in infant and adult rhesus monkeys. *Brain* 1983;**106**:675–705

39. Alkadhi H, Kollias S S, Crelier G R, *et al.* Plasticity of the human motor cortex in patients with arteriovenous malformations: a functional MR imaging study. *Am J Neuroradiol* 2000;**21**:1423–33

40. Raz E, Tinelli E, Guidetti G, *et al.* Neuroplastic changes in the brain: a case of two successive adaptive changes within the motor cortex. *J Neuroimag* 2009;

41. Berger H. Uber das Elektrenkephalogram des Menschen. *Arch Psychiatr Nervenkr* 1929;**87**:527–70

42. Garreffa G, Bianciardi M, Hagberg G E, *et al.* Simultaneous EEG-fMRI acquisition: how far is it from being a standardized technique? *Magn Reson Imaging* 2004;**22**:1445–55

43. Di Bonaventura C, Carni M, Diani E, *et al.* Drug resistant ADLTE and recurrent partial status epilepticus with dysphasic features in a family with a novel LGI1 mutation: electroclinical, genetic, and EEG/fMRI findings. *Epilepsia* 2009;**50**:2481–6

44. Di Bonaventura C, Vaudano A E, Carnì M, *et al.* EEG/fMRI study of ictal and interictal epileptic activity: methodological issues and future perspectives in clinical practice. *Epilepsia* 2006;**47**(Suppl 5):52–8

45. Lemieux L, Allen P J, Franconi F, Symms M R, Fish D R. Recording of EEG during fMRI experiments: patient safety. *Magn Reson Med* 1997;**38**:943–52

46. Dempsey M F, Condon B. Thermal injuries associated with MRI. *Clin Radiol* 2001;**56**:457–65

47. Krakow K, Allen P J, Symms M R, *et al.* EEG recording during fMRI experiments: image quality. *Hum Brain Mapp* 2000;**10**:10–15

48. Bénar C, Aghakhani Y, Wang Y, *et al.* Quality of EEG in simultaneous EEG-fMRI for epilepsy. *Clin Neurophysiol* 2003;**114**:569–80

49. Lemieux L, Salek-Haddadi A, Josephs O, *et al.* Event-related fMRI with simultaneous and continuous EEG: description of the method and initial case report. *Neuroimage* 2001;**14**:780–7

50. Bénar C G, Gross D W, Wang Y, *et al.* The BOLD response to interictal epileptiform discharges. *NeuroImage* 2002;**17**:1182–92

51. Bagshaw A P, Aghakhani Y, Bénar C -G, *et al.* EEG-fMRI of focal epileptic spikes: analysis with multiple haemodynamic functions and comparison with gadolinium-enhanced MR angiograms. *Hum Brain Mapp* 2004;**22**:179–92

Chapter 3

Electrophysiological assessment in multiple sclerosis

Letizia Leocani and Giancarlo Comi

Electrophysiological measures, mainly standard multimodal evoked potentials (EPs), have been used for the assessment of central nervous system (CNS) function in multiple sclerosis (MS). Their abnormalities correspond well with clinical involvement of the pathways being investigated and also provide information on the nature of the pathologic process such as demyelination or axonal loss. Several studies have assessed their value in the diagnosis, monitoring, and prediction of the course of MS. Other measures, such as the analysis of spontaneous and induced brain oscillatory activity, cognitive potentials, or studies of motor cortical excitability and mapping of motor representation using transcranial magnetic stimulation (TMS), may provide useful information about the pathophysiology of MS and related features such as cognitive involvement or fatigue. This chapter will review the application and usefulness of standard EPs and other neurophysiological techniques in MS.

Standard evoked potentials (EPs)
Evoked potentials in MS diagnosis and assessment of disease activity

Multimodal EPs (visual, somatosensory, auditory, motor) provide functional information on eloquent CNS pathways. In MS, demyelination and axonal block or axonal loss lead to EP abnormalities such as delayed latency, morphological abnormalities, and an increased refractory period. A well-preserved wave morphology together with relevant latency delay is suggestive of a demyelinating disorder [1], although none of these abnormalities is specific to MS. The use of EPs in the diagnosis of MS has been greatly reduced by the advent of magnetic resonance imaging

(MRI), since although EPs can detect subclinical CNS involvement, their sensitivity to brain lesions is much lower compared to that of MRI [2]. On one hand, MRI is clearly superior to EPs in detecting supratentorial lesions since plaques are preferentially located in periventricular regions and do not affect sensory and motor pathways. On the other hand, EPs can be abnormal only if their corresponding pathway is involved. This characteristic, which makes them useful in the objective observation of subtle symptoms or signs, limits their value in detecting asymptomatic lesions. The low sensitivity of EPs to asymptomatic lesions, important for meeting the criteria of spatial dissemination, also explains their limited value in the prediction of conversion to MS in clinically isolated syndromes. For example, in patients with optic neuritis, the prognostic value of EPs has been shown to be poor when compared with MRI [3, 4], although it increased when including lower limb somatosensory [4] and both somatosensory and motor [5] EPs. This may be explained by the fact that lower limb motor and somatosensory EPs are the most frequently abnormal tests in the general MS population [6] and the more sensitive in revealing subclinical white matter lesions, probably since they assess the longest CNS pathway, and are thus more susceptible to being involved by CNS lesions. Differently from brain involvement, showing a clear superiority of MRI, EPs have been shown equally sensitive to MRI in the identification of optic nerve involvement, both in symptomatic eyes and in detecting subclinical lesions [7]. Their capability of detecting subclinical abnormalities may be explained by the fact that, at examination of the retinal nerve fiber layer at the optic disk, more than 50% of neural tissue must be lost before a visual defect is clinically evident [8]. Moreover, the high sensitivity

---

Multiple Sclerosis: Recovery of Function and Neurorehabilitation, eds. J. Kesselring, G. Comi, and A. J. Thompson. Published by Cambridge University Press. © Cambridge University Press 2010.

of visual EPs in the initial stages of the disease could be explained by a high susceptibility of this pathway, as suggested by pathological studies [9]. For these reasons, visual EPs may still be considered an easily available, low-cost alternative to optic nerve MRI for the detection of subclinical lesions and for the confirmation of previous or ongoing optic neuritis. These features, together with the additional information on the underlying pathologic process (demyelination or axonal involvement) make visual EPs particularly useful in some cases in the diagnostic phase of the disease.

Concerning the possibility of detecting new lesions, this is important both in the diagnostic stage for the confirmation of temporal dissemination, and, after the diagnosis, in the assessment of disease activity and of drug effects. Considering that EPs are very sensitive in detecting symptomatic lesions, we may say that their importance is highest for the confirmation of a relapse in patients complaining of vague or transitory symptoms. Conversely, in asymptomatic patients, especially in the early stages of the disease, the yield of EPs in detecting new lesions is quite low. We may conclude that EPs have a poor value in the assessment of disease activity in MS, by reason of their limited global sensitivity. More recent methods for recording EPs such as multifocal visual evoked potentials (VEPs) [10, 11] and triple stimulation technique [12] have been proposed for the quantification of optic and corticospinal damage, respectively. In a cross-sectional study on multifocal VEPs in 26 MS patients, a good correlation was found with conventional VEPs, together with a higher detection of subclinical abnormalities [10]. In that study, the reproducibility of abnormal findings in order to exclude false-positive results was not assessed. However, the finding of a good topographic correspondence between multifocal VEPs and retinal fiber layer thickness at optic coherence tomography in 50 MS patients with a history of optic neuritis [11] seems very promising. Although amplitude and area measurement of standard motor evoked potentials (MEPs) has been proposed to be more sensitive compared to central motor conduction time [13], the majority of studies reported that the former measure adds little to the latter [12, 14]. The triple stimulation technique has been proposed as a more sensitive method for detecting a reduced number of functioning corticospinal fibers as compared with conventional amplitude measurements of MEPs [12, 14]. Other TMS measures of motor pathways, such as intracortical excitation and inhibition [14, 15], transcallosal conduction and ipsilateral silent period [14, 16, 17], mapping of motor cortex representation [18], modulation of response amplitudes by exercise [14, 19], seem more suitable for the study of the physiopathology of MS and related dysfunction and/or reorganization within the motor system. Another potentially useful application of TMS stimulation in MS is to achieve neuromodulation: preliminary reports suggest improvement of spasticity [20], urinary dysfunction [21], and hand dexterity [22] after treatment with repetitive TMS. In the somatosensory modality, the use of laser-evoked EPs for assessment of the spinothalamic pathway may increase the sensitivity in MS patients compared with standard EPs from electrical stimulation alone [23], the latter being more suitable for investigating the lemniscal pathway [24]. Measures of intracortical conduction such as long-latency sensorimotor reflexes, which have been reported as more sensitive compared with separate measurement of the corresponding somatosensory and motor pathways in a group of 23 patients at acute phases of MS [25], need to be replicated.

Evoked potentials in measuring disease progression and treatment response in MS

Even though the EPs provide information confined to eloquent pathways, thus being of limited value in the diagnosis of multiple sclerosis, this feature is an advantage when assessing functional involvement of MS patients [26]. In fact, EPs are strictly related to function, as reflected by the correlation between their abnormalities and symptoms and signs in the corresponding somatosensory [24], pyramidal [27], visual [28], and brainstem [29] systems. In the visual modality, EP amplitudes have also been reported to correlate with lesion length [30], with MRI measures of optic nerve area [31], and with retinal layer fiber thickness in optic coherence tomography [32]. Motor cross-sectional studies have also demonstrated that global multimodal EP measures correlate with clinical disability [6, 33] measured with the expanded disability status scale (EDSS) [34], and that single-modality EPs correlate with the corresponding functional system [6]. Finally, EPs are more frequently and severely abnormal in patients with a longer disease duration and disability, both at multimodal [6, 35] and motor [14] assessments.

There have been some attempts to monitor disease progression over time and to assess the effects of therapy, with controversial results [1], with the rationale that ongoing demyelination and axonal loss are reflected by progressive latency increase and amplitude reduction or morphological disruption of the main EP waveforms. A main limitation to this approach, besides the increased waveform variability in MS patients [1], is constituted by a floor effect in patients with very low disability (due to the low sensitivity of EPs to subclinical lesions) aimed at a ceiling effect in the most severe patients. In fact, after the main components of a given EP have been lost at confirmed examination after 6 months to rule out transient conduction block [1] it becomes impossible to detect additional involvement of the corresponding pathway. For that reason, non-parametric conventional scores may be useful in order to take into account the severity of morphological abnormality and the number of absent EP components within the same modality [1, 6]. In a longitudinal study, combined visual and motor EPs have been shown to correlate with expanded disability status scale (EDSS) over a 2-year follow-up, with better correlation at the final observation; changes over time were also significant. Similar findings have been reported in a cohort of 84 patients followed for about 4 years [6] and in 37 patients with early MS followed for 2 years [36]. Moreover, abnormalities in multimodal EPs may be predictive of future development of disability [6, 35, 36], especially in the early stages of the disease [35, 36], suggesting that EPs could be useful in the identification of patients with initial, subclinical involvement of eloquent pathways, which are important in determining the development of disability. In the visual system, in another longitudinal study in patients after unilateral optic neuritis, visual EPs were able to detect progressively improving nervous conduction despite little recovery in visual function, possibly related to remyelination or ion channel reorganization in the demyelinated region, together with subtle worsening of conduction in the fellow asymptomatic eye, possibly indicating an insidious demyelinating process which, although accompanied by worsening of contrast sensitivity [37] would have been undetected by clinical examination alone. Improvement after optic neuritis has been shown also at multifocal VEPs in 12 patients [38] over a period of 6–56 months; however, comparison data with standard VEPs were not provided. Evoked potentials have also been used for assessing the effects of treatment with contrasting results [1, 14]. In a 3-year controlled study, the effects of azathioprine in chronic–progressive MS, associated or not associated with steroids, were measured using multimodal EPs [39]. A significant effect on VEP and somatosensory evoked potentials (SEP) in favor of the active treatment group was observed 1 year before corresponding differences were seen clinically. In another study, a significant correlation between changes of a composite EP score and changes of disability has been found in a clinical trial evaluating the efficacy of methylprednisolone in acute MS [40]. Improved latency of visual EPs after interferon-1b treatment has also been reported [41]. Prolonged central motor conduction time during a relapse has been shown to improve after steroid treatment together with clinical improvement [14]. In a 6-month follow-up of 15 early MS patients undergoing interferon beta-1a treatment, the number of abnormalities in MEPs, when considering both central conduction time and amplitude measurements, was predictive of disability at 6 months [42]. Interestingly enough, in the latter study amplitude of MEPs, and not latency, was significantly changed after treatment, suggesting that the sensitivity to change of composite scores may improve when both amplitude and latency measures are included. This is also indicated by changes in triple stimulation technique (TST) amplitudes to TMS 5 days after treatment of acute MS exacerbation with methylprednisolone [43], again with no changes in central motor conduction. In addition, studies of treatment effects on fatigue in MS patients have reported improvement of amplitude and shape of resting MEPs after 4-aminopyridine [44] or of post-exercise amplitudes of MEPs after interferon beta-1a [45]. Decreased intracortical inhibition and increased intracortical facilitation following fatigue treatment with 3,4-diaminopyridine in 12 MS patients has also been found [46].

Globally considered, EPs seem more valuable for monitoring and predicting disability in MS patients rather than for making the diagnosis and detecting disease activity.

Electrophysiological assessment of higher brain function

Cognitive impairment is a common feature in multiple sclerosis, generally with a typical pattern of subcortical dementia [47], at least partially related to reduction of cortico-cortical and cortico-subcortical connections. Advanced analysis of the electroencephalogram (EEG) and event-related potentials (ERPs) may provide information on cognitive functions.

Cognitive potentials

Event-related potentials – particularly the P300 wave to oddball paradigm (required to distinguish rare stimuli from frequent stimuli within a series) – constitute an objective electrophysiological index of cognitive function. Their latency and amplitude are respectively related to the speed of cognitive processing and to the amount of synchronized neurons participating in a given task. An increased latency of P300 has been reported in MS [48–51] with differential involvement according to disease course [52, 53], related to brain lesion load [50, 54], disability [52], and the degree of cognitive involvement [51]. Event-related potentials have been used for monitoring MS evolution and the effects of treatment. In a double-blind study design [55], the effects of high-dose intravenous methylprednisolone were investigated in 44 patients with clinically active MS. The latency of P300 was significantly shortened after treatment and not after placebo. Two longitudinal studies assessed P300 in MS patients after treatment with interferon beta [56, 57]. Gerschlager et al. [56] did not report significant changes in P300 parameters after 1 year of interferon beta-1b therapy in 14 MS patients, but showed development of abnormal ERPs after 1 year in three patients without detectable clinical changes. Flechter et al. [57] reported reduced P300 latency and amplitude after 1 year of interferon beta-1b in 16 patients. A predictive role of P300 on positive response has been suggested by a longitudinal study on 33 MS patients complaining of fatigue treated with modafinil. These findings suggest the possibility of a future role of ERPs in monitoring cognitive drug effects in clinical trials. As for other types of cognitive impairments and dementia, the low sensitivity and specificity of ERPs to the standard oddball paradigm could be also attributed to the fact that this task is relative and not very specific concerning the cognitive domain investigated. Event-related potentials to tasks more oriented towards particular cognitive domains such as working memory [58, 59, 60], emotional responses [61], or preattentional auditory information processing [16] could add sensitivity and specificity concerning the type of neuropsychological involvement. However, these reports generally involved small samples and non-homogeneous methodologies across studies, so they need further replication and validation.

EEG oscillatory activity

The EEG, which is the expression of multiple neuronal network interactions, affected by white matter damage, may be used as an indicator of the global status of such interactions [1]. Computerized analysis of EEG rhythms allows the investigation of cortico-subcortical networks underlying brain oscillatory activity at rest and during specific tasks. Although studies using this type of methodology in MS are generally confined to the investigation of the physiopathology of the disease and are not used in the diagnosis or monitoring of the disease, they can add information on brain mechanisms underlying cognitive involvement or other phenomena such as fatigue. On the other hand, their application to MS allows a deeper knowledge of mechanisms underlying brain oscillations, through the relationship between specific clinical dysfunction and the corresponding pattern of EEG abnormality. Spectral analysis of the EEG has revealed abnormalities in 40–79% of MS patients [62], mainly an increase of slow frequencies and decrease of the alpha band, which are related to cognitive dysfunctions. Other studies reported increased power of faster frequencies in MS patients compared with controls but data analyzed were obtained during performance of cognitive tasks rather than during rest [63, 64]. Spectral power and coherence of EEG have been analyzed in a group of 28 MS patients with or without cognitive impairment assessed by a battery of neuropsychological tests [26]. Cognitively impaired MS patients had a significant increase of theta power over the frontal regions and a diffuse coherence decrease not found in cognitively intact patients; moreover, coherence was negatively correlated with the amount of subcortical lesion load, suggesting cortico-cortical disconnection as a possible common substrate for the development both of cognitive impairment and of coherence decrease. Reduced inter-hemispheric coherence has also been shown with magneto-EEG (MEG), unrelated to disability and to brain global, subcortical, and corpus callosum MRI lesion load [65]. Another MEG study focusing on the rolandic region found reduced functional connectivity of signals recorded after somatosensory stimulation within the hand area slightly correlated with brain lesion load [66]. However, these EEG parameters have not yet proved adequately sensitive to allow clinical utilization of the techniques.

The reactivity of EEG brain rhythms may also be investigated during cognitive or motor tasks. Voluntary movement results from the complex interaction between different cortical and subcortical circuits. Analysis of event-related desynchronization (ERD) and synchronization (ERS) [67] of mu and beta sensorimotor rhythms provides information on the dynamic pattern of cortical activation and idling occurring during motor activity. In physiological conditions, mu and beta ERD are observed over the sensorimotor regions before and during voluntary movement and are considered as sign of cortical activation. After movement execution, ERD is replaced by ERS, more consistently for the beta band [67–69], in correspondence with a period of corticospinal inhibition [70]. The impact of brain damage in MS on the efficiency of cortical processes underlying motor programming, as assessed by mu ERD, has been studied in a group of 34 MS patients undergoing MRI scans for quantification of lesions. Contralateral sensorimotor ERD onset did not significantly differ between the whole group of MS patients and normal subjects but was significantly delayed in patients with a higher brain lesion load [71]. These findings suggested that functional cortico-cortical and cortico-subcortical connections underlying the expression of ERD during programming of voluntary movement are disrupted by the MS-related pathological process [71]. This study, performed on patients without clinically evident impairment of the upper limb, has not been replicated. Moreover, correlations between ERD parameters and MRI involvement of specific cortico-subcortical anatomical pathways were not evaluated. Another study [72] focused on the relationship between ERD/ERS and fatigue, a subjective sense of tiredness and exaustion already present at rest. Fatigue can be present in up to 70% of MS patients, even in the earliest phases of the disease, when patients still have a mild disability [73]. Several mechanisms have been hypothesized to play a role in the physiopathology of fatigue, from immune factors, to depression, to corticospinal involvement [74]. Nevertheless, the finding of slowed complex reaction times, in MS patients complaining of fatigue, unrelated to slowed conduction along primary afferent or efferent pathways [75], as well as abnormal frontal and basal ganglia metabolism [76], suggested a role of

circuitries involved in motor planning. The impact of fatigue on the efficiency of motor control circuitries, measured by ERD/ERS, has been evaluated in MS patients in the early stages without clinical disability, subdivided into two groups according to the presence or absence of subjective fatigue [72] assessed using a conventional subjective scale [77]. MS patients with fatigue showed enhanced beta ERD over the anterior midline region, correlated with severity of fatigue in the whole MS group. Increased ERD in MS patients with fatigue over midline frontal regions is consistent with overactivity of the supplementary motor area (SMA) on functional MRI in a similar group of patients performing hand movement [78]. MS patients complaining of fatigue also had reduced post-movement sensorimotor beta Hz ERS, negatively correlated with the fatigue score, suggesting that inhibitory circuits acting on the motor cortex after movement termination may also be involved in the pathophysiological mechanism of fatigue in MS [72]. An alternative suggestion for these findings is a possible abnormal balance between cortical excitation and inhibition from cortico-cortical disconnection. Once again, not only do these findings need to be replicated, but the specificity and sensitivity of ERD/ERS parameters in assessing fatigue in MS and the involvement of specific brain circuits have not been evaluated.

To date, the most reliable neurophysiological tool for the assessment of nervous function in MS is represented by standard EPs. They have proven to be not very useful in the diagnosis of the disease and in the detection of disease activity. However, their value in providing objective evaluation of the nervous function represents an expansion of the neurological examination, which can be useful for confirmation of dubious relapses in patients complaining of vague symptoms. Moreover, they may provide information on the demyelinating nature of the pathological process, thus possibly contributing in some cases to the diagnostic process. In the early phases, neurophysiological tests revealing involvement of eloquent nervous pathways may also predict future progression to clinically definite MS, while during the course of the disease they may be helpful in monitoring disability and in testing treatment effects, due to their correlation with the degree of nervous dysfunction. For these purposes, standardization within and between laboratories is essential.

The goal of quantifying mental dysfunction in MS is a complex task. With this aim, some neurophysiological descriptors such as the analysis of brain oscillations and cognitive potentials could be employed, but their sensitivity and specificity in MS need to be assessed. However, these methods have proven valuable in the investigation of the physiopathology of MS and related involvement of higher brain functions.

References

1. Comi G, Leocani L, Locatelli T, Medaglini S, Martinelli V. Electrophysiological investigations in multiple sclerosis dementia. *Electroencephalogr Clin Neurophysiol* 1999;**50**(Suppl):480–5

2. Comi G, Filippi M, Martinelli V, *et al.* Brain magnetic resonance imaging correlates of cognitive impairment in multiple sclerosis. *J Neurol Sci* 1993;**115**:S66–S73

3. Filippini G, Comi G C, Cosi V, *et al.* Sensitivities and predictive values of paraclinical tests for diagnosing multiple sclerosis. *J Neurol* 1994;**241**:132–7

4. Ghezzi A, Martinelli V, Torri V, *et al.* Long-term follow-up of isolated optic neuritis: the risk of developing multiple sclerosis, its outcome, and the prognostic role of paraclinical tests. *J Neurol* 1999;**246**:770–5

5. Simó M, Barsi P, Arányi Z. Predictive role of evoked potential examinations in patients with clinically isolated optic neuritis in light of the revised McDonald criteria. *Mult Scler* 2008;**14**:472–8

6. Leocani L, Rovaris M, Boneschi F M, *et al.* Multimodal evoked potentials to assess the evolution of multiple sclerosis: a longitudinal study. *J Neurol Neurosurg Psychiatry* 2006;**77**:1030–5

7. Davies M B, Williams R, Haq N, Pelosi L, Hawkins C P. MRI of optic nerve and postchiasmal visual pathways and visual evoked potentials in secondary progressive multiple sclerosis. *Neuroradiology* 1998;**40**:765–70

8. Quigley H A, Addicks E M. Quantitative studies of retinal nerve fiber layer defects. *Arch Ophthalmol* 1982;**100**:807–14

9. Dawson J. The histology of disseminated sclerosis. *Trans R Soc Edinb* 1916;**50**:517–740

10. Klistorner A, Fraser C, Garrick R, Graham S, Arvind H. Correlation between full-field and multifocal VEPs in optic neuritis. *Doc Ophthalmol* 2008;**116**:19–27

11. Klistorner A, Arvind H, Nguyen T, *et al.* Multifocal VEP and OCT in optic neuritis: a topographical study of the structure–function relationship. *Doc Ophthalmol* 2009;**118**:129–37

12. Humm A M, Magistris M R, Truffert A, Hess C W, Rösler K M. Central motor conduction differs between acute relapsing–remitting and chronic progressive multiple sclerosis. *Clin Neurophysiol* 2003;**114**:2196–203

13. Gagliardo A, Galli F, Grippo A, *et al.* Motor evoked potentials in multiple sclerosis patients without walking limitation: amplitude vs. conduction time abnormalities. *J Neurol* 2007;**254**:220–7

14. Chen R, Cros D, Curra A, *et al.* The clinical diagnostic utility of transcranial magnetic stimulation: report of an IFCN committee. *Clin Neurophysiol* 2008; **119**:504–32

15. Conte A, Lenzi D, Frasca V, *et al.* Intracortical excitability in patients with relapsing–remitting and secondary progressive multiple sclerosis. *J Neurol* 2009; **256**: 933–8

16. Jung J, Morlet D, Mercier B, Confavreux C, Fischer C. Mismatch negativity (MMN) in multiple sclerosis: an event-related potentials study in 46 patients. *Clin Neurophysiol* 2006;**117**:85–93

17. Lenzi D, Conte A, Mainero C, *et al.* Effect of corpus callosum damage on ipsilateral motor activation in patients with multiple sclerosis: a functional and anatomical study. *Hum Brain Mapp* 2007;**28**:636–44

18. Thickbroom G W, Byrnes M L, Archer S A, Kermode A G, Mastaglia F L. Corticomotor organization and motor function in multiple sclerosis. *J Neurol* 2005;**252**:765–71

19. Perretti A, Balbi P, Orefice G, *et al.* Post-exercise facilitation and depression of motor evoked potentials to transcranial magnetic stimulation: a study in multiple sclerosis. *Clin Neurophysiol* 2004;**115**: 2128–33

20. Centonze D, Koch G, Versace V, *et al.* Repetitive transcranial magnetic stimulation of the motor cortex ameliorates spasticity in multiple sclerosis. *Neurology* 2007;**68**:1045–50

21. Centonze D, Petta F, Versace V, *et al.* Effects of motor cortex rTMS on lower urinary tract dysfunction in multiple sclerosis. *Mult Scler* 2007;**13**:269–71

22. Koch G, Miano R, Boffa L, Finazzi-Agrò E. Effects of motor cortex rTMS on lower urinary tract dysfunction in multiple sclerosis. *Mult Scler* 2007;**13**:269–71

23. Spiegel J, Hansen C, Baumgärtner U, Hopf H C, Treede R D. Sensitivity of laser-evoked potentials versus somatosensory evoked potentials in patients with multiple sclerosis. *Clin Neurophysiol* 2003;**114**: 992–1002

24. Leocani L, Martinelli V, Natali-Sora M G, Rovaris M, Comi G. Somatosensory evoked potentials and sensory involvement in multiple sclerosis: comparison with clinical findings and quantitative sensory tests. *Mult Scler* 2003;**9**:275–9

25. Bonfiglio L, Rossi B, Sartucci F. Prolonged intracortical delay of long-latency reflexes: electrophysiological evidence for a cortical dysfunction in multiple sclerosis. *Brain Res Bull* 2006;**69**:606–13

26. Leocani L, Locatelli T, Martinelli V, *et al.* Electroencephalography coherence analysis in multiple sclerosis: correlation with clinical, neurophysiological, and MRI findings. *J Neurol Neurosurg Psychiatry* 2000;**69**:192–8

27. van der Kamp W, Maertens de Noordhout A, Thompson P D, *et al.* Correlation of phasic muscle strength and corticomotoneuron conduction time in multiple sclerosis. *Ann Neurol* 1991;**29**:6–12

28. Frederiksen J L, Petrera J. Serial visual evoked potentials in 90 untreated patients with acute optic neuritis. *Surv Ophthalmol* 1999;**44**:S54–62

29. Soustiel J F, Hafner H, Chistyakov A V, *et al.* Brainstem trigeminal and auditory evoked potentials in multiple sclerosis: physiological insights. *Electroencephalogr Clin Neurophysiol* 1996;**100**:152–7

30. Youl B D, Turano G, Miller D H, *et al.* The pathophysiology of acute optic neuritis: an association of gadolinium leakage with clinical and electrophysiological deficits. *Brain* 1991;**114**:2437–50

31. Trip S A, Schlottmann P G, Jones S J, *et al.* Optic nerve atrophy and retinal nerve fibre layer thinning following optic neuritis: evidence that axonal loss is a substrate of MRI-detected atrophy. *NeuroImage* 2006;**31**:286–93

32. Trip S A, Schlottmann P G, Jones S J, *et al.* Retinal nerve fiber layer axonal loss and visual dysfunction in optic neuritis. *Ann Neurol* 2005;**58**:383–91

33. Fuhr P, Borggrefe-Chappuis A, Schindler C, Kappos L. Visual and motor evoked potentials in the course of multiple sclerosis. *Brain* 2001;**124**:2162–8

34. Kurtzke J F. Rating neurologic impairment in multiple sclerosis: an expanded disability status scale (EDSS). *Neurology* 1983;**33**:1444–52

35. Kallmann B A, Fackelmann S, Toyka K V, Rieckmann P, Reiners K. Early abnormalities of evoked potentials and future disability in patients with multiple sclerosis. *Mult Scler* 2006;**12**:58–65

36. Jung P, Beyerle A, Ziemann U. Multimodal evoked potentials measure and predict disability progression in early relapsing–remitting multiple sclerosis. *Mult Scler* 2008;**14**:553–6

37. Brusa A, Jones S J, Plant G T. Long-term remyelination after optic neuritis: a 2-year visual evoked potential and psychophysical serial study. *Brain* 2001;**124**:468–79

38. Yang E B, Hood D C, Rodarte C, *et al.* Improvement in conduction velocity after optic neuritis measured with the multifocal VEP. *Invest Ophthalmol Vis Sci* 2007;**48**:692–8

39. Nuwer M R, Packwood J W, Myers L W, Ellison G W. Evoked potentials predict the clinical changes in a multiple sclerosis drug study. *Neurology* 1987;**37**: 1754–61

40. La Mantia L, Eoli M, Milanese C, *et al.* Double-blind trial of dexamethasone versus methylprednisolone in multiple sclerosis acute relapses. *Eur Neurol* 1994;**34**:199–203

41. Anlar O, Kisli M, Tombul T, Ozbek H. Visual evoked potentials in multiple sclerosis before and after two years of interferon therapy. *Int J Neurosci* 2003;**113**:483–9

42. Feuillet L, Pelletier J, Suchet L, *et al.* Prospective clinical and electrophysiological follow-up on a multiple sclerosis population treated with interferon beta-1a: a pilot study. *Mult Scler* 2007;**13**:348–56

43. Humm A M, Z'Graggen W J, Bühler R, Magistris M R, Rösler K M. Quantification of central motor conduction deficits in multiple sclerosis patients before and after treatment of acute exacerbation by methylprednisolone. *J Neurol Neurosurg Psychiatry* 2006;**77**:345–50

44. Rossini P M, Pasqualetti P, Pozzilli C, *et al.* Fatigue in progressive multiple sclerosis: results of a randomized, double-blind, placebo-controlled, crossover trial of oral 4-aminopyridine. *Mult Scler* 2001;**7**:354–8

45. White A T, Petajan J H. Physiological measures of therapeutic response to interferon beta-1a treatment in remitting–relapsing MS. *Clin Neurophysiol* 2004;**115**:2364–71

46. Mainero C, Inghilleri M, Pantano P, *et al.* Enhanced brain motor activity in patients with MS after a single dose of 3,4-diaminopyridine. *Neurology* 2004;**62**:2044–50

47. Rao S M. Neuropsychology of multiple sclerosis. *Curr Opin Neurol* 1995;**8**:216–20

48. Gil R, Zai L, Neau J P, *et al.* Event-related auditory evoked potentials and multiple sclerosis. *Electroencephalogr Clin Neurophysiol* 1993;**88**:182–7

49. Aminoff J C, Goodin D S. Long-latency cerebral event-related potentials in multiple sclerosis. *J Clin Neurophysiol* 2001;**18**:372–7

50. Piras M R, Magnano I, Canu E D, *et al.* Longitudinal study of cognitive dysfunction in multiple sclerosis: neuropsychological, neuroradiological, and neurophysiological findings. *J Neurol Neurosurg Psychiatry* 2003;**74**:878–85

51. Magnano I, Aiello I, Piras M R. Cognitive impairment and neurophysiological correlates in MS. *J Neurol Sci* 2006;**245**:117–22

52. Ellger T, Bethke F, Frese A, *et al.* Event-related potentials in different subtypes of multiple sclerosis: a cross-sectional study. *J Neurol Sci* 2002;**205**:35–40

53. Gonzalez-Rosa J J, Vazquez-Marrufo M, Vaquero E, *et al.* Differential cognitive impairment for diverse forms of multiple sclerosis. *BMC Neurosci* 2006;**19**:7–39

54. Sailer M, Heinze H J, Tendolkar I, *et al.* Influence of cerebral lesion volume and lesion distribution on event-related brain potentials in multiple sclerosis. *J Neurol* 2001;**248:**1049–55

55. Filipovic S R, Drulovic J, Stojsavlievic N, Levic Z. The effects of high-dose intravenous methylprednisolone on event-related potentials in patients with multiple sclerosis. *J Neurol Sci* 1997;**152:**147–53

56. Gerschlager W, Beisteiner R, Deecke L, *et al.* Electrophysiological, neuropsychological and clinical findings in multiple sclerosis patients receiving interferon beta-1b: a 1-year follow-up. *Eur Neurol* 2000;**44:**205–9

57. Flechter S, Vardi J, Finkelstein Y, Pollak L. Cognitive dysfunction evaluation in multiple sclerosis patients treated with interferon beta-1b: an open-label prospective 1-year study. *Isr Med Assoc J* 2007;**9:**457–9

58. Nagels G, D'hooge M B, Vleugels L, *et al.* P300 and treatment effect of modafinil on fatigue in multiple sclerosis. *J Clin Neurosci* 2007;**114:**33–40

59. Pelosi L, Geesken J M, Holly M, Hayward M, Blumhardt L D. Working memory impairment in early multiple sclerosis: evidence from an event-related potential study of patients with clinically isolated myelopathy. *Brain* 1997;**120:**2039–58

60. Papageorgiou C C, Sfagos C, Kosma K K, *et al.* Changes in LORETA and conventional patterns of P600 after steroid treatment in multiple sclerosis patients. *Prog Neuropsychopharmacol Biol Psychiatry* 2007;**31:**234–41

61. Haiman G, Pratt H, Miller A. Brain responses to verbal stimuli among multiple sclerosis patients with pseudobulbar effect. *J Neurol Sci* 2008;**27:**137–47

62. Leocani L, Comi G. Neurophysiological investigations in multiple sclerosis. *Curr Opin Neurol* 2000;**13:**255–61

63. Vasquez-Marrufo M, Gonzalez-Rosa J J, Vaquero E, *et al.* Quantitative electroencephalography reveals different physiological profiles between benign and remitting-relapsing multiple sclerosis patients. *BMC Neurology* 2008;**8:**44

64. Vasquez-Marrufo M, Gonzalez-Rosa J J, Vaquero E, Duque P. Abnormal ERPS and high frequency bands power in multiple sclerosis. *Int J Neurosci* 2008;**118:**27–38

65. Cover K S, Vrenken H, Geurts J J G, *et al.* Multiple sclerosis patients show a highly significant decrease in alpha band interhemispheric synchronization measured using MEG. *Neuroimage* 2006;**29:**783–8

66. Tecchio F, Zito G, Zappasodi F, *et al.* Intracortical connectivity in multiple sclerosis: a neurophysiological approach. *Brain* 2008;**131:**1783–92

67. Pfurtscheller G. Central beta rhythm during sensorimotor activities in man. *Electroencephalogr Clin Neurophysiol* 1981;**5:**253–64

68. Leocani L, Toro C, Magnanotti P, Zhuang P, Hallett M. Event-related coherence and event-related desynchronization/synchronization in the 10 Hz and 20 Hz EEG during self-paced movements. *Electroencephalogr Clin Neurophysiol* 1997;**104:** 199–206

69. Leocani L, Toro C, Zhuang P, Gerloff C, Hallett M. Event-related desynchronization in reaction time paradigms: a comparison with event-related potentials and corticospinal excitability. *Clin Neurophysiol* 2001;**112:**923–30

70. Chen R, Yassen Z, Cohen L G, Hallet M. The time course of corticospinal excitability in reaction time and self-paced movements. *Ann Neurol* 1998; **44:**317–25

71. Leocani L, Rovaris M, Martinelli-Boneschi F, *et al.* Movement preparation is affected by tissue damage in multiple sclerosis: evidence from EEG event-related desynchronization. *Clin Neurophysiol* 2005;**116:** 1515–19

72. Leocani L, Colombo B, Magnani G, *et al.* Fatigue in multiple sclerosis is associated with abnormal cortical activation to voluntary movement: EEG evidence. *Neuroimage* 2001;**13:**1186–92

73. Krupp L B, Alvarez L A, LaRocca N G, Scheinberg L C. Fatigue in multiple sclerosis. *Arch Neurol* 1988;**45:** 435–7

74. Comi G, Leocani L, Rossi P, Colombo B. Physio-pathology and treatment of fatigue in multiple sclerosis. *J Neurol* 2001;**248:**174–9

75. Sandroni P, Walker C, Starr A. "Fatigue" in patients with multiple sclerosis: motor pathway conduction and event-related potentials. *Arch Neurol* 1992; **49:**517–24

76. Roelcke U, Kappos L, Lechner-Scott J, *et al.* Reduced glucose metabolism in the frontal cortex and basal ganglia of multiple sclerosis patients with fatigue: an ^{18}F-fluorodeoxyglucose positron emission tomography study. *Neurology* 1997;**48:**1566–71

77. Krupp L, LaRocca N, Muir-Nash J, Steinberg A. The fatigue severity scale: application to patients with multiple sclerosis and systemic lupus erythematosus. *Arch Neurol* 1989;**46:**1121–3

78. Filippi M, Rocca M A, Colombo B, *et al.* Functional magnetic resonance imaging correlates of fatigue in multiple sclerosis. *NeuroImage* 2002;**15:** 559–67

Functional magnetic resonance imaging monitoring of therapeutic interventions in multiple sclerosis

Massimo Filippi and Maria A. Rocca

Introduction

Several studies of patients with different neurological conditions, e.g., stroke, have unambiguously demonstrated that functional magnetic resonance imaging (fMRI) represents a powerful tool to monitor recovery of function following central nervous system (CNS) damage. More recently, the validity of this technique for assessing the longitudinal changes of brain activations after specific therapeutic interventions, i.e., rehabilitative and pharmacological, has also been assessed. Despite this, only a few studies have used fMRI for monitoring therapeutic interventions in multiple sclerosis (MS).

This chapter summarizes the main issues that should be addressed when planning a longitudinal fMRI study specifically aimed at monitoring clinical recovery, either natural or modified by treatment, in patients with MS. A specific focus is devoted to fMRI changes observed with learning in healthy individuals. This provides a model for understanding the way in which brain structure and function can change with injury. Finally, the main results obtained in patients with MS are illustrated.

Issues to be addressed

Although studies of healthy individuals have shown that longitudinal fMRI scans have a good reproducibility [1–3], caution must be exercised when interpreting fMRI results obtained from diseased people because various factors, including abnormalities of the blood oxygenation level dependent (BOLD) effect related to the presence of inflammatory lesions, can affect data reliability across sessions. Clearly, this problem is likely to influence results obtained from MS patients during the acute phases of the disease or

those patients with a significant inflammatory burden, as revealed by post-contrast T1-weighted images.

In clinically stable patients and those outside the acute stage of a relapse but who might need rehabilitation, the main issues to be addressed are related to the set-up of the experimental design, since the results from any fMRI study are only as reliable as the care with which the experiment is constructed and executed. Among the factors that should be considered during the set-up of an fMRI experiment aimed at monitoring longitudinal changes of activations in MS patients (but also in patients with other neurological diseases), the following need to be considered carefully.

Patient selection

Usually, MS patients have heterogeneous clinical characteristics, which result from the involvement of different functional systems by macro- and microscopic structural damage. Clearly, the experimental question will drive the criteria for patient selection. However, to reduce as much as possible disease-related variability and to achieve meaningful and interpretable results, it is desirable to enroll patients with similar clinical characteristics, including the clinical disease phenotype. The inconvenience of such an approach is that the results obtained, despite being robust, are usually not generalizable outside the selected group.

Task performance

In longitudinal studies of recovery, between-subject differences in performance abilities at baseline as well as differences in recovery outcomes might confound fMRI results. Similarly, task performance is likely to vary in the same patient during recovery. Several

Multiple Sclerosis: Recovery of Function and Neurorehabilitation, eds. J. Kesselring, G. Comi, and A. J. Thompson.
Published by Cambridge University Press. © Cambridge University Press 2010.

strategies have been suggested to have each patient performing the same task during the entire study period, including the investigation of an active motor task with different levels of difficulty, which always requires the same effort from individual subjects [4], the performance of passive tasks, and the imagination of movements [5, 6]. The use of passive tasks is supported by the fact that there are reciprocal projections between the motor and the related sensory cortices; hence, patterns of brain activation that reflect local field potentials from presynaptic activity primarily [7], even with entirely passive movements, may identify those brain regions involved in active voluntary movements. This hypothesis has indeed been confirmed by fMRI studies of healthy controls which have demonstrated that activations associated with active and passive hand movements are similar in localization and size [8, 9].

An attractive approach, which would allow the investigation of severely impaired patients with no bias from task performance, is the exploration of the so-called resting-state networks (RSN) activity [10]. At "rest" (i.e., in the absence of external stimulation), the brain is organized in multiple active subsystems, resembling specific neuroanatomical networks, such as the motor, the visual, and the dorsal and ventral attention systems [11, 12]. To date, a few preliminary studies [13, 14] have investigated low-frequency functional fluctuations in MS, showing abnormal connectivity inside the motor network in patients compared with controls.

Task characteristics

Several variables have been shown to influence the observed patterns of movement-associated cortical activations in healthy subjects during motor task execution, including movement rate, which has been positively correlated with the recruitment of the contralateral primary sensorimotor cortex (SMC) [15], supplementary motor area (SMA) [16], and ipsilateral cerebellar cortex [17]; force, as suggested by the load-dependent effect observed in the primary SMC [15, 18]; and movement complexity, which has been shown to modulate activity of the primary SMC [19, 20], SMA, and premotor cortex [21], as well as several regions of the parietal lobes [15].

The majority of the experiments of the sensorimotor system are conducted using a "block" design, in which periods of 15–30 seconds of activity are

followed by periods of rest. Considering the between- and within-subject variability of clinical impairment, it is arguable that MS patients might experience difficulties in maintaining the same rate and force during the entire block acquisition. One way to overcome this issue is to use an event-related design in which the inter-trial interval is long enough for the task to be performed repetitively without increasing the sense of effort [4]. In addition, to reduce as much as possible variability of task performance, a simple rather than a complex task should be used.

Monitoring of task execution

Accurate monitoring of task performance during fMRI experiments is critical in order to have interpretable fMRI results. In patients with motor deficits, involuntary or mirror movements can occur. Several strategies have been proposed to control for these movements, including recording behavior during a pre-scan rehearsal, or using instrumentation that is compatible with the MRI setting. While the first approach provides some idea of whether a task can be performed correctly, the second provides objective parameters that can be incorporated into image analysis as a covariate.

Cortical reorganization during motor training and motor skill learning

Changes of brain activation that occur during recovery after CNS damage need to be interpreted in the context of changes observed in the healthy brain with learning. Psychophysiological studies have demonstrated that the acquisition of motor skills follows two distinct stages. The first is a fast-learning stage during which considerable improvement in performance can be observed within a single training session; the second is a later, slow-learning stage, during which further gains can be observed across several sessions of practice [20]. Karni et al. [20] used a simple finger-opposition task during which healthy individuals were trained over the course of several weeks and were scanned at weekly intervals using fMRI. Repetition of the task after 3 weeks of practice showed that there was a significant larger activation of the contralateral primary SMC as compared with the activation obtained with a control, untrained finger-opposition sequence. These results support the notion that motor practice induces recruitment of additional

M1 units into a local network specifically representing the motor-trained sequence. These findings are in agreement with the demonstration that, in healthy individuals, the recruitment of the primary SMC can be modified by previous activities, such as playing musical instruments [22, 23] or racquets [24]. In the previous experiment, changes in primary SMC recruitment were also observed in the early scan session, reflecting a sort of initial habituation-like effect, in which the second sequence performed in a set evoked a smaller response than that of the first sequence [20].

While there is agreement that learning of relatively complex motor tasks is associated with increased activation of the contralateral primary SMC, the evaluation of activation patterns associated with repetition of simple movements gave conflicting results, since some studies reported reductions and others increases of task-related activations [1, 20, 25, 26]. These discrepancies among studies might be related to variability in number and length of sessions on length of training, as well in the way motor performance was monitored. Recent evidence suggests that the repetition of a simple sequence within a brief time window typically results in a reduced recruitment of the primary SMC, due to habituation [1, 20, 26]. In addition, a change in the degree of activation of the parietal lobe in healthy volunteers has also been described after motor training [26].

Dynamic activation changes during acquisition of motor skills have also been seen in different regions of the basal ganglia [27]. In detail, the dorsal parts of the putamen and the more rostral striatal areas have been shown to be active only during the early learning stage. In contrast, activation of the posteroventral regions of the putamen and globus pallidus increases with practice.

Functional MRI to monitor therapeutic interventions in MS

The notion that in patients with MS the presence and effectiveness of brain plasticity might make an important contribution to recovery from relapses and in limiting the accumulation of irreversible disability is supported by the results derived from several studies which investigated the motor, visual, and cognitive systems in patients with different disease phenotypes (see Chapter 11).

Only a few studies have assessed dynamic changes of the brain patterns of activations in MS patients.

Pantano et al. [28] evaluated longitudinal (time interval of 15–26 months) changes of activation of the motor system in 18 clinically stable patients with early relapsing–remitting (RR) MS and nine matched controls during the performance of a self-paced sequential finger-opposition movement with the right hand. The MS patients exhibited greater bilateral activation than controls in both fMRI studies. At follow-up, the MS patients showed a reduction in functional activity of the ipsilateral SMC and the contralateral cerebellum. No significant difference between the two fMRI studies was observed in controls. Activation changes in ipsilateral motor areas correlated inversely with age, extent and progression of T1 lesion load, and occurrence of a new relapse, suggesting that younger patients with less structural brain damage and a favorable clinical course demonstrate brain plasticity that follows a more lateralized pattern of brain activations.

Dynamic functional changes have also been described in MS patients following an acute relapse involving the motor system [29, 30]. Both these studies demonstrated that short-term cortical changes are mainly characterized by the recruitment of pathways of the unaffected hemisphere. Recovery of function of the primary SMC of the affected hemisphere was found in patients with clinical improvement, while in patients without clinical recovery, there was persistent recruitment of the primary SMC of the unaffected hemisphere, suggesting that the restoration of function of motor areas of the affected hemisphere might be a critical factor for a favorable recovery. In agreement with the results of studies in patients with chronic and sub-acute stroke [31], these findings also suggest that activation of regions in the unaffected (ipsilateral) cerebral hemisphere may not be necessary for recovery and might, rather, represent a phenomenon of maladaptive cortical reorganization.

The notion that over-recruitment of a given network might not always be beneficial, and, in some cases, even detrimental is also supported by a longitudinal, short-term (4 days) study of motor-related fMRI changes in RRMS patients complaining of reversible fatigue after administration of interferon beta-1a [32]. Compared to patients without fatigue, those with reversible, drug-induced fatigue showed an association between a fatigue score and the extent of recruitment of the frontothalamic circuitry.

As well as occurring spontaneously with brain injury, dynamic changes in representation of functions also can be induced by treatments. At present, only a limited number of studies have applied fMRI to monitoring drug or training effects in patients with MS. Parry *et al.* [33] tested the acute (after 150 minutes) administration of rivastigmine, a central cholinesterase inhibitor, on the patterns of brain activation during the performance of the counting Stroop task in five MS patients and four healthy controls. Before treatment administration, compared to controls, MS patients had increased recruitment of left prefrontal regions and decreased recruitment of right frontal regions and basal ganglia. After treatment administration, a relative normalization of the abnormal Stroop-associated brain activations was observed in patients, while no change in the pattern of brain activations was found in any of the healthy controls. Mainero *et al.* [34] combined fMRI and transcranial magnetic stimulation to investigate motor cerebral activity in 12 MS patients after a single oral dose of 3,4-diaminopyridine, a potassium channel blocker, which is known to improve fatigue and motor function. Motor-related brain activations were increased in the ipsilateral primary SMC and SMA under 3,4-diaminopyridine than under placebo, suggesting that this treatment may modulate brain motor activity in patients with MS, probably by enhancing excitatory synaptic transmission.

Only one study [35] has evaluated changes of motor network activations after motor training in a group of nine MS patients with mild motor impairment in the right upper limb in comparison with nine matched healthy controls. In all the subjects, fMRI was acquired before and after 30 minutes of training. The training period consisted of flexion movements of the right thumb visually cued at 1 Hz frequency. Before training, MS patients had a more prominent activation of the contralateral dorsal premotor cortex during thumb movements when compared to controls. After training, unlike the control group, MS patients did not exhibit task-specific reductions in activation of the contralateral primary SMC and adjacent parietal association cortices. The absence of training-dependent reductions in activation supports the notion that MS patients have a decreased capacity to optimize recruitment of the motor network with practice. The results of this study do not allow correlation of fMRI changes with clinical recovery, since the study was cross-sectional and included exclusively patients with a good clinical performance. However, these workers have suggested a mechanism, which had not been considered previously (i.e., impairment of training-dependent plasticity), that might influence the outcome of rehabilitative treatments.

Only recently has the potential of fMRI in prospective multi-center studies been studied in an international collaborative effort [36]. With this aim, 56 MS patients and 60 age-matched, healthy controls have been recruited and studied at eight sites during the performance of a simple motor task. Compared to controls, MS patients had more significant activations bilaterally in several regions of the sensorimotor network. In the same cohort, abnormalities of effective connectivity have also been described [37]. These findings suggest that large multi-center fMRI studies of diseased people are feasible. Clearly, this sets the stage for large-scale trials of neurorehabilitation and neuroprotection in MS to be monitored using fMRI.

Conclusion

The extensive application of fMRI to the assessment of brain functional plasticity in patients with MS has undoubtedly contributed to improving the understanding of the mechanisms responsible for the recovery of function in this disease. Functional MRI studies assessing therapeutic intervention in MS are still lacking; however, previous "natural history" studies in MS patients, as well as studies in healthy individuals, have certainly set the stage for the application of this technique in the fields of rehabilitation and clinical pharmacology. Such an approach is likely to provide important results which might guide future therapeutic strategies. In this perspective, it is worth mentioning that, despite motor rehabilitation being widely used in clinical practice to treat MS patients with motor impairment, a standardized procedure is not commonly applied. Considering the costs of motor rehabilitation and its impact on healthcare resources, it is critical to define the utility of a given treatment, as well as the persistence of its benefits.

References

1. Loubinoux I, Carel C, Alary F, *et al.* Within-session and between-session reproducibility of cerebral sensorimotor activation: a test–retest effect evidenced with functional magnetic resonance imaging. *J Cereb Blood Flow Metab* 2001;**21**:592–607

2. Mattay V S, Frank J A, Santha A K, *et al.* Whole-brain functional mapping with isotropic MR imaging. *Radiology* 1996;**201**:399–404

3. Yetkin FZ, McAuliffe TL, Cox R, Haughton VM. Test–retest precision of functional MR in sensory and motor task activation. *Am J Neuroradiol* 1996;**17**:95–8

4. Ward NS, Newton JM, Swayne OB, *et al.* Motor system activation after subcortical stroke depends on corticospinal system integrity. *Brain* 2006;**129**:809–19

5. Decety J, Perani D, Jeannerod M, *et al.* Mapping motor representations with positron emission tomography. *Nature* 1994;**371**:600–2

6. Porro CA, Francescato MP, Cettolo V, *et al.* Primary motor and sensory cortex activation during motor performance and motor imagery: a functional magnetic resonance imaging study. *J Neurosci* 1996;**16**:7688–98

7. Logothetis NK, Pauls J, Augath M, *et al.* Neurophysiological investigation of the basis of the fMRI signal. *Nature* 2001;**412**:150–7

8. Reddy H, Floyer A, Donaghy M, Matthews PM. Altered cortical activation with finger movement after peripheral denervation: comparison of active and passive tasks. *Exp Brain Res* 2001;**138**:484–91

9. Reddy H, Narayanan S, Woolrich M, *et al.* Functional brain reorganization for hand movement in patients with multiple sclerosis: defining distinct effects of injury and disability. *Brain* 2002;**125**:2646–57

10. Fox MD, ME Raichle. Spontaneous fluctuations in brain activity observed with functional magnetic resonance imaging. *Nat Rev Neurosci* 2007;**8**:700–11

11. Biswal B, Yetkin FZ, Haughton VM, Hyde JS. Functional connectivity in the motor cortex of resting human brain using echo-planar MRI. *Magn Reson Med* 1995;**34**:537–41

12. Damoiseaux JS, Beckmann CF, Arigita EJ, *et al.* Reduced resting-state brain activity in the "default network" in normal aging. *Cereb Cortex* 2008;**18**:1856–64

13. Lowe MJ, Phillips MD, Lurito JT, *et al.* Multiple sclerosis: low-frequency temporal blood oxygen level-dependent fluctuations indicate reduced functional connectivity: initial results. *Radiology* 2002;**224**:184–92

14. De Luca M, Smith S, De Stefano N, *et al.* Blood oxygenation level dependent contrast resting state networks are relevant to functional activity in the neocortical sensorimotor system. *Exp Brain Res* 2005;**167**:587–94

15. Wexler BE, Fulbright RK, Lacadie CM, *et al.* An fMRI study of the human cortical motor system response to increasing functional demands. *Magn Reson Imaging* 1997;**15**:385–96

16. Deiber MP, Honda M, Ibañez V, *et al.* Mesial motor areas in self-initiated versus externally triggered movements examined with fMRI: effect of movement type and rate. *J Neurophysiol* 1999;**81**:3065–77

17. VanMeter JW, Maisog JM, Zeffiro TA, *et al.* Parametric analysis of functional neuroimages: application to a variable-rate motor task. *NeuroImage* 1995;**2**:273–83

18. Dettmers C, Fink GR, Lemon RN, *et al.* Relation between cerebral activity and force in the motor areas of the human brain. *J Neurophysiol* 1995;**74**:802–15

19. Schlaug G, Knorr U, Seitz R. Inter-subject variability of cerebral activations in acquiring a motor skill: a study with positron emission tomography. *Exp Brain Res* 1994;**98**:523–34

20. Karni A, Meyer G, Jezzard P, *et al.* Functional MRI evidence for adult motor cortex plasticity during motor skill learning. *Nature* 1995;**377**:155–8

21. Rao SM, Binder JR, Bandettini PA, *et al.* Functional magnetic resonance imaging of complex human movements. *Neurology* 1993;**43**:2311–18

22. Jancke L, Shah NJ, Peters M. Cortical activations in primary and secondary motor areas for complex bimanual movements in professional pianists. *Brain Res Cogn Brain Res* 2000;**10**:177–83

23. Krings T, Topper R, Foltys H, *et al.* Cortical activation patterns during complex motor tasks in piano players and control subjects: a functional magnetic resonance imaging study. *Neurosci Lett* 2000;**278**:189–93

24. Pearce AJ, Thickbroom GW, Byrnes ML, Mastaglia FL. Functional reorganization of the corticomotor projection to the hand in skilled racquet players. *Exp Brain Res* 2000;**130**:238–43

25. Dirnberger G, Duregger C, Lindinger G, Lang W. Habituation in a simple repetitive motor task: a study with movement-related cortical potentials. *Clin Neurophysiol* 2004;**115**:378–84

26. Morgen K, Kadom N, Sawaki L, *et al.* Kinematic specificity of cortical reorganization associated with motor training. *NeuroImage* 2004;**21**:1182–7

27. Lehéricy S, Benali H, Van de Moortele PF, *et al.* Distinct basal ganglia territories are engaged in early and advanced motor sequence learning. *Proc Natl Acad Sci USA* 2005;**102**:12 566–71

28. Pantano P, Mainero C, Lenzi D, *et al.* A longitudinal fMRI study on motor activity in patients with multiple sclerosis. *Brain* 2005;**128**:2146–53

29. Reddy H, Narayanan S, Matthews PM, *et al.* Relating axonal injury to functional recovery in MS. *Neurology* 2000;**54**:236–9

30. Mezzapesa DM, Rocca MA, Rodegher M, Comi G, Filippi M. Functional cortical changes of the sensorimotor network are associated with clinical recovery in multiple sclerosis. *Hum Brain Mapp* 2008;**29**:562–73

31. Calautti C, Baron JC. Functional neuroimaging studies of motor recovery after stroke in adults: a review. *Stroke* 2003;**34**:1553–66

32. Rocca M A, Agosta F, Colombo B, *et al.* fMRI changes in relapsing–remitting multiple sclerosis patients complaining of fatigue after IFNβ-1a injection. *Hum Brain Mapp* 2007;**28**:373–82

33. Parry A M, Scott R B, Palace J, *et al.* Potentially adaptive functional changes in cognitive processing for patients with multiple sclerosis and their acute modulation by rivastigmine. *Brain* 2003;**126**:2750–60

34. Mainero C, Inghilleri M, Pantano P, *et al.* Enhanced brain motor activity in patients with MS after a single dose of 3,4-diaminopyridine. *Neurology* 2004; **62**:2044–50

35. Morgen K, Kadom N, Sawaki L, *et al.* Training-dependent plasticity in patients with multiple sclerosis. *Brain* 2004;**127**:2506–17

36. Wegner C, Filippi M, Korteweg T, *et al.* Relating functional changes during hand movement to clinical parameters in patients with multiple sclerosis in a multi-centre fMRI study. *Eur J Neurol* 2008; **15**:113–22

37. Rocca M A, Absinta M, Valsasina P, *et al.* Abnormal connectivity of the sensorimotor network in patients with MS: a multicenter fMRI study. *Hum Brain Mapp* 2009;**30**:2412–25

How to measure the effects of rehabilitation

Stefan J. Cano and Alan J. Thompson

Introduction

In recent years, the importance of evaluating the impact of rehabilitation on multiple sclerosis (MS) has become clear. However, health cannot be measured directly and instead indicators are used to represent clinical outcomes. Increasingly, outcome measures in the form of rating scales are used to score aspects of disease (e.g., symptoms) or elicit patients' opinions about aspects of health (e.g., health-related quality of life). This chapter explores the key issues surrounding measuring the effects of rehabilitation using such outcome measures. It has three aims:

- to describe the principles underlying rehabilitation including assessment, treatment planning, and methods of evaluating effectiveness
- to introduce the science behind rating scales to help MS rehabilitation clinicians choose appropriate outcome measures
- to highlight important considerations for current and future approaches to measuring the effects of rehabilitation.

Rehabilitation in MS

There can be few neurological conditions that pose the range and complexity of problems seen in MS [1] and for which the rehabilitation philosophy is more appropriate [2]. Quite apart from uncertainty about the cause and an incomplete understanding of its pathophysiology, particularly in relation to the development of irreversible disability, medications that can modify the course of the condition are still at a relatively early stage in development. This is a condition that affects people in their early adult years, and its hallmarks are those of variability and unpredictability with the only certainty being that, in time, it will cause moderate to severe disability in the majority of those affected by it. It can, and usually does, affect most parts of the central nervous system producing a complex array of symptoms which interact with each other to create challenging management issues.

The acute events or relapses, the hallmark of MS, come without warning and result in an unpredictable level of dysfunction and recovery. For most, at some point in the condition, there is an insidious progression which robs them of their mobility, independence, and often autonomy. From a social perspective, this condition is associated with high levels of unemployment and results in breakdown in relationships and a high incidence of mood disorders with an increased risk of suicide. While there is no underestimating the challenge of managing such a diverse condition, the rehabilitation philosophy provides a structure which can be useful at every stage of the condition.

Philosophy and principles

The philosophy of rehabilitation, which emphasizes patient education and self-management, is ideally suited to meet the complex and variable needs of MS. Rehabilitation aims to improve independence and quality of life by maximizing ability and participation. It has been defined by the World Health Organization as "an active process by which those disabled by injury or disease achieve a full recovery or if a full recovery is not possible realize their optimal physical, mental and social potential and are integrated into their most appropriate environment." It has also been appropriately described as an educational process that aims to increase ability, participation, and autonomy and to improve functional independence and quality of life. Reflecting on these definitions, it is clear that the philosophy of rehabilitation is as appropriate to

Multiple Sclerosis: Recovery of Function and Neurorehabilitation, eds. J. Kesselring, G. Comi, and A. J. Thompson.
Published by Cambridge University Press. © Cambridge University Press 2010.

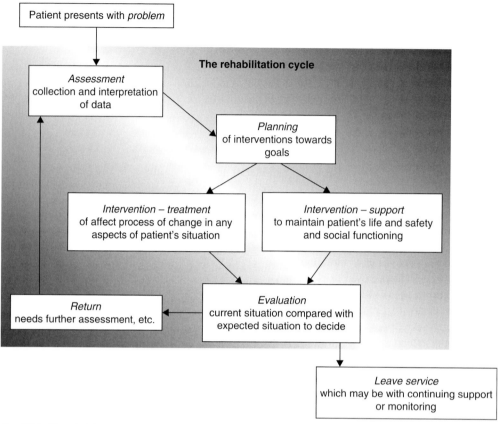

Fig. 15.1. The rehabilitation process. (From Thompson [6], courtesy of Professor D Wade, reproduced in *Clinical Neurology*, ed. T J Fowler and J W Scadding, Arnold, 2003, p 553.)

chronic progressive conditions such as MS as it is to the management of the sequelae of acute events affecting the brain, e.g., stroke and traumatic injury, or the spinal cord [3, 4].

Delivering a comprehensive rehabilitation service requires clear structure and process and these should be driven by explicit clinical standards [5]. The essential components of successful rehabilitation, all of which are underpinned by the involvement of the patient include:

(1) expert interdisciplinary assessment and problem definition;
(2) treatment planning (goal-oriented programs) and delivery;
(3) evaluation of effectiveness and reassessment (Fig. 15.1).

Interdisciplinary assessment

Patients with complex disability in whom multiple factors affecting functional performance present as a single problem will benefit from comprehensive assessment by a rehabilitation team. The term "interdisciplinary" implies an integrated approach in which the individual experts work together, often in joint sessions, towards a set of agreed goals. Team members have a fuller understanding of other members' roles and skills and can work together in a holistic way. The advantage of such an assessment is that different disciplines identify different contributory causes and can develop a coordinated plan that addresses all of them. For example, poor mobility in a patient with MS may relate to weakness, spasticity, poor balance, pain, and cognitive difficulties, requiring expert input from medical, nursing, physiotherapy, occupational therapy, and neuropsychology practitioners.

The necessary structure for such team-working is provided by the World Health Organization's international classification of impairments, disabilities, and handicaps (ICIDH) revised in 2001 as the International Classification of Functioning, Disability and

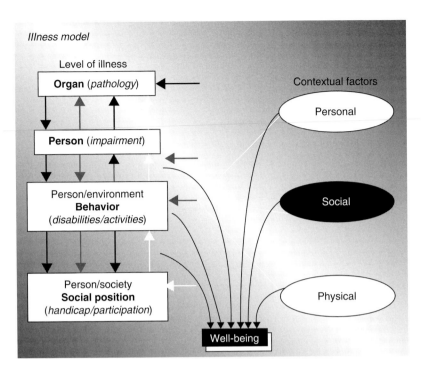

Illness model

Fig. 15.2. Illness model incorporating levels of impact based on World Health Organization, contextual factors, and their complex interactions. (From Thompson [6], courtesy of Professor D Wade, reproduced in *Clinical Neurology*, ed. T J Fowler and J W Scadding, Arnold, 2003, p 552.)

Health (ICF) [7]. The overall aim of this classification is to provide a unified and standard language and framework for the description of health and health-related states. The ICF classifies functioning at the level both of body/body part and of the whole person, and emphasizes that disablement and functioning are outcomes of interactions between health conditions and personal and contextual factors (social and physical environment) (Fig. 15.2).

Treatment planning

The treatment plan is shaped around goal-setting, a core skill for rehabilitation professionals. There is a small but growing literature on the evidence base for goal-setting. There are a number of key elements to goal-setting including the goals themselves which should be SMART (specific, measurable, achievable, relevant, and time limited) [8]. The benefits of goal-setting can be moderated by factors such as the individual's commitment to the goal, the importance of the goal to them, and their belief that the goal can be attained (self-efficacy). These factors underline the importance of the patients' involvement in the goal-setting and rehabilitation process [9–11]. In a recent

study evaluating patient involvement in goal-setting [11], 201 patients were recruited from an inpatient neurological rehabilitation unit. The study was an AB block design with each block lasting 3 months, over an 18-month period. Patients ($n = 100$) recruited in phase A were involved in standard goal-setting. Patients ($n = 101$) recruited in phase B were involved in setting their own goals. Phase B patients were provided with a workbook to help them define and prioritize their own goals. Outcomes included patients' perceptions of the relevance of goal-setting, autonomy within the process, functional outcomes, and number, type, and outcome of goals. Results showed that there were no differences between the two groups in functional outcomes. However, phase B patients reported significantly more participation-related goals, more relevant goals, and greater autonomy and satisfaction with goal-setting. Phase B patients also set fewer goals, and achieved a higher proportion of those goals.

Recent systematic reviews suggest that goal-setting improves patients' adherence to treatment regimes and improves patient performance in some specific situations, though translating this into improved outcomes is inconsistent [12].

Table 15.1 Goal-based outcome measures

Outcome Measure	Author	Date	Description
Self-Identified Goals Assessment (SIGA)	Melville and Nelson [14]	2001	Developed from research in older people, this is designed for occupational therapists to use with clients in sub-acute rehabilitation and nursing homes. It is the only goal-based outcome measure that provides a protocol to elicit patient-identified goals, based on an exploratory interview. Each goal is assigned a rating 0 (unable to do) – 10 (can do) on a visual analog scale. Post-therapy intervention the patient rates their performance and change scores are compared.
Goal Attainment Scaling (GAS)	Kirusek et al. [15]	1994	A five-point scale. The expected outcome (goal) is assigned the position of zero on the scale. Better than expected and much better than expected levels of outcome are +1 and +2 respectively. Worse than expected and much worse are –I and –2. A high level of skill is needed on the part of the therapist to quantify various levels of goal achievement. This has been used in a variety of settings, demonstrating acceptable inter-rater reliability and concurrent validity [19].
Canadian Occupational Performance Measure (COPM)	Baptiste et al. [16]	1993	Designed for occupational therapists to use with clients to set goals. Standardized instrument with semi-structured interview format that elicits patient-identified goals and quantitative patient ratings of these goals. Change scores between assessment and reassessment are the most meaningful scores derived from this assessment.
Self Assessment of Occupational Functioning (SAOF)	Baron and Curtin [17]	1990	Based on the Model of Human Occupation [20] which promotes collaborative treatment planning between patient and occupational therapist. This instrument elicits written responses to predetermined items.
Satisfaction with Performance Questionnaire	Yerxa and Baum [18]	1986	Quantitative scale of satisfaction with performance in daily occupations and community living. The scores highlight areas of decreased satisfaction with performance. Goals are negotiated between the therapist and patient on that basis.

Source: Courtesy of Dr. E. D. Playford, Institute of Neurology, Queen Square, London.

Evaluation of effectiveness

The effectiveness of rehabilitation can be viewed from several different perspectives including goal achievement, detectable changes on measures of disability, participation, and health-related quality of life. However, it is also important to appreciate that it may be much harder to measure many of the less obvious benefits of rehabilitation which relate to improving the patient's understanding, coping skills, and self-efficacy [13].

Measuring goal effectiveness

In response to the need for goals to be specific and measurable a variety of goal-based outcome measures have been developed (Table 15.1). The usefulness of these measures depends on how closely they link in to the goal-setting process. This seems to be a sound approach warranting further work to determine reliability and sensitivity as a measuring tool [21]. Goal achievement may also be audited as part of an integrated care pathway which has also been shown to be quite effective in the appropriate setting [22].

Measuring outcome

Evaluating the outcome from interventions at any stage of MS is extremely challenging but also of the greatest importance if there is to be ongoing improvement in the process and impact of rehabilitation [23].

Evaluating the effect on the patient requires the use of outcome measures that are scientifically sound (reliable, valid, and responsive) and clinically useful (short, simple, etc.) [24]. The measure must be appropriate to the sample under study and the intervention being evaluated. In the case of neurorehabilitation, the potential effects are not expected at the levels of pathology and impairment but rather in improving activity and participation (ICF) and in enhancing the broader, more patient-oriented areas of quality of life, coping skills, and self-efficacy. It is particularly important that the perspective of the patient is incorporated into the measure in a scientifically sound manner.

The standard outcome measure in therapeutic trials in MS, Kurtzke's expanded disability status scale (EDSS), is inappropriate for evaluating rehabilitation not only because of its scientific limitations (particularly poor responsiveness) but also because it does not measure many of the relevant areas, such as fatigue and cognition, and does not incorporate the perspective of the patient [25]. Consequently, a number of generic measures of disability/ability (Barthel Index, BI) [26], Functional Independence Measure (FIM) [27], Functional Independence Measure/Functional Assessment Measure (FIM/FAM) [28], participation/handicap (London Handicap Scale, LHS) [29], and health-related quality of life (The Short Form 36 Health Survey Questionnaire, SF-36) [30] have been used in MS rehabilitation (Table 15.2). Generic measures have the advantage of being able to compare outcome across a range of different conditions but may not be able to detect specific aspects of any given condition and may therefore lack responsiveness.

More recently, a number of MS-specific measures have been developed that are currently undergoing evaluation. These address disability (UK Disability Scale [48]; MS Functional Composite – PASAT, nine-hole peg test, and 10-meter timed walk), health-related quality of life which incorporates the patients' perspective (MS Quality of Life Inventory, Functional Assessment of MS, FAMS [49], MS QoL 54 [44]; Leeds QoL Scale; [50]; and specific aspects of MS (Multiple Sclerosis Impact Scale, MSIS-29); measuring the physical and psychological impact of MS [42, 51–53]; 12-Item MS Walking Scale (MSWS-12) [43]; and the 88-Item Multiple Sclerosis Spasticity Scale (MSSS-88) [46].

The measures that have received the most attention (and evaluation) include the FAMS, MS QoL 54, MSIS-29, and MSWS-12 [54]. Whereas the first two measures are derived from oncology and generic scales respectively, the MSIS-29 and MSWS-12 have been extensively evaluated in a number of MS centers worldwide. They have been shown to be a reliable, valid measure which is responsive to change and the MSIS-29 has been shown to compare favorably to the MS Functional Composite [42, 43, 51–53, 55–57]. Importantly these scales can also be used with proxies of patients with MS in both cross-sectional and longitudinal studies – a valuable attribute in the more severely disabled and cognitively impaired population [58, 59].

Measures: science and selection

Researchers in MS rehabilitation frequently have to choose one scale from among many potential candidates [60]. Unfortunately, no one measure is applicable to all situations. Measures should be clinically useful and scientifically sound. Clinical usefulness refers to the successful incorporation of an instrument into clinical practice and its appropriateness to the study sample. Scientific soundness refers to the demonstration of reliable, valid, and responsive measurement of the outcome of interest. Clinical usefulness does not guarantee scientific soundness, and vice versa.

When considering the quality of a rating scale we recommend examining at least six measurement properties: data quality, scaling assumptions, acceptability, reliability, validity, and responsiveness (Table 15.3).

Data quality

Indicators of data quality, such as percent item non-response and percent computable scores, determine the extent to which an instrument can be incorporated into a clinical setting. These indicators, like all psychometric properties, vary across samples [61]. If the measure is patient-report, these indicators reflect respondents' understanding and acceptance of a measure and help to identify items that may be irrelevant, confusing, or upsetting to patients [61]. If the measure is clinician-report, these indicators reflect the ability to incorporate a measure into a clinical setting. When there are large amounts of missing data for items scores for scales cannot be reliably estimated.

Table 15.2 Levels of measurement and examples of generic and MS-specific measures

Term	Definition	Outcome measures	
		Generic	MS-specific
Impairment	Clinical signs/symptoms resulting from nervous system damage		Functional system of EDSS [37] MS Functional Composite Scale (T25 FW, 9HP, PASAT) [38]
Disability (Ability)	Limitations on activities of daily living from neurological impairment	Barthel Index (BI) [26] Functional Independence Measure [27]/ Functional Assessment Measure (FIM/FAM) [28]	Guy's Neurological Disability Scale (GNDS) [39] MS Impairment Scale (MSIS) [40]
Handicap (Participation)	Social and environmental consequences from impairment and disability	London Handicap Scale (LHS) [29]	Environmental Status Scale (ESS) [41]
Health-related quality of life (QoL)	The satisfaction that people have with health-related dimensions of life, from their own perspective	Short Form-36 (SF-36) [30] Nottingham Health Profile [31] Sickness Impact Profile [32]	MS Impact Scale, MS Walking Scale [42, 43] MSQoL54[a], Functional Assessment of MS QoL Instrument (FAMS) [44][a], MS QoL Inventory (MSQLI)[a], Functional Assessment of MS
Emotional well-being		General Health Questionnaire [33]	
Symptoms, e.g., fatigue	Overwhelming sense of tiredness or exhaustion in excess of what might be expected from level of activity	Fatigue Impact Scale [34] Fatigue Severity Scale [35]	MS-Specific Fatigue Scale [45]
Spasticity	Velocity-dependent increase in tonic stretch reflexes	Ashworth Scale [36]	MS Spasticity Scale (MSSS-88) [46]

Notes: [a]Developed from existing scales.
Source: From [47] *Multiple Sclerosis: The Guide to Treatment and Management*, 6th edn, 2006, eds. C H Polman, A J Thompson, T J Murray, A C Bowling, J H Noseworthy, Demos Medical Publishing, New York, p 72.

Scaling assumptions

Tests of scaling assumptions determine whether it is legitimate to generate scores for an instrument using the algorithms proposed by the developers. Items can be summed without weighting or standardization when they measure at the same point on the scale (have similar mean scores), contribute similarly to the variance of the total score (have similar variances), measure a common underlying construct (the items must be internally consistent), and are correctly grouped into scales (hypothesized item groupings

are supported by techniques including factor analysis and examination of item convergent and discriminant validity) [62].

Targeting

Targeting is the extent to which the spectrum of health measured by a scale matches the distribution of health in the study sample and is determined simply by examining score distributions [63]. Ideally, the observed scores from a sample should span the entire range of the scale, the mean score should be

Table 15.3 Key features of some of the core psychometric requirements with brief definitions

Psychometric property	Definition
Data quality	Completeness of data and score distributions
Scaling assumptions	Items in a scale should measure a common underlying construct Items in a scale should contain a similar proportion of information concerning the construct being measured Items should be correctly grouped into scales
Targeting	The extent to which a scale is acceptable as a measure for the sample
Reliability	
Internal consistency	The extent to which items in a scale measure the same construct
Test–retest reproducibility	The stability of a scale between repeat administrations of the scale on two occasions
Validity	
Content validity	The extent to which the content of a scale is representative of the conceptual domain it is intended to cover
Construct validity	Accumulation of evidence that the scale measures a single construct, that items can be combined to form a summary score, and that subscales measure distinct but related constructs
Responsiveness	Ability of a scale to detect clinically significant change

near the scale mid-point, and floor and ceiling effects (percent of the sample having the minimum and maximum score respectively) should be small. McHorney and Tarlov recommend floor and ceiling effects should be <15% [64].

Reliability

The reliability of a measure is the degree to which it is free from random error. If no random error is present, the reliability is 1.0; this number approaches zero as the relative amount of random error increases. Reliability is an important property of a rating scale, because it is essential to establish that any changes observed in patient groups are due to the intervention or disease and not to problems in the measure [65]. In general, there are two approaches commonly used to evaluate the reliability of rating scales: internal consistency and test–retest.

Internal consistency is a function of the number of items and their covariation within a scale measuring a construct (e.g., symptoms, psychological functioning) [66]. It can be assessed in a number of different ways. However, Cronbach's coefficient alpha [67] is the most commonly used to estimate the reliability of a measured based on internal consistency. The criterion

for adequate reliability is Cronbach's alpha coefficient >0.80 [67].

The second approach commonly used to evaluate reliability is test–retest or reproducibility. This form of reliability assesses whether a measure yields the same results on repeated applications, when respondents have not changed on the construct being measured. For continuous data, the intraclass correlation coefficient (ICC) is often computed to estimate test–retest reliability, in order to assess the extent to which individuals who scored high on the initial assessment also tend to score high on the repeated assessment, and vice versa [68]. The criterion for adequate reliability is ICC > 0.80 [69].

Validity

In contrast to reliability, validity is, in general, the extent to which an instrument measures what it intends to measure. Validity involves gathering information in the process of developing or using a measure relevant to its specific purpose or set of purposes. There are two main types of validity that are particularly relevant to health measurement: content validity and construct validity.

Content validity refers to how well a measure covers important parts of the health components that are required for the measure's intended purpose.

In order to evaluate content validity, qualitative methods are used as opposed to statistical criteria, using evidence (e.g., literature, expert opinion, patients' views) obtained during the development of the measure [70].

Construct validity involves specifying the dimensions of a construct, and the expected relations of the dimensions to each other, both internally and externally [71]. Construct validity is evaluated by hypothesizing how a measure should perform and confirming or not these hypotheses [66]. One of the most common ways to assess this in health measurement is "convergent and discriminant validity"; the former offers convergent evidence that the measure is related to other measures (or other variables) of the same construct on theoretical grounds, and the latter provides discriminant evidence that the measure is not related to other distinct constructs [72].

Responsiveness

If a new measure is to be used in evaluating the effects of a given intervention (e.g., interferon beta in MS), the responsiveness of the measure needs to be evaluated. Responsiveness, a type of validity, can be considered as the ability of a measure to detect significant change over time, such as an indication of a therapeutic effect or a meaningful reduction in symptoms from the patient's perspective. It is an important property of a measure that is used to evaluate change over time [69]. To be useful, the user of a rating scale must know the degree to which a measure can detect differences in outcomes that are important [68].

There are two major components to responsiveness: "internal" and "external" [73]. Internal responsiveness is the ability of the scales of a measure to detect change over a set time period. The three most common ways of calculating this are: effect size [74], t-test comparisons, and the responsiveness statistic [75]. However, this type of responsiveness only provides a statistically significant change over time which may not be synonymous with clinically important change [74]. Therefore, "external responsiveness" is used to reflect the extent to which change in a measure relates to corresponding change in a reference clinical or health status measure. External responsiveness of an instrument can be calculated by comparing to a reference measure that is regarded as an accepted indication of change [73], and can be expressed in terms of receiver operating characteristics, correlation, and regression models. Cohen defined an effect size of 0.20 as small, one of 0.50 as moderate, and one of 0.80 or greater as large [74].

Considerations for current and future approaches to measuring rehabilitation effectiveness

Current approaches

The importance of appropriately measuring the effectiveness of treatments on health outcomes are starting to becoming increasingly recognized as important [76–78]. Of particular relevance are the recommendations currently being finalized by the US Food and Drug Administration (FDA) concerning patient reported rating scales used in clinical trials, to satisfy minimum performance standards that we have described above and that will have implications for all types of rating scales, not just those that are patient reported [79]. So, why is this important? An illustration of some of our own work and experiences over the last 15 years may help to support the argument.

First, we would suggest that MS research continues to use outcome measures proven scientifically poor. This is clearly illustrated through even the most superficial of literature reviews. For example, using PubMed we identified randomized control trials (RCTs) in MS published over a 20-year period (1987–2007). Of the 68 relevant articles, we found that 59% of these had used a rating scale. However, only six (15%) of those articles had included scales that had any supporting psychometric evidence.

Second, many widely used scales do not meet basic psychometric assumptions. For example, the Medical Outcomes Study 36-item Short Form Health Survey (SF-36) [77] is the most widely used generic measure of health status in clinical research, and has been widely used in MS research. As such, it is widely used in neuroscience research as it generally perceived to be a "validated" tool. However, our own research has raised concerns about its use in neurological disorders (summarized in Table 15.4) [80–84]. In particular, there is a consistent finding in all of the studies that show the physical (PCS) and mental component summary scores (MCS) not to be valid indicators of physical and mental health. Despite this, we were able to identify 490 studies of neurologic diseases that have used the SF-36. Of these, 322 (66%) report the PCS and MCS scores.

Finally, statistical adequacy does not automatically confirm clinical validity. One good example from

Table 15.4 Summary of our previous research into the SF-36 in six neurologic conditions

	MS	Stroke	PD	CD	ALS	Cx spine
SF-36 scales						
Physical functioning	N	Y	Y	Y	Y	N
Role–physical	N	N	N	N	N	N
Bodily pain	N	N	Y	Y	Y	Y
General health	Y	Y	N	Y	Y	Y
Vitality	Y	Y	Y	Y	Y	Y
Social functioning	Y	Y	N	Y	Y	Y
Role–emotional	N	N	N	N	N	N
Mental health	Y	Y	Y	Y	Y	Y
Physical component score	N	N	N	N	N	N
Mental component score	N	N	N	N	N	N

Notes: Y, psychometric evidence supporting use; N, psychometric evidence against use.
MS, multiple sclerosis; PD, Parkinson's disease; CD, cervical dystonia; ALS, amyotrophic lateral sclerosis; Cx spine, people undergoing cervical spinal surgery.

our own research focused on the most widely used fatigue rating scale currently available (currently used in over 70 studies). We conducted two independent phases of research. In the first phase, we carried out qualitative evaluations of validity through expert opinion ($n = 30$ neurologists, therapists, nurses, and clinical researchers). The second phase involved a standard quantitative psychometric evaluation ($n = 333$ MS patients). The findings from Phase 2 implied that the fatigue measure in question was reliable and valid. However, the Phase 1 qualitative study did not support either the content or face validity. In fact, expert opinion agreed with the scale placement of only 23 items (58%), and classified all of its 40 items as non-specific to fatigue (further information available from authors).

Our research findings support the need for the stringent quantitative and qualitative requirements in the FDA draft guidelines. Researchers in MS still use rating scales proven to be scientifically weak, or report scores for scales that are not valid. Scales continue to be developed without adequate recourse to recognized methods of scale construction, and widely used scales do not meet even the most basic psychometric assumptions. It is vital that awareness of the critical role played by rating scales increases. They must be proven to be clinically meaningful and scientifically rigorous for valid interpretations of clinical studies. As

such, more clinicians need to be formally trained in rating scale methods to ensure that health measurement develops clinically meaningful scales, and journal editors, reviewers, and grant-giving bodies should include, or have direct access to, people with expertise in rating scale development and evaluation.

Future approaches

Health outcomes measurement is a rapidly growing field, and techniques that could be applied to improve measuring the effectiveness of MS rehabilitation are being rapidly developed and advanced.

Two such approaches are Rasch measurement [85] and Item Response Theory (IRT) [86] methods that are being increasingly used in outcome measure development as a means to increase the clinical utility of new rating scales for individual patients. Fundamentally, these methods differ from traditional psychometric approaches as their focus is the relationship between a person's measurement and their probability of responding to an item, rather than the relationship between a person's measurement and their observed scale total score. This leads to the legitimate summing of items to produce total scores and in turn the total scores produce interval-level measures from ordinal level rating scale data [87, 88], which improves the accuracy with which we can measure clinical change. In addition, these methods provide estimates for patients (and items) that are independent of the sampling distribution of items (and patients). Among other benefits, this allows for accurate estimates suitable for individual person measurement. This can help to directly inform patient monitoring, management, and treatment. Other advantages include item banking, scale equating, computerized scale administration, and the handling of missing data [89–91].

Conclusions

The effectiveness of MS rehabilitation can be measured from several different perspectives including goal achievement, detectable changes on measures of disability, participation, and health-related quality of life. As such, there are number of clinician- and patient-reported outcome measures available for measuring different aspects of effectiveness. When assessing available scales, MS rehabilitation clinicians should evaluate their clinical usefulness and scientific soundness with respect to a particular study. There are a number of scientific criteria relating to the reliability, validity, and responsiveness of outcome measures that should be checked for, and importantly these are now becoming formal requirements for their use in clinical research. Finally, the introduction of new health measurement methods will pave the way for more informative, detailed assessments of the effectiveness of MS rehabilitation. Clinicians and researchers should start to familiarize themselves with these methods in order to maximize their potential.

References

1. Kesselring J, Beer S. Symptomatic therapy and neurorehabilitation in multiple sclerosis. *Lancet Neurol* 2005;**4**:643–52

2. Thompson A J (ed). *Neurological Rehabilitation of Multiple Sclerosis*. London: Taylor & Francis, 2006

3. Ward C D, Phillips M, Smith A, *et al*. Multidisciplinary approaches in progressive neurological disease: can we do better? *J Neurol Neurosurg Psychiatry* 2003;**74** (Suppl 4):8–12

4. Thompson A J. Neurorehabilitation in multiple sclerosis: foundations, facts and fiction. *Curr Opin Neurol* 2005;**18**:267–71

5. Turner-Stokes L, Williams H, Abraham R, *et al*. Clinical standards for inpatient specialist rehabilitation services in the UK. *Clin Rehab* 2000;**14**:468–80

6. Thompson A J. Neurological rehabilitation. In: Fowler T J, Scadding J W, eds. Clinical neurology. London: Arnold, 2003:551–6

7. World Health Organization. *International classification of functioning, disability and health* (ICIDH2). http://www3.who.int/icf/icftemplate.cfm

8. Locke E A, Latham G P. Building a practically useful theory of goal setting and task motivation: a 35-year odyssey. *Am Psychol* 2002;**57**:705–17

9. Holliday R C, Antoun M, Playford E D. A survey of goal-setting methods used in rehabilitation. *Neurorehab Neural Repair* 2005; **19**:227–31

10. Holliday R C, Ballinger C, Playford E D. Goal setting in neurological rehabilitation: patient's perspective. *Disabil Rehabil* 2007;**29**:389–94

11. Holliday R C, Cano S J, Freeman J A, Playford E D. Should patients participate in clinical decision making? An optimized balance block design controlled study of goal setting in a rehabilitation unit. *J Neurol Neurosurg Psychiatry* 2007;**78**:576–80

12. Levack W M M, Taylor K, Siegert R J, *et al*. Is goal-planning in rehabilitation effective? A systematic review. *Clin Rehab* 2006;**20**:739–55

13. Edwards S G M, Playford E D, Hobart J C, *et al*. Comparison of physician outcome measures and patients' perception of benefits of inpatient neurorehabilitation. *BMJ* 2002;**324**:1493

14. Melville L, Nelson D. The Melville–Nelson occupational therapy evaluation system for skilled nursing facilities and sub-acute rehabilitation, 2001. www.mco.edu/allh/OT/melville-nelson.html

15. Kirusek T J, Smith A, Cardillo J E. Goal attainment scaling: applications theory and measurement. Hillsdale, NJ: Lawrence Erlbaum, 1994

16. Baptiste S, Law M, Pollock N, *et al*. Canadian Occupational Performance Measure (COPM). *World Fed Occup Ther Bull* 1993;**28**:47–51

17. Baron K B, Curtin C. A manual for use with the self assessment of occupational functioning. Chicago, IL: University of Illinois, 1990

18. Yerxa E, Baum S. Engagement in daily occupations and life satisfaction among young people with spinal cord injuries. *Occup Ther J Res* 1986;**6**:272–83

19. Emmerson G J, Neely M A. Two adaptable, valid, and reliable data-collection measures: goal attainment scaling and the semantic differential. *Counsel Psychologist* 1988;**16**:261–71

20. Kielhofner G. Model of human occupation: theory and application. 2nd ed. Philadelphia, PA: Lippincott Williams Wilkins, 1995

21. Hurn J, Kneebone I, Cropley M. Goal setting as an outcome measure: a systematic review. *Clin Rehab* 2006;**20**:756–72

22. Rossiter D A, Edmondson A, Al-Shahi R, *et al.* Integrated care pathways in multiple sclerosis rehabilitation: completing the audit cycle. *Mult Scler* 1998;**4**:85–9

23. Thompson A J. The effectiveness of neurological rehabilitation in multiple sclerosis. *J Rehab Res Develop* 2000;**37**:455–61

24. Hobart J C, Lamping D L, Thompson A J. Evaluating neurological outcome measures: the bare essentials. *J Neurol Neurosurg Psychiatry* 1996;**60**:127–30

25. Hobart J C, Freeman J A, Thompson A J. Kurtzke scales revisited: the application of psychometric methods to clinical intuition. *Brain* 2000;**123**:1027–40

26. Mahoney F l, Barthel D W. Functional evaluation: the Barthel Index (BI). *Maryland State Med J* 1965; **14**:61–5

27. Granger C V, Cotter A C, Hamilton B B, *et al.* Functional assessment scales: a study of persons with multiple sclerosis. *Arch Phys Med Rehab* 1990;**71**:870–5

28. Hobart J, Lamping D, Freeman J, *et al.* Measuring neurology: is bigger better? Comparative measurement properties of the functional independence measure (FIM) and Barthel index. *Neurology* 1997;**48**:A235

29. Harwood R H, Rogers A, Dickinson E, *et al.* Measuring handicap: London Handicap Scale – a new outcome measure for chronic disease. *Qual Health Care* 1994;**3**:11–16

30. Ware J E, Sherbourne C D. The MOS 36-item short form health survey (SF-36). 1. Conceptual framework and item selection. *Med Care* 1992;**30**:473–83

31. Hunt S M, McKenna S P, McEwen J, Williams J, Papp E. The Nottingham Health Profile: subjective health status and medical consultations. *Soc Sci Med* 1981;**15**:221–9

32. Bergner M, Bobbitt R A, Carter W B, *et al.* The Sickness Impact Profile: development and final revision of a health status measure. *Med Care* 1981;**19**:787–805

33. Goldberg D, Hillier V F. A scaled version of the general health questionnaire. *Psychol Medi* 1979; **9**:139–45

34. Fisk J D, Pontefract A, Ritvo P G, *et al.* The impact of fatigue on patients with multiple sclerosis. *Canad J Neurol Sci* 1994;**21**:9–14

35. Krupp L B, LaRocca N C, Muir-Nash J, *et al.* The fatigue severity scale applied to patients with multiple sclerosis and systemic lupus erythematosus. *Arch Neurol* 1989;**46**:1121–3

36. Ashworth B. Preliminary trial of carisoprodal in multiple sclerosis. *Practitioner* 1964;**192**:540–2

37. Kurtzke J F. Rating neurologic impairment in multiple sclerosis: an expanded disability status scale (EDSS). *Neurology* 1983;**33**:1444–52

39. Sharrack B, Hughes R A C. The Guy's Neurological Disability Scale (GNDS): a new disability measure for multiple sclerosis. *Multiple Sclerosis* 1999; **5**:223–233

40. Ravnborg M, Gronbech-Jensen M, Jonsson A. The MS impairment scale: a pragmatic approach to the assessment of impairment in patients with multiple sclerosis. *Mult Scler* 1997;**3**:31–42

41. Stewart G, Kidd D, Thompson A J. The assessment of handicap: an evaluation of the Environmental Status Scale. *Disabil Rehab* 1995;**17**:312–16

42. Hobart J C, Lamping D L, Fitzpatrick R, Riazi A, Thompson A J. The Multiple Sclerosis Impact Scale (MSIS-29): a new patient-based outcome measure. *Brain* 2001;**124**:962–73

43. Hobart J C, Riazi A, Lamping D L, Fitzpatrick R, Thompson A J. Measuring the impact of MS on walking ability: the 12-item MS walking scale (MSWS-12). *Neurology* 2003;**60**; 31–6

44. Vickrey B G, Hays R D, Harooni R, *et al.* A health-related quality of life measure for multiple sclerosis. *Qual Life Res* 1995;**4**:187–206

45. Krupp L B, Coyle P K, Doscher C, *et al.* Fatigue therapy in multiple sclerosis: results of a double-blind randomized parallel trial of amantadine, pemoline, and placebo. *Neurology* 1995;**45**:1956–61

46. Hobart J C, Riazi A, Thompson A J, *et al.* Getting the measure of spasticity in MS: the MS Spasticity Scale (MSSS-89). *Brain* 2006;**129**:224–34

47. Polman C H, Thompson A J, Murray T J, *et al.* (eds). Multiple sclerosis: the guide to treatment and management. 6th ed. New York, Demos Medical Publishing Multiple Sclerosis International Foundation: 2006

48. Expanded Disability Status Scale (EDSS). Available online at www.mstrust.org.uk

49. Cella D F, Dineen K, Arnason B, *et al.* Validation of the functional assessment of multiple sclerosis quality of life instrument. *Neurology* 1996;**47**:129–39

50. Ford H L, Gerry E, Tennant A, *et al.* Developing a disease specific quality of life measure for people with multiple sclerosis. *Clin Rehab* 2001;**15**:247–58

51. Riazi A, Hobart J C, Lamping D L, Fitzpatrick R, Thompson A J. Multiple sclerosis impact scale (MSIS-29): reliability and validity in hospital-based samples. *J Neurol Neurosurg Psychiatry* 2002;**73**:701–4

52. Hobart J C, Riazi A, Lamping D L, Fitzpatrick R, Thompson A J. Improving the evaluation of therapeutic interventions in multiple sclerosis:

development of a patient-based outcome measure. *Health Technol Assess* 2004;**8**(9):1–60

53. Hobart J C, Riazi A, Lamping D L, Fitzpatrick R, Thompson A J. How responsive is the Multiple Sclerosis Impact Scale (MSIS-29)? A comparison with other self-report scales. *J Neurol Neurosurg Psychiatry* 2005;**76**:1539–43

54. Fischer J S, LaRocca N G, Miller D M, *et al.* Recent developments in the assessment of quality of life in multiple sclerosis (MS). *Mult Scler* 1999;**5**:251–9

55. McGuigan C, Hutchinson M. The Multiple Sclerosis Impact Scale (MSIS-29) is a reliable and sensitive measure. *J Neurol Neurosurg Psychiatry* 2004;**75**:266–9

56. Hoogervorst J N P, Jelles B, Polman C H, *et al.* Multiple Sclerosis Impact Scale (MSIS-29): relation to established measures of impairment and disability. *Mult Scler* 2004;**10**:569–74

57. Costelloe L, O'Rourke K, Kearney H, *et al.* Does the patient know best? Significant change in the multiple sclerosis impact scale (MSIS-29 physical) over four years. *Mult Scler* 2006;**12**:S86, P328 (ECTRIMS 2006 abstract)

58. Van der Linden F A H, Kragt J J, Klein M, *et al.* Psychometric evaluation of the multiple sclerosis impact scale (MSIS-29) for proxy use. *J Neurol Neurosurg Psychiatry* 2005;**76**:1677–81

59. Van der Linden F A H, Kragt J J, Hobart J C, *et al.* Longitudinal proxy measurements in multiple sclerosis: agreements between patients and their partners on the impact of MS on daily life over a period of two years. *Mult Scler* 2006;**12**:S86, P330 (ECTRIMS 2006 abstract)

60. Wade D T. *Measurement in Neurological Rehabilitation*. Oxford: Oxford University Press, 1992

61. McHorney C A, Ware J E J, Lu J F R, Sherbourne C D. The MOS 36-Item Short-Form Health Survey (SF-36). III. Tests of data quality, scaling assumptions and reliability across diverse patient groups. *Med Care* 1994;**32**:40–66

62. Ware J E J, Harris W J, Gandek B, Rogers B W, Reese P R. MAP-R for windows: multitrait/multi-item analysis program – revised user's guide. Boston, MA: Health Assessment Laboratory, 1997

63. Lohr K N, Aaronson N K, Alonso J, *et al.* Evaluating quality of life and health status instruments: development of scientific review criteria. *Clin Ther* 1996;**18**:979–92

64. McHorney C A, Tarlov A R. Individual-patient monitoring in clinical practice: are available health status surveys adequate? *Qual Life Res* 1995;**4**:293–307

65. Fitzpatrick R, Davey C, Buxton M J, Jones D R. Evaluating patient-based outcome measures for use in clinical trials. *Health Technol Assess* 1998;**2**(14). www.ncchta.org/project/934.asp

66. Hays R D, Anderson R, Revicki D A. Psychometric considerations in evaluating health-related quality of life measures. *Qual Life Res* 1993;**2**:441–9

67. Cronbach L J. Coefficient alpha and the internal structure of tests. *Psychometrika* 1951;**16**:297–334

68. Deyo R A, Diehr P, Patrick D L. Reproducibility and responsiveness of health status measures: statistics and strategies for evaluation. *Control Clin Trials* 1991;**12**:142s–158s

69. Nunnally J C, Bernstein I H. Psychometric theory. 3rd ed. New York: McGraw-Hill, 1994

70. Cronbach L J. Validity on parole: how can we go straight? *New Direct Testing Meas* 1980;**5**:99–108

71. Kaplan R M, Bush J W, Barry C C. Health status: types of validity and the index of well-being. *Health Serv Res* 1976;**11**(Winter):478–507

72. Campbell D T, Fiske D W. Convergent and discriminant validation by the multitrait–multimethod matrix. *Psychol Bull* 1959;**56**:81–105

73. Husted J, Cook R, Farewell V, Gladman D. Methods for assessing responsiveness: a critical review and recommendations. *J Clin Epidemiol* 2000;**53**:459–68

74. Kazis L E, Anderson J J, Meenan R F. Effect sizes for interpreting changes in health status. *Med Care* 1989;**27**(3 suppl):S178–S189

75. Guyatt G H, Walter S, Norman G. Measuring change over time: assessing the usefulness of evaluative instruments. *J Chron Dis* 1987;**40**:171–8

76. Food and Drug Administration. Patient reported outcome measures: use in medical product development to support labeling claims, 2006. www.fda.gov/cber/gdlns/prolbl.pdf

77. European Medicines Agency. Reflection paper on the regulatory guidance for the use of the health-related quality of life (HRQL) measures in the evaluation of medicinal products. London: European Medicines Agency, 2006

78. Revicki D. FDA draft guidance and health-outcomes research. *Lancet* 2007;**369**:540–2

79. Ware J E J, Snow K K, Kosinski M, Gandek B. SF-36 Health Survey manual and interpretation guide. Boston, MA: Nimrod Press, 1993

80. Hobart J C, Freeman J A, Lamping D L, Fitzpatrick R, Thompson A J. The SF-36 in multiple sclerosis (MS): why basic assumptions must be tested. *J Neurol Neurosurg Psychiatry* 2001;**71**:363–70

81. Hobart J C, Williams L, Moran K, Thompson A J. Quality of life measurement after stroke: uses and abuses of the SF-36. *Stroke* 2002;**33**:1348–56

82. Jenkinson C, Hobart J C, Chandola T, *et al.* Use of the short form health survey (SF-36) in patients with amyotrophic lateral sclerosis: tests of data quality, score reliability, response rate and scaling assumptions. *J Neurol* 2002;**249**:178–83

83. Cano S, Thompson A, Fitzpatrick R, *et al.* Evidence-based guidelines for using the Short Form 36 in cervical dystonia. *Mov Disord* 2006;**22**:122–7

84. Hagell P, Törnqvist A, Hobart J. Testing the SF-36 in Parkinson's disease: implications for reporting rating scale data. *J Neurol Neurosurg Psychiatry* 2008;**255**:246–54

85. Rasch G. Probabilistic models for some intelligence and attainment tests. Copenhagen: Danish Institute for Education Research, 1960

86. Lord F M, Novick M R. Statistical theories of mental test scores. Reading, MA: Addison-Wesley, 1968

87. Wright B D, Stone M H. Best test design: Rasch measurement. Chicago: MESA, 1979

88. Wright B D, Linacre J M. Observations are always ordinal: measurements, however, must be interval. *Arch Phys Med Rehab* 1989;**70**:857–60

89. Wainer H, Dorans N J, Flaugher R, *et al.* (eds). Computerized adaptive testing: a primer. Hillsdale, NJ: Lawrence Erlbaum, 1990

90. Revicki D, Cella D. Health status assessment for the twenty-first century: item response theory, item banking and computer adaptive testing. *Qual Life Res* 1997;**6**:595–600

91. Linacre J. Computer-adaptive testing: a methodology whose time has come. In: Chae S, Kang U, Jeon E, Linacre J, eds. Development of computerized middle school achievement tests. Seoul: Komesa Press, 2000:1–58

Chapter 6

Value and limits of rehabilitation in multiple sclerosis

Serafin Beer

Introduction

Multiple sclerosis must be regarded as a highly complex disease. The complexity is illustrated by the various underlying pathologies (inflammation, axonal loss, demyelination, dystrophy) and the highly variable course with different disease patterns (relapsing–remitting, secondary progressive, primary progressive MS). This variability together with an almost unpredictable change of disease activity makes an accurate evaluation and appropriate management a very difficult task. In the long term, the majority of MS patients will gradually accumulate pathological changes at different sites of the central nervous system (CNS) leading to a broad pattern of symptoms and functional deficits and disabilities with complex interferences. Uncertainty of the highly variable and unpredictable course of disease makes it difficult for the affected patients coping with the disease [1].

Immunomodulatory therapies (interferon beta, glatirameracetate, mitoxantrone, natalizumab) have been shown to significantly decrease relapse rate and the appearance of new lesions, and also to some extent to slow clinical progression in patients with relapsing–remitting and, less markedly, in secondary progressive MS [2, 3]. A substantial number of MS patients with primary progressive course (15–20%), however, do not respond to immunomodulatory agents. In addition, existing symptoms and functional deficits are not reversed, and in general, progression can only be delayed but not completely stopped by these therapies [4, 5]. Thus, accumulation of deficits and disabilities continues, even though at a lower rate. Symptomatic therapies have been shown to be helpful, reducing or alleviating certain complaints and functional deficits. Drug treatment for most prevalent and disabling symptoms (fatigue, paralysis, ataxia, etc.), however, is generally not very effective or not available. Finally, use of immunomodulatory drugs and symptomatic treatment may have a negative impact on function and quality of life due to disabling side effects [6].

Even taking into account the positive effects of drug treatments and patients with a benign course (10%) [7], the majority of MS patients will therefore experience a gradual decline in personal activities, social participation, and quality of life [8]. About 50% of MS patients will lose their mobility within 15 years after disease onset, with a high unemployment rate of up to 80%, many of them losing their jobs within the first 5 years after disease onset [9, 10]. The progression of disability, especially the deterioration of cognitive functions and neuropsychiatric symptoms, has also an important negative impact on quality of life of caregivers [11]. Considering the early onset of disease (mean 28–32 years), MS patients are afflicted with these dramatic changes during a generally very important and active period of live (third to fifth decade), with a biographic disruption of affected persons and their families in terms of employment and income [10]. Due to their long survival time (median over 40 years) [12], MS patients and their relatives have to bear the burden of disease for a very long time-span. The early appearance and high prevalence of disabilities and unemployment in this population also has a significant negative impact on socio-economic areas. Yearly direct and indirect costs for MS patients are estimated to average €18 000 in patients with lower disabilities (expanded disability status scale [EDSS] < 4.0), €36 500 in patients with moderate disabilities (EDSS 4.0–6.5), and €62 000 in patients with severe disabilities (EDSS > 7.0), disability level correlating closely with costs, incapacity to work, and quality of life [13, 14].

Multiple Sclerosis: Recovery of Function and Neurorehabilitation, eds. J. Kesselring, G. Comi, and A. J. Thompson.
Published by Cambridge University Press. © Cambridge University Press 2010.

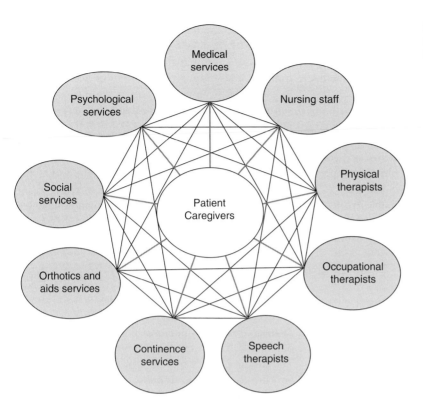

Fig. 16.1. Patient-centered, multidisciplinary network in MS rehabilitation.

Conceptual value of rehabilitation

Considering the complex impact of MS on different personal, social, and economic aspects of life, and despite the undisputed benefit of disease-modifying therapies, there is a continuing need for an individualized comprehensive, multidisciplinary long-term management, which constitutes the basic concept of rehabilitation (Fig. 16.1).

Rehabilitation is an active process aimed at enabling persons with disabilities to reach or maintain their optimal physical, sensory, intellectual, psychological, and social functional level, providing them with the tools they need to attain independence and self-determination. Another important key issue is to provide disabled people with relevant information for appropriate informed decisions [15]. The aim of rehabilitation is thus to allow disabled people to live with the highest possible independence and best quality of life within the limits of the disease [16]. Considering this definition and goals, rehabilitation should be based on a comprehensive, multidisciplinary, patient-centered, goal-oriented approach. Measures targeting at these aims are: assessment of physical, psychological, and social needs of the individual and

environment (context factors); assisting physical, psychological, and social adaptation to disability and handicap; facilitating independence in daily activities; maximizing life satisfaction for both patient and carers; empowering the person; and prevention of secondary complications [17]. Specific education and counseling of patients (and carers) about the disease, treatment options, and learning strategies for coping with it and managing it, as well as suitable use of health and social services, are other important components [18]. All measures should be embedded in a long-term perspective with individualized specific goals, depending on disease characteristics in respect of the needs of the individual, and the demands of the environment. This can only be assured by a coordinated timely delivery of interventions, which in general necessitates a multidisciplinary approach.

Rehabilitation can be evaluated at different levels [19]: (1) the broadest concept of service delivery; (2) packages of comprehensive care; (3) individual components of the package; and (4) the intrinsic elements of the rehabilitation process. Even though growing evidence exists for the benefit of some specific rehabilitation services, packages of comprehensive care and their individual components, other intrinsic elements are still poorly validated [19].

In general, there is a wide consensus concerning essential requirements and components of rehabilitation in MS, even though there are still some controversies in this respect [18, 20]. Appropriate patient selection, together with timing and mode of rehabilitation, taking into account level of disability as personal and environmental requirements, are considered as key issues for successful planning and performing rehabilitation measures in MS patients [16]. Setting of specific, measurable, attainable, realistic (relevant), and timely (SMART) goals together with affected patients and caregivers before starting the rehabilitation process is another important issue in this respect.

Timing and scheduling rehabilitation measures during disease course

As the need for rehabilitative treatment, packages of care, and specific treatment modalities change during the course of MS, it seems reasonable to schedule interventions based on the stage of disease [16, 21, 22].

Maintenance of functioning as a possible goal of rehabilitation emphasizes the need for *early evaluation of MS patients for rehabilitation measures*. Preservation of functions is generally achieved easier and more reliably than restoration of lost abilities. In MS patients *without or with only minor functional deficits (EDSS 0–2.5)*, therefore, measures should aim to maintain or optimize physical and mental capabilities. Education and performance of an individually tailored physical training has shown to be an effective and cost-effective intervention [23]. In patients with *moderate functional impairments (EDSS 3–5.5)* realistic and relevant goals would be to improve or maintain mobility or reduce spasticity. In these patients, in general assisted physiotherapy together with other specific treatment modalities and if required adaptation of technical aids is needed. Intensity of measures at this stage depends on the level of impairments and disabilities and the specific goals: the higher the target, the higher the treatment intensity needed. In MS patients with *moderate to severe functional limitations (EDSS 6–7.5)* the main target consists in maintenance of wheelchair mobility and highest possible independence in daily activities. In general, regular low-intensity treatment accompanied

by endurance and strengthening measures is appropriate for the majority of these patients. At this stage of disease, careful instruction of patients for self-training and optimal adaptation of technical aids is particularly important for avoiding secondary complications. In mostly bedridden *MS patients with severe functional limitations (EDSS 8–9.5)*, rehabilitation measures should aim to maintain range of movement and mobility, to reduce the need for care, and especially to prevent secondary complications (i.e., contractures, pressure sores, pain, respiratory problems). In addition to assisted treatment modalities, counseling and instruction of caregivers for regular movement exercises and prevention of complications is crucial.

All patients should be assessed at regular intervals for goal attainment or deterioration, and for the possible need to adapt treatment regime.

Even though there is a good evidence for some of these treatment measures, impact and efficacy of others are based only on lower levels of evidence. Thus, these recommendations proposed above should be considered as a framework, which should be adapted to the patient's needs and to availability of rehabilitation services.

Mode of rehabilitation service delivery

Inpatient, outpatient, and home-based treatment are possible settings for delivery of rehabilitation services, which should be selected in consideration of the disease characteristics as well as of individual and environmental needs, and the availability of services. In general, MS patients with more complex functional deficits and disabilities need multidisciplinary rehabilitation treatment, which is best assured in an inpatient setting. Outpatient multidisciplinary treatment may be an alternative; however, sometimes it is not feasible for logistic reasons. Another advantage of inpatient rehabilitation is higher intensity of treatment, and nursing care round the clock, especially important for severely disabled MS patients. In addition, inpatient treatment allows MS patients to devote their limited resources to active therapies alternating with resting intervals, thus avoiding exhaustion by additional daily duties. Finally, more severely disabled MS patients, who do not respond to outpatient treatment, may profit more from inpatient treatment [24]. Negative aspects of inpatient treatment are the higher costs, and the unfamiliar environment and style of everyday life, which may influence negatively the transfer of improvement when the patient returns to the community.

Outpatient and especially home-based treatment have several advantages in this respect, as patients can perform their treatment programs in their normal environment with a more realistic background. Another positive aspect is the involvement and close collaboration with the family and caregivers. On the other hand, multimodal outpatient or home-based treatment and close interdisciplinary team approach is generally difficult to set up outside of areas with specialized MS centers.

Factors influencing outcome of rehabilitation

The outcome of rehabilitation can be influenced by various factors: in a preliminary multiple regression analysis, Langdon and Thompson found a correlation with disability level on admission, verbal intelligence, and cerebellar function [25]. A recent analysis of a large MS patient group by Grasso and co-workers found a two- to threefold higher improvement in patients with low to moderate disability in contrast to patients with a severe disability level [26]. In addition, duration of disease, sphincter disturbances, and severe cognitive deficits were negatively correlated with improvement. These findings emphasize the importance of early evaluation and admission of MS patients for rehabilitation in order to maximize functional recovery [26].

Supposed mode of action of rehabilitation in MS

Functional magnetic resonance imaging (MRI) studies suggest that some functional cortical reorganization, which is thought to play an important role in recovery after acute brain lesions, also occurs in MS [27]. It is, however, not clear whether this functional change in MS patients reflects compensatory adaptive changes (altered use pattern) or functional restoration as a response to progressing brain injury [28]. A recent study by Thickbroom and co-workers studying central motor conduction in MS patients suggests the presence of central adaptive processes to compensate and maintain task performance [29]. These compensatory mechanisms seem to be more pronounced in the early phases of disease [30]. A putative disease-modifying

effect of exercise training was discussed by Heesen and co-workers [31], based on some preliminary data: clinical studies, however, failed to demonstrate any benefit on disease activity or on disease course [32].

Thus, in addition to direct or indirect specific effects of treatment modalities, the benefit of rehabilitation in MS seems to rely in a great part on improved compensation, adaptation, coping, and reconditioning. Furthermore, information and instruction of patients and caregivers, together with a better use of medical and social resources, contribute to their coping better with disease and disability, thereby improving quality of life of patients with MS and their caregivers. Some of these non-specific factors may also explain the observed long-term benefits of rehabilitation [32].

Value of multidisciplinary rehabilitation

Since the first study, published by Feigenson and co-workers in 1981, *multidisciplinary inpatient rehabilitation* has been shown to be a valuable and effective treatment in MS patients [24, 33–36]. The best evidence for the benefit of this treatment regimen came from a study by Freeman and co-workers, who could demonstrate in a randomized clinical trial a significant improvement of disability, handicap, and quality of life by a multidisciplinary inpatient rehabilitation treatment [37]. In accordance with earlier studies [34, 37], the same group could show a long-term effect of this inpatient rehabilitation outlasting the treatment phase by several months despite progression of disease [32].

A recent randomized double-blind controlled trial published by Storr and co-workers, however, failed to demonstrate any significant benefit [38]. The authors argued that lack of formalized evaluation of the need for rehabilitation, bias in recruitment, and differences between the two groups as difficulties in quantifying the efficacy of multidisciplinary rehabilitation that may have influenced the results.

Grasso *et al.* investigated the impact of different factors on the outcome of inpatient multidisciplinary rehabilitation: they found that disease duration, basal EDSS score, cognitive status, and sphincter disturbances were negatively associated with effectiveness of treatment [26].

The efficacy of *outpatient multidisciplinary rehabilitation* was first described by DiFabio and co-workers [39]: in a prospective, longitudinal, randomized study a significant reduction in the frequency of symptoms and in particular of fatigue could be observed in MS patients after an outpatient multidisciplinary treatment (physiotherapy, occupational therapy, individual counseling, 1 day per week over 1 year) in comparison to a control group. Another randomized controlled trial published by Patti and co-workers examined the effect of a short multidisciplinary treatment in MS patients with chronic progressive disease: after an individualized multidisciplinary outpatient rehabilitation (6 weeks) a significant improvement in disability was demonstrated in the treatment group, while impairment level remained unchanged [40].

The best evidence for the effectiveness of multidisciplinary rehabilitation exists for patients with chronic progressive MS, whereas evidence is less convincing for relapsing–remitting MS. Two newer studies, however, have suggest that multidisciplinary rehabilitation (outpatient or inpatient) may also be useful in relapsing–remitting MS, especially in patients with incomplete recovery from relapses with moderate to severe disability [41, 42].

The value of *home-based management* was investigated by Pozzilli *et al.* [43]: in comparison to standard hospital care, multidisciplinary home-based support of MS patients was shown to be superior in respect of different domains of quality of life (general health, bodily pain, role–emotional, social functioning).

Consistent with the conclusions of a systematic Cochrane review by Khan and co-workers [44], one can summarize that there is strong evidence from clinical trials that multidisciplinary inpatient rehabilitation of MS patients can lead to improvement in activity and participation, even though there is no measurable reduction in impairment (assessed by EDSS). For high-intensity outpatient and home-based programs, the actual value is less clear, with limited evidence for short-term improvements in symptoms and disability, participation, and quality of life. Another important conclusion from these studies is that patients with all forms of MS should undergo regular specialized evaluation and follow-up to assess their need for appropriate rehabilitation intervention, and that mode and setting of the rehabilitation treatment (inpatient, outpatient, community) should be individualized based upon patients' specific needs [44].

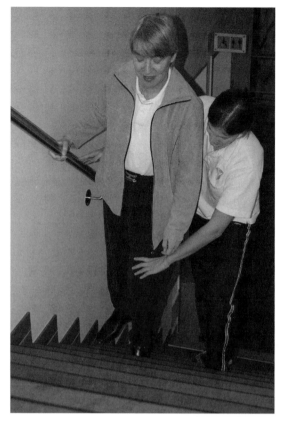

Fig. 16.2. Physical therapy.

Value of specific treatment modalities

It is well known that physical activity is low in MS patients compared to non-disabled persons, the activity level depending both on disease characteristics and disability and on employment status and environmental factors [45–47]. Improving or restoring physical abilities therefore is a key issue in rehabilitation of MS patients. In a longitudinal survey of MS patients, Stuifbergen *et al.* found a negative correlation between changes of functional limitations with physical activity and quality of life [48], supporting the importance of continued physical activity and exercise for persons with MS over the course of the disease. The authors concluded that exercise interventions may have substantial long-term effects on decreasing functional limitations and enhancing quality of life for people with MS.

Physical therapy aims at improvement of motor functions (coordination, fine movements), balance and gait, and reduction of spasticity (Fig. 16.2). Physical treatment should be accompanied by comprehensive counseling of MS patients and caregivers. Another important task, generally covered by physical therapists in close collaboration with orthotics and medical technicians, is adaptation and the supply of technical equipment (splints, orthotic devices, walking aids, wheelchair): interdisciplinary evaluation is helpful in significantly reducing abandonment of equipment [49].

Good evidence exists that *intensive, individualized physical therapy* (inpatient or outpatient) leads to a significant improvement in disability, mobility, and in some aspects of quality of life [50, 51], with a reduction of risk of falls [51]. The effect, however, seems to be of short duration, being no longer detectable after 8 and 9 weeks, respectively.

Aerobic training has shown to significantly improve aerobic capacity, strength, some psychomental factors (anxiety, depression), and level of activity [52, 53].

In a recent review, Dalgas and co-workers discussed the value of *endurance and resistance training*: they found good evidence that MS patients can tolerate and benefit from endurance training at low to moderate intensity, whereas, due to limited studies, evidence was rather low for resistance training [54]. Guttierez and co-workers [55], however, could demonstrate a significant gain in muscle strength and improvement of gait after an 8-week strengthening training. One important finding of these trials is that no persistent deterioration of symptoms occurred after training sessions.

Van den Berg and co-workers could demonstrate in a first pilot trial a positive effect of aerobic *treadmill training*, showing a significant increase of walking velocity [56]. In a pre–post analysis, the same research group found a significant improvement in walking impairments and in cardiovascular deconditioning, thereby potentially reducing effort and fatigue in MS [57].

Most of the studies mentioned have been investigating the effect of physical training mainly in ambulatory MS patients with low or moderate disabilities (EDSS < 6.5).

In our own randomized pilot trial, the impact of *robot-assisted gait training* in patients with severe walking disabilities (EDSS 6.0–7.5) was investigated (Fig. 16.3). Despite some limitations, pre–post analysis indicated more benefit of this new assisted active therapy compared with conventional walking training in this patient group with significant gain in walking

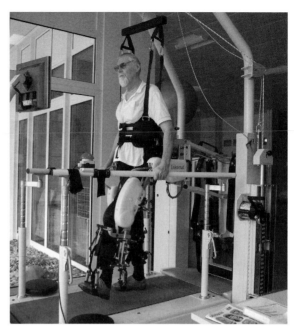

Fig. 16.3. Robot-assisted gait training for patients with severe walking disabilities.

speed, endurance, and strength [58]. One reason for these findings may be that individually adjusted body weight support and assisted leg movements may lessen central fatigability in MS patients with severe walking disabilities, allowing a longer effective treatment time, higher intensity, and higher speed compared to conventional over-ground walking. In a group of stroke patients Husemann and co-workers found some evidence suggesting a significant increase of muscle mass during robot-assisted training as compared to conventional walking training [59].

In a randomized controlled trial, McAuley and co-workers demonstrated that a formal *instruction of an efficacy-enhancement exercise condition* was beneficial for exercise adherence, well-being, and affective responses to exercise, patients in the intervention group attending more exercise sessions, and reporting higher levels of well-being and exertion, and feeling better following exercise than individuals in the standard care condition [23].

There are only few studies that compare physical therapy with aerobic training: Rasova *et al.* found that neurophysiologically based physiotherapy or a combined training (physiotherapy plus aerobic training) were associated with significant improvement in impairment and fatigue, whereas aerobic training lead only to improvement in some spiro-ergometric parameters [60]. Another small trial comparing aerobic training with physical therapy found a greater benefit for aerobic training in improving maximum exercise tolerance and walking capacity in MS patients with mild to moderate disability [61].

Another possible physical approach is *cooling therapy* in thermosensible patients with Uhthoff phenomenon [62]. Beenakker *et al.* could demonstrate a significant reduction of fatigue and an improvement in postural stability and muscle strength in ten heat-sensitive MS patients wearing a cold vest with active cooling (7 °C, 60 minutes) in comparison to wearing a placebo cooling suit [62]. Preliminary data from another cross-over study using a tight-cuff passive cooling garment prototype suggest an improvement in a timed walking test, leg strength, fine-motor skills, and subjective benefits [63]. Another small trial investigated the impact of a pre-cooling bath (16 °C, 30 minutes, lower body regions) in reducing motor fatigue during consecutive physical training [64]. These functional improvements after cooling are probably due to partial restoration of central motor conduction capacities in demyelinated fibers [65]. Taking into account experimental and clinical data, pre-cooling or cooling during and after therapy may increase the effect of active physical training in thermosensitive MS patients.

For other physical treatment options (*hippotherapy, aquatic therapy*) there are no controlled studies investigating the effect: horse-riding therapy is thought to diminish spasticity by rhythmic activation of trunk muscles and to stabilize postural control in ataxic patients [66]; *aquatic therapy* may be helpful in reducing spasticity and facilitating training of movements [67, 68].

For *occupational therapy (ergotherapy)* in MS only a few, mainly open-labeled, non-controlled, studies exist indicating some a positive effect of ergotherapy (tone modulating measures, specific training of manual and practical functions) on muscle function, range of movement, and activities of daily living [69, 70]. Another specific intervention was investigated by Mathiowetz and co-workers: in a randomized controlled study an *energy conservation course* led to reduced fatigue impact and to increased self-efficacy together with improvement of some aspects of quality of life [71].

As aphasia is rare in MS, specific *speech therapy* is rarely necessary. In patients with dysarthrophonia,

however, speech training together with exercises of respiration may help to improve the capacity to articulate. Furthermore, in analogy to stroke patients, training of swallowing with triggering of reflexes swallowing process and compensatory measures as an adaptation to consistency of food and liquids may help to improve the process of swallowing and reduce the risk of aspirations [72, 73].

Severely disabled, bedridden MS patients are at high risk for pulmonary infections, due to swallowing disturbances together with insufficient respiratory function and reduced coughing. In this patient group, *respiratory training* may help to improve respiratory function and cough reflex [74].

Bladder symptoms are particularly incapacitating in activities of daily living. Urgency is often made worse by motor disabilities potentially impeding to reach the toilet in due time. Complementary to drug treatment, *pelvic floor training* together with specific instruction for self-training may help to improve bladder symptoms improving incontinence, urgency, and frequency significantly [75]. Incomplete bladder voiding can be treated by an *external bladder stimulator* (Queen Square stimulator), which may lead to a significant reduction of resting urinary volume [76, 77].

The value of *cognitive training* was investigated in two studies demonstrating a benefit in specifically trained cognitive aspects (attention, learning) [78, 79]. Another study, however, could not demonstrate any benefit of cognitive training: in this study intervention was limited to instructing patients in self-training without formal neuropsychological therapy [80]. The testing group without cognitive intervention experienced a reduction of quality of life after 8 months; therefore neuropsychological evaluation on its own without therapeutic intervention should be avoided.

In MS patients suffering from depressive symptoms *psychological–psychiatric therapy* may add a beneficial effect to drug treatment with antidepressants [81]. A recent systematic review found, despite the diversity of interventions, reasonable evidence that *cognitive behavioral approaches* are beneficial in the treatment of depression, and helping MS patients to adjust to and cope with the disease [1]. Effective support and treatment of neuropsychiatric symptoms and cognitive dysfunctions are also important from the perspective of caregivers: Figved and co-workers identified neuropsychiatric symptoms and cognitive dysfunctions as the two main causes for distress and loss of quality of life in caregivers of MS patients [11].

Finally *group therapies* may enhance motivation, social interaction, and participation of patients, even though formal validation of the impact is lacking.

Specific problems and limitations of rehabilitation in MS

Despite increasing knowledge and better understanding of the value of specific measures and treatment programs, appropriate evaluation of the impact of rehabilitation in MS remains a challenging task. The different disease patterns, together with unpredictable changes in disease activity and functional performance within days or even hours, make an accurate validation of rehabilitation measures in MS particularly difficult. Selection of a homogeneous group of MS patients allowing accurate differentiation of natural history of disease from actual effect of rehabilitation treatment is still a challenge. Even selection of a "stable" group of patients without a change in disease activity during the last few months does not exclude the influence of natural fluctuations on outcome. This may be the main reason for the difficulties in performing scientifically sound studies, and the *still limited evidence of some aspects of rehabilitation in MS*. It is not only of scientific interest to measure outcome with the proper instruments but it also contributes to evaluation of the efficacy of different treatment modalities and to adaptation and development of new treatment options [82].

Considering the huge impact on affected MS patients and their families, comprehensive evaluation of rehabilitation should include the *patient's and caregiver's perspectives*. Recently, a first systematic survey was published, defining the different domains of caregiving tasks in a large group of caregivers and MS patients in Australia [83]. Another study published by Sweetland and co-workers analyzed patients' needs in vocational rehabilitation, identifying distinct ways of giving support in the workplace [85].

In general, *knowledge about comprehensive rehabilitation* in MS patients and health professionals not directly involved in the rehabilitation process seems still to be rather limited. In a recent study investigating the measures helpful for patients in meeting their current needs, rehabilitation therapies were indicated by only 9%, compared to 29% undergoing

medical treatment [84]. The need for rehabilitation, socio-environmental support, and non-professional care, however, increases with greater disease impact.

Proper patient selection is a particular problem in MS rehabilitation. As shown in a recent randomized trial [38], selecting patients for multidisciplinary rehabilitation only by chance without formal evaluation of the *necessity and specific goals* seems not to be appropriate, as this study failed to demonstrate any significant benefit. This negative finding reflects also the importance of *active cooperation and motivation* on the results of rehabilitation measures. As most treatments are aiming at improving personal activities, patients lacking required ability and will to cooperate probably cannot profit from an active rehabilitation program. Interventions in later stages of the disease, especially in severely disabled bedridden patients, therefore, are generally limited to education of caregivers for regular mobilization and for preventing secondary complications. The same limitations must be considered in MS patients with severe comorbidities, precluding active physical training.

Another limitation concerns the stage of the disease, and especially progressive cognitive decline during the disease course. As stated above, the major benefit of rehabilitation is thought to be due to improved compensation, adaptation, coping, and reconditioning. Even though the specific role of functional brain reorganization in the rehabilitation of MS patients is still not clear, recent functional MRI data suggest that brain activation and *compensatory processes are limited in cognitively severely impaired MS patients* compared to mildly or moderately affected patients, characterized by decreased additional recruitment of brain regions [30]. A multiregression analysis by Grasso and co-workers indicated that disease duration, EDSS score, and cognitive status are negatively correlated with effectiveness of rehabilitation treatment [26]. Another study using virtual reality testing demonstrated impaired short-term motor learning in MS patients [86]. Thus rehabilitation of MS patients with severe cognitive disturbances seems to be of limited value due to the lack of compensatory processes and lower learning abilities.

Even though some experimental data suggest a positive influence of improved physical activity on disease activity [31], clinical studies have shown continuous progression of disease and functional deficits (measured by EDSS) after rehabilitation treatment

[32, 50]. Thus, rehabilitation measures seem to have *no measurable beneficial effect on disease activity or on disease course itself.*

Two specific problems in rehabilitation of MS patients are *motor fatigue* and *thermosensitivity*. For decades, MS patients were told to avoid any physical activity, which was thought to deteriorate functions and progression of disease. One reason for this assumption was Uhthoff's phenomenon [62], which may bring on or deteriorate symptoms due to increased body temperature or during physical activities in thermosensitive patients by a disruption of central conduction in demyelinated fibers [65, 87]. The reason for central motor fatigue in MS patients is less clear. The inability of MS patients to maintaining strength during a strenuous task has been attributed to a recruitment failure of central motor pathways [88]. Experimental data, however, suggest that frequency- and use-dependent conduction block occurs in demyelinated fibers and even persists for a certain period [87]. Thus, intensive continuing physical activities may bear a certain risk of inducing recruitment and conduction failures in MS patients. In addition, as functional capacity decreases during strenuous activities, high-intensity training may reduce the effectiveness of physical treatment due to central fatigue. Thus, physical training in MS patients should be individually adapted and *limited to low to moderate intensity* [54]. Respecting these limitations, physical training is beneficial in MS patients with no risk of persisting deterioration [89, 90].

Due to its personnel-intensive structure multidisciplinary rehabilitation is generally cost-intensive, limiting it to countries with higher economic power. *Cost–benefit analysis* of rehabilitation in MS has still to be evaluated. In a first study Feigenson and co-workers estimated that the yearly costs per patient could be reduced substantially by inpatient rehabilitation from US$25 000 to US$19 000 due to lower need for care [24]. Pozzilli *et al.* found some benefit of home-based management in reducing costs slightly as a result of lower rate of hospital admissions (mean – €822/patient/year) [43]. Considering the findings of Kobelt and co-workers indicating a close correlation of total costs with disability [14], even a slight reduction of disability by rehabilitation measures might lead to significant savings in the long-term care of MS patients.

References

1. Thomas P W, Thomas S, Hillier C, Galvin K, Baker R. Psychological interventions for multiple sclerosis. *Cochrane Database Syst Rev* 2006;CD004431

2. Stuart W H, Cohan S, Richert J R, Achiron A. Selecting a disease-modifying agent as platform therapy in the long-term management of multiple sclerosis. *Neurology* 2004;**63**:S19–27

3. Wiendl H, Toyka K V, Rieckmann P, *et al.* Basic and escalating immunomodulatory treatments in multiple sclerosis: current therapeutic recommendations. *J Neurol* 2008;**255**:1449–63

4. The PRISMS Study Group, PRIMS-4: long-term efficacy of interferon-B-1a in relapsing MS. *Neurology* 2001;**56**:1628–36

5. Polman C H, O'Connor P W, Havrdova E, *et al.* A randomized, placebo-controlled trial of natalizumab for relapsing multiple sclerosis. *N Engl J Med* 2006;**354**:899–910

6. Tremlett H L, Oger J. Ten years of adverse drug reaction reports for the multiple sclerosis immunomodulatory therapies: a Canadian perspective. *Mult Scler* 2008;**14**:94–105

7. Sayao A L, Devonshire V, Tremlett H. Longitudinal follow-up of "benign" multiple sclerosis at 20 years. *Neurology* 2007;**68**:496–500

8. Paltamaa J, Sarasoja T, Wikstrom J, Malkia E. Physical functioning in multiple sclerosis: a population-based study in central Finland. *J Rehab Med* 2006;**38**:339–45

9. Weinshenker B G. Natural history of multiple sclerosis. *Ann Neurol* 1994;**36**(Suppl):S6–11

10. Green G, Todd J, Pevalin D. Biographical disruption associated with multiple sclerosis: using propensity scoring to assess the impact. *Soc Sci Med* 2007;**65**:524–35

11. Figved N, Myhr K M, Larsen J P, Aarsland D. Caregiver burden in multiple sclerosis: the impact of neuropsychiatric symptoms. *J Neurol Neurosurg Psychiatry* 2007;**78**:1097–102

12. Grytten Torkildsen N, Lie S A, Aarseth J H, Nyland H, Myhr K M. Survival and cause of death in multiple sclerosis: results from a 50-year follow-up in Western Norway. *Mult Scler* 2008;**14**:1191–8

13. Patwardhan M B, Matchar D B, Samsa G P, *et al.* Cost of multiple sclerosis by level of disability: a review of literature. *Mult Scler* 2005;**11**:232–9

14. Kobelt G, Berg J, Lindgren P, Fredrikson S, Jonsson B. Costs and quality of life of patients with multiple sclerosis in Europe. *J Neurol Neurosurg Psychiatry* 2006;**77**:918–26

15. World Health Organization. Community based rehabilitation: a strategy for rehabilitation, equalization of opportunities, poverty reduction and social inclusion of people with disabilities. Geneva: WHO, 2004

16. Kesselring J, Beer S. Symptomatic therapy and neurorehabilitation in multiple sclerosis. *Lancet Neurol* 2005;**4**:643–52

17. Kesselring J. Long-term rehabilitation in multiple sclerosis. In: Siva A, Kessselring J, Thompson A J, eds. Frontiers in multiple sclerosis. London: Martin Dunitz, 1999:243–52

18. Thompson A J. Multidisciplinary approach. In: Hawkins C P, Wolinsky J S, eds. *Principles of Treatment in Multiple Sclerosis*. London: Butterworth Heinemann, 2000:299–315

19. Thompson A. The effectiveness of neurological rehabilitation in multiple sclerosis. *J Rehab Res Devel* 2000;**37**:455–61

20. Freeman J A, Thompson A J. Rehabilitation in multiple sclerosis. In: Noseworthy J H, McDonald W I, ed. *Multiple Sclerosis* 2nd edn. Oxford: Butterworth-Heinemann, 2003;63–107

21. Freeman J, Ford H, Mattison P, Thompson A. Developing MS healthcare standards: evidence-based recommendations for service providers. London: Multiple Sclerosis Society of Great Britain and Northern Ireland and the MS Professional Network, 2002

22. Beer S, Schluep M, Steinlin Egli R, Vuadens P, Wiederkehr M. Ambulante Physiotherapie bei MS. MS Info. *Schweiz Mult Skler Gesell* 2004;4:8

23. McAuley E, Motl R W, Morris K S, *et al.* Enhancing physical activity adherence and well-being in multiple sclerosis: a randomized controlled trial. *Mult Scler* 2007;**13**:652–9

24. Feigenson J S, Scheinberg L, Catalano M, *et al.* The cost-effectiveness of multiple sclerosis rehabilitation: a model. *Neurology* 1981;**31**:1316–22

25. Langdon D W, Thompson A J. Multiple sclerosis: a preliminary study of selected variables affecting rehabilitation outcome. *Mult Scler* 1999;**5**:94–100

26. Grasso M G, Troisi E, Rizzi F, Morelli D, Paolucci S. Prognostic factors in multidisciplinary rehabilitation treatment in multiple sclerosis: an outcome study. *Mult Scler* 2005;**11**:719–24

27. Rocca M A, Falini A, Colombo B, *et al.* Adaptive functional changes in the cerebral cortex of patients with nondisabling multiple sclerosis correlate with the extent of brain structural damage. *Ann Neurol* 2002; **51**:330–9

28. Cifelli A, Matthews P M. Cerebral plasticity in multiple sclerosis: insights from fMRI. *Mult Scler* 2002;**8**:193–9

29. Thickbroom G W, Sacco P, Faulkner D L, Kermode A G, Mastaglia F L. Enhanced corticomotor excitability with dynamic fatiguing exercise of the lower limb in multiple sclerosis. *J Neurol* 2008;**255**:1001–5

30. Penner I K, Opwis K, Kappos L. Relation between functional brain imaging, cognitive impairment and cognitive rehabilitation in patients with multiple sclerosis. *J Neurol* 2007;**254**(Suppl 2):53–7

31. Heesen C, Romberg A, Gold S, Schulz K H. Physical exercise in multiple sclerosis: supportive care or a putative disease-modifying treatment. *Expert Rev Neurother* 2006;**6**:347–55

32. Freeman J A, Langdon D W, Hobart J C, Thompson A J. Inpatient rehabilitation in multiple sclerosis: do the benefits carry over into the community? *Neurology* 1999;**52**:50–6

33. Greenspun B, Stineman M, Agri R. Multiple sclerosis and rehabilitation outcome. *Arch Phys Med Rehab* 1987;**68**:434–7

34. Francabandera F L, Holland N J, Wiesel-Levison P, Scheinberg L C. Multiple sclerosis rehabilitation: inpatient vs. outpatient. *Rehab Nurs* 1988;**13**:251–3

35. Aisen M L, Sevilla D, Fox N. Inpatient rehabilitation for multiple sclerosis. *J Neurol Rehab* 1996;**10**:43–6

36. Kidd D, Thompson A J. Prospective study of neurorehabilitation in multiple sclerosis. *J Neurol Neurosurg Psychiatry* 1997;**62**:423–4

37. Freeman J A, Langdon D W, Hobart J C, Thompson A J. The impact of inpatient rehabilitation on progressive multiple sclerosis. *Ann Neurol* 1997;**42**:236–44

38. Storr L K, Sorensen P S, Ravnborg M. The efficacy of multidisciplinary rehabilitation in stable multiple sclerosis patients. *Mult Scler* 2006;**12**:235–42

39. Di Fabio R P, Soderberg J, Choi T, Hansen C R, Schapiro R T. Extended outpatient rehabilitation: its influence on symptom frequency, fatigue, and functional status for persons with progressive multiple sclerosis. *Arch Phys Med Rehabil* 1998;**79**:141–6

40. Patti F, Ciancio M R, Cacopardo M, *et al.* Effects of a short outpatient rehabilitation treatment on disability of multiple sclerosis patients: a randomized controlled trial. *J Neurol* 2003;**250**:861–6

41. Craig J, Young C A, Ennis M, Baker G, Boggild M. A randomized controlled trial comparing rehabilitation against standard therapy in multiple sclerosis patients receiving intravenous steroid treatment. *J Neurol Neurosurg Psychiatry* 2003;**74**:1225–30

42. Liu C, Playford E D, Thompson A J. Does neurorehabilitation have a role in relapsing–remitting multiple sclerosis? *J Neurol* 2003;**250**:1214–18

43. Pozzilli C, Brunetti M, Amicosante A M, *et al*. Home based management in multiple sclerosis: results of a randomized controlled trial. *J Neurol Neurosurg Psychiatry* 2002;**73**:250–5

44. Khan F, Turner-Stokes L, Ng L, Kilpatrick T. Multidisciplinary rehabilitation for adults with multiple sclerosis. *Cochrane Database Syst Rev* 2007; CD006036

45. Motl R W, McAuley E, Snook E M. Physical activity and multiple sclerosis: a meta-analysis. *Mult Scler* 2005;**11**:459–63

46. Doerksen S E, Motl R W, McAuley E. Environmental correlates of physical activity in multiple sclerosis: a cross-sectional study. *Int J Behav Nutr Phys Activ* 2007;**4**:49

47. Motl R W, Snook E M, McAuley E, Scott J A, Hinkle M L. Demographic correlates of physical activity in individuals with multiple sclerosis. *Disabil Rehab* 2007;**29**:1301–4

48. Stuifbergen A K, Blozis S A, Harrison T C, Becker H A. Exercise, functional limitations, and quality of life: a longitudinal study of persons with multiple sclerosis. *Arch Phys Med Rehab* 2006;**87**:935–43

49. Verza R, Carvalho M L, Battaglia M A, Uccelli M M. An interdisciplinary approach to evaluating the need for assistive technology reduces equipment abandonment. *Mult Scler* 2006;**12**:88–93

50. Solari A, Filippini G, Gasco P, *et al*. Physical rehabilitation has a positive effect on disability in multiple sclerosis patients. *Neurology* 1999;**52**:57–62

51. Wiles C M, Newcombe R G, Fuller K J, *et al*. Controlled randomized crossover trial of the effects of physiotherapy on mobility in chronic multiple sclerosis. *J Neurol Neurosurg Psychiatry* 2001; **70**:174–9

52. Petajan J H, Gappmaier E, White A T, *et al*. Impact of aerobic training on fitness and quality of life in multiple sclerosis. *Ann Neurol* 1996;**39**:432–41

53. Mostert S, Kesselring J. Effects of a short-term exercise training program on aerobic fitness, fatigue, health perception and activity level of subjects with multiple sclerosis. *Mult Scler* 2002;**8**:161–8

54. Dalgas U, Stenager E, Ingemann-Hansen T. Multiple sclerosis and physical exercise: recommendations for the application of resistance-, endurance- and combined training. *Mult Scler* 2008;**14**:35–53

55. Gutierrez G M, Chow J W, Tillman M D, *et al*. Resistance training improves gait kinematics in persons with multiple sclerosis. *Arch Phys Med Rehab* 2005;**86**:1824–9

56. van den Berg M, Dawes H, Wade D T, *et al*. Treadmill training for individuals with multiple sclerosis: a pilot randomized trial. *J Neurol Neurosurg Psychiatry* 2006;**77**:531–3

57. Newman M A, Dawes H, van den Berg M, *et al*. Can aerobic treadmill training reduce the effort of walking and fatigue in people with multiple sclerosis: a pilot study. *Mult Scler* 2007;**13**:113–19

58. Beer S, Aschbacher B, Manoglou D, *et al*. Robot-assisted gait training in multiple sclerosis: a pilot randomized trial. *Mult Scler* 2008;**14**:231–6

59. Husemann B, Muller F, Krewer C, Heller S, Koenig E. Effects of locomotion training with assistance of a robot-driven gait orthosis in hemiparetic patients after stroke: a randomized controlled pilot study. *Stroke* 2007;**38**:349–54

60. Rasova K, Havrdova E, Brandejsky P, *et al*. Comparison of the influence of different rehabilitation programmes on clinical, spirometric and spiroergometric parameters in patients with multiple sclerosis. *Mult Scler* 2006;**12**:227–34

61. Rampello A, Franceschini M, Piepoli M, *et al*. Effect of aerobic training on walking capacity and maximal exercise tolerance in patients with multiple sclerosis: a randomized crossover controlled study. *Phys Ther* 2007;**87**:545–55; discussion 555–9

62. Beenakker E A, Oparina T I, Hartgring A, *et al*. Cooling garment treatment in MS: clinical improvement and decrease in leukocyte NO production. *Neurology* 2001;**57**:892–4

63. Meyer-Heim A, Rothmaier M, Weder M, *et al*. Advanced lightweight cooling-garment technology: functional improvements in thermosensitive patients with multiple sclerosis. *Mult Scler* 2007;**13**:232–7

64. White A T, Wilson T E, Davis S L, Petajan J H. Effect of precooling on physical performance in multiple sclerosis. *Mult Scler* 2000;**6**:176–80

65. Humm A M, Beer S, Kool J, *et al*. Quantification of Uhthoff's phenomenon in multiple sclerosis: a magnetic stimulation study. *Clin Neurophysiol* 2004;**115**:2493–501

66. Künzle, U. Schweizer Studie über die Wirksamkeit der Hippotherapie-K bei Multiple-Sklerose-Patienten Hippotherapie. Berlin: Springer, 2000:359–81

67. Gamper U N. Wasserspezifische Bewegungstherapie und Training. Stuttgart: Gustav Fischer, 1995

68. Kesiktas N, Paker N, Erdogan N, *et al*. The use of hydrotherapy for the management of spasticity. *Neurorehab Neural Repair* 2004;**18**:268–73

69. Baker N A, Tickle-Degnen L. The effectiveness of physical, psychological, and functional interventions in treating clients with multiple sclerosis: a meta-analysis. *Am J Occup Ther* 2001;**55**:324–31

70. Steultjens E M, Dekker J, Bouter L M, *et al.* Occupational therapy for multiple sclerosis. *Cochrane Database Syst Rev* 2003;CD003608

71. Mathiowetz V G, Finlayson M L, Matuska K M, Chen H Y, Luo P. Randomized controlled trial of an energy conservation course for persons with multiple sclerosis. *Mult Scler* 2005;**11**:592–601

72. Prosiegel M, Heintze M, Wagner-Sonntag E, *et al.* Schluckstörungen bei neurologischen Patienten: eine prospektive Studie zu Diagnostik, Störungsmustern, Therapie und Outcome. *Nervenarzt* 2002;**73**:364–70

73. Squires N. Dysphagia management for progressive neurological conditions. *Nurs Stand* 2006;**20**:53–7

74. Gosselink R, Kovacs L, Ketelaer P, Carton H, Decramer M. Respiratory muscle weakness and respiratory muscle training in severely disabled multiple sclerosis patients. *Arch Phys Med Rehab* 2000;**81**:747–51

75. Vahtera T, Haaranen M, Viramo-Koskela A L, Ruutiainen J. Pelvic floor rehabilitation is effective in patients with multiple sclerosis. *Clin Rehab* 1997;**11**:211–19

76. Dasgupta P, Haslam C, Goodwin R, Fowler C J. The 'Queen Square bladder stimulator': a device for assisting emptying of the neurogenic bladder. *Br J Urol* 1997;**80**:234–7

77. Prasad R S, Smith S J, Wright H. Lower abdominal pressure versus external bladder stimulation to aid bladder emptying in multiple sclerosis: a randomized controlled study. *Clin Rehab* 2003;**17**:42–7

78. Plohmann A M, Kappos L, Ammann W, *et al.* Computer assisted retraining of attentional impairments in patients with multiple sclerosis. *J Neurol Neurosurg Psychiatry* 1998;**64**:455–62

79. Chiaravalloti N D, DeLuca J, Moore N B, Ricker J H. Treating learning impairments improves memory performance in multiple sclerosis: a randomized clinical trial. *Mult Scler* 2005;**11**:58–68

80. Lincoln N B, Dent A, Harding J, *et al.* Evaluation of cognitive assessment and cognitive intervention for people with multiple sclerosis. *J Neurol Neurosurg Psychiatry* 2002;**72**:93–8

81. Kesselring J. Rehabilitation in MS is effective. *Int Mult Scler J* 2001;**8**:68–71

82. Kesselring J. Neurorehabilitation in multiple sclerosis: what is the evidence base? *J Neurol* 2004;**251**(Suppl 4): 25–9

83. Pakenham K I. The nature of caregiving in multiple sclerosis: development of the caregiving tasks in multiple sclerosis scale. *Mult Scler* 2007;**13**:929–38

84. Forbes A, While A, Taylor M. What people with multiple sclerosis perceive to be important to meeting their needs. *J Adv Nurs* 2007;**58**:11–22

85. Sweetland J, Riazi A, Cano S J, Playford E D. Vocational rehabilitation services for people with multiple sclerosis: what patients want from clinicians and employers. *Mult Scler* 2007;**13**:1183–9

86. Leocani L, Comi E, Annovazzi P, *et al.* Impaired short-term motor learning in multiple sclerosis: evidence from virtual reality. *Neurorehab Neural Repair* 2007;**21**:273–8

87. Smith K J, McDonald W I. The pathophysiology of multiple sclerosis: the mechanisms underlying the production of symptoms and the natural history of the disease. *Phil Trans R Soc Lond B* 1999;**354**:1649–73

88. Sheean G L, Murray N M F, Rothwell J C, Miller D H, Thompson A J. An electrophysiological study of the mechanism of fatigue in multiple sclerosis. *Brain* 1997; **120**:299–315

89. Smith R M, Adeney-Steel M, Fulcher G, Longley W A. Symptom change with exercise is a temporary phenomenon for people with multiple sclerosis. *Arch Phys Med Rehab* 2006;**87**:723–7

90. Bjarnadottir O H, Konradsdottir A D, Reynisdottir K, Olafsson E. Multiple sclerosis and brief moderate exercise: a randomised study. *Mult Scler* 2007;**13**:776–82

Prognosis in neurorehabilitation

Angelo Ghezzi and Annalisa Rizzo

The primary goal of rehabilitation in a disease like multiple sclerosis (MS), causing progressive disability and loss of functional independence, should be the improvement of function in order to maximize adaptation and to improve life activities [1–3].

There is empirical evidence that rehabilitation is useful in MS patients, improving functional independence; however, its effectiveness has not been proven in large clinical trials. With respect to the assessment of the efficacy of drugs, where the end points can be clearly defined (e.g., reduction of relapse rate), as well as the characteristics of the agent (dose, route of administration) and the methods of assessment (e.g., relapse count, expanded disability status scale [EDSS] evaluation), with the possibility of randomizing patients to an active drug or placebo in a double-blind study, the conduction of clinical trials in neurorehabilitation is more complex and difficult, for these main reasons:

- it is not easy to standardize the input and to measure its effect on the recipient;
- it is difficult to have a reliable, responsive, accepted, and clinically and scientifically sound measure to assess the outcome;
- it is not feasible to administer a placebo and to conduct a double-blind design.

Moreover, in contrast to a drug that is passively taken, in rehabilitation the patients actively participate in an individualized education–training program tailored to specific needs, with their physical, cognitive, and emotional characteristics, in a close interaction with the treating team. For these reasons the general rules of clinical trials cannot easily be adopted in this field of medicine. At present specific and accepted guidelines are not available regarding the intensity and duration of rehabilitation, and there is no consensus on the tool with which to measure the outcome of rehabilitation. Different measures can be used, covering important aspects of the disease, such as impairment, disability, handicap, quality of life, goal achievement, coping skills, and self-sufficiency [1], and obviously the choice of the instrument, its sensitivity, and its appropriateness can necessarily affect the possibility of detecting changes induced by the treatment. In a recent paper, aiming to evaluate the most evaluative outcome measure for MS, de Groot et al. [4] used several scales related to MS involvement – physical functioning, mental health, social functioning, and general health – in a cohort of 156 recently diagnosed MS patients, and found that SF-36 physical functioning and the Rehabilitation Activities Profile occupation subscale were the most sensitive scales for detecting changes associated to MS.

In spite of these complex methodological problems, efforts have been made to demonstrate that neurorehabilitation has a beneficial effect in MS patients, improving neurological disability and independence.

- **Freeman et al.** [5] included 66 progressive MS patients in a short-period rehabilitation program, using subjects on a waiting list for rehabilitation as controls. At the end of the treatment period the handicap and disability scores inproved significantly compared to controls. The benefits were maintained in the follow-up: the improvement in disability and handicap for 6 months, the improvement in emotional well-being for 7 months, the improvement in quality of life for 10 months.
- **Solari et al.** [6] assigned 50 ambulatory MS patients to 3 weeks of inpatient physical rehabilitation (study treatment) or exercises

Multiple Sclerosis: Recovery of Function and Neurorehabilitation, eds. J. Kesselring, G. Comi, and A. J. Thompson. Published by Cambridge University Press. © Cambridge University Press 2010.

performed at home (control treatment), and found an improvement in disability and mental components of health-related quality of life perception at 3 and 9 weeks, whereas the impairment remained unchanged.

- **Jorger et al.** [7] treated 90 male and 196 female MS patients for a period of 28 days and observed a gain in the Extended Barthel Index (EBI) ranging from 0.85 per week in subjects with a baseline score of 30–39 to 0.18 for those with a score of 60–64; the gain was 0.74 and 0.58 respectively for subjects with basal EBI of 40–49 and 50–59.
- **Mosert and Kesselring** [8] included 37 MS patients in a short-term training program, consisting of five 30-minute sessions of graded bicycle exercise each week for 4 weeks, and found a significant improvement of aerobic threshold, activity levels, health perception measures, and reduced fatigue.
- **Patti et al.** [9] evaluated the effect of a 6-week individualized program of outpatient rehabilitation in 58 primary/secondary progressive MS patients, compared to 53 control subjects, in a randomized controlled trial; at the end of the treatment period disability was significantly improved in treated compared to control patients, while the level of impairment did not change. The benefits were maintained for a further 6 weeks.
- **Romberg et al.** [10] randomized subjects with mild to moderate MS to receive an exercise program consisting of resistance training for 6 weeks ($n = 47$), or no intervention. At 6 months the exercising subjects showed improvement of MS Functional Score, whereas control subjects showed deterioration. On the contrary the effect on the EDSS, Functional Independence Measure (FIM), MSQoL-54 and depression (Center for Epidermiological Studies Depression Scale [CES-D]) was poor. There are some other data suggesting that exercise is recommended during all stages of the disease, with a beneficial effect on mood, well-being, and quality of life [11].
- **Newman et al.** [12] investigated the effect of treadmill walking at an aerobic training intensity in 16 MS patients, and found a reduced effort of walking and fatigue, concluding that this intervention can be useful for some people with MS. A positive effect of aerobic exercise was also

demonstrated by Suraka et al. [13] in a study where 47 patients were randomized to exercise whereas another 48 MS controls continued their normal living.
- **Storr et al.** [14], differently from previous reports, did not observe a different outcome in 38 patients who received a comprehensive multidisciplinary rehabilitation treatment for an average of 35.5 days, compared to 52 control subjects who received no treatment.

The process of adaptation is a key point in rehabilitation, during the different phases of the disease: at onset, when subjects face the impact of diagnosis; during the first stages of the disease, when relapses occur, with a negative psychological effect and, in spite of the low level of disability, the strong influence of MS on family and social life; in the subsequent chronic progressive phase, when disability increases and the effect of restriction is severe [2]. For these reasons efforts should be made to improve health behavior and quality of life. This approach has been evaluated in a randomized clinical trial [15] in which 61 female MS patients were randomized to receive an intervention consisting of an educational program intended to promote changes of lifestyle, to increase self-abilities, to manage stressful events, and to improve mind–body interaction. Another 60 subjects served as controls. After the intervention program had lasted for 8 weeks, followed by bimonthly telephone calls, subjects showed an improvement in their adaptation and mental health, compared with controls.

Prognosis

Once it is accepted that rehabilitation is useful in MS, an important question is to verify whether its effect is influenced by clinical variables or other possible prognostic factors. Only a few studies have investigated this topic; however, there are data suggesting that, among clinical variables, cognitive impairment, cerebellar dysfunction, and the severity of the disease (disease duration, EDSS score) have a negative effect on rehabilitation.

Langdon and Thompson [16] evaluated the effects of an individually designed goal-oriented program formulated by a multidisciplinary team, including physiotherapy, occupational therapy and nursing input, speech and language therapy, social work, and psychological assistance, in a group of 38 MS patients. The evaluation included several measures of neurological impairment, physical disability, cognitive impairment, and emotional distress. The median FIM motor score on admission was 59; after a 3-week rehabilitation program, the median FIM motor gain was six points. The median FIM cognitive score on admission was 35 and was unchanged at the end of the treatment period. Changes of FIM motor scored were correlated with demographic, neurological, cognitive, and emotional variables. It was found that cognitive function and cerebellar involvement were correlated with a poor outcome. Attention, recall memory, and executive functions are frequently affected in subjects with cognitive impairment and can give a reason for the negative effect of cognitive impairment on rehabilitation: this study, in particular, showed that Wechsler Adult Intelligence Scale-Revised (WAIS-R) vocabulary score was statistically correlated with changes in FIM motor score, suggesting the role of verbal communication in the rehabilitation process. As expected on the basis of its disabling effect, cerebellar dysfunction was also associated with a poor prognosis.

Grasso *et al.* [17] correlated the effect of rehabilitation, measured by means of EDSS, Barthel Index, and Rivermead Mobility Index, with EDSS, cognitive impairment, and disease duration, in a cohort of 230 consecutive patients. There was no change in EDSS but both Barthel Index and Rivermead Mobility Index increased at the end of the treatment period, indicating a clinical improvement: 124 subjects improved on Barthel Index and 113 on Rivermead Mobility Index. The outcome of rehabilitation was negatively influenced by basal EDSS, cognitive impairment, and disease duration.

According to the definition that the final goal of rehabilitation is to improve adaptation in relation to the specific needs of the individual patient in an individualized goal-oriented program, the treatment can have a poor effect because of a deficient implementation of the program. According to Freeman [3], the outcome of rehabilitation is related to a number of key principles:

- comprehensive and accurate assessment of factors contributing to the problem;
- multidisciplinary teamwork;
- programs tailored to meet individual needs;
- establishment of mutually agreed patient-centered goals;
- regular review, taking into account that both the disease and the needs can change with time.

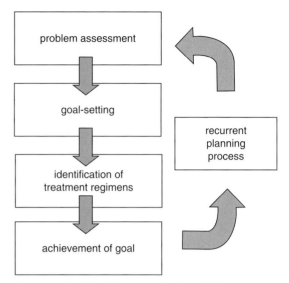

Fig. 17.1. Flowchart illustrating a flexible rehabilitation program which measures the results and effects of intervention.

The first step in rehabilitation consists in the identification of factors that can contribute to impairment of mobility and to restriction of patient's ability to participate in family, social, vocational, and leisure activities [3]. They include:

- physical problems, such as motor and sensory impairment, fatigue, ataxia, urinary and sexual disturbances, speaking, eating, swallowing dysfunction;
- psychological problems, such as cognitive impairment, depression, motivation;
- environmental causes, for example climate, physical barriers, but also socio-cultural and economic impediments.

The second step moves from the evaluation of needs to determine the goal of intervention. A multidisciplinary team can help to identify clear, realistic, and achievable goals.

The third step involves the implementation of specific procedures of intervention, addressed at the level of impairment, alleviating neurological signs and symptoms, but broadened to environmental factors that contribute to reducing the patient's activities [3]. The rehabilitation program should be realized in a flexible way, periodically measuring the results and the effect of intervention (Fig. 17.1). Many circumstances can affect the outcome, as summarized in Table 17.1.

Table 17.1 Steps and pitfalls of the rehabilitation program

Steps	Pitfalls
Step 1 Assessment of problems	Is the assessment accurate? • is the problem misunderstood? • depression, emotional, family problems? • more cognitive difficulties? • fatigue? • deterioration of neurological condition after the assessment?
Step 2 Identification of the goal	Is the goal appropriate? • too difficult? • timescale too ambitious? • not relevant to patient's lifestyle? • lack of motivation? • too complex or not clearly defined?
Step 3 Planning of intervention	Is the intervention appropriate? • treatment not related to goal? • lack of consistency of intervention? • team not coordinated? • more specialists needed? • number of sessions insufficient? • lack of resources?

Conclusions

In spite of many methodological problems, there are data suggesting that rehabilitation is useful in MS patients.

Cognitive impairment, disease duration, EDSS, and cerebellar and sphincter dysfunction seem to be correlated to a poor outcome.

The rehabilitation program can improve the adaptation, life activities, and finally the quality of life if tailored to specific, meaningful, and consistent needs of patients, verifying during its development the accuracy of patient assessment, the correct identification of goals, and the appropriateness of interventions.

References

1. Kesselring J. Neurorehabilitation in multiple sclerosis: what is the evidence-base? *J Neurol* 2004;**251**(Suppl 4): 25–9

2. Thompson AJ. Neurorehabilitation in multiple sclerosis: foundations, facts and fictions. *Curr Opin Neurol* 2005;**18**:267–71

3. Freeman JA. Improving mobility and functional independence in persons with multiple sclerosis. *J Neurol* 2001;**248**:255–9

4. De Groot V, Beckerman H, Uitdehaag BMJ, *et al.* The usefulness of evaluative outcome measures in patients with multiple sclerosis. *Brain* 2006;**129**:2648–59

5. Freeman JA, Langdon DW, Hobart JC, Thompson AJ. The impact of inpatient rehabilitation on progressive multiple sclerosis. *Ann Neurol* 1997;**42**:236–44

6. Solari A, Filippini G, Gasco P, *et al.* Physical rehabilitation has a positive effect on disability in multiple sclerosis patients. *Neurology* 1999;**52**:57–62

7. Jorger M, Beer S, Kesselring J. Impact of neurorehabilitation on disability in patients with acutely and chronically disabling diseases of the nervous system measured by the Extended Barthel Index. *Neurorehab Neural Repair* 2001;**15**:15–22

8. Mosert S, Kesselring J. Effects of a short-term exercise training program on aerobic fitness, fatigue, health perception and activity level of subjects with multiple sclerosis. *Mult Scler* 2002;**8**:161–8

9. Patti F, Ciancio MR, Cacopardo M, *et al.* Effect of a short outpatient rehabilitation treatment on disability of multiple sclerosis patients: a randomized controlled trial. *J Neurol* 2003;**250**:861–6

10. Romberg A, Virtanen A, Ruutiainen J. Long-term exercise improves functional impairment but not quality of life in multiple sclerosis. *J Neurol* 2005;**252**:839–45

11. Sutherland G, Andersen MB. Exercise and multiple sclerosis: physiological, psychological and quality of life issues. *J Sports Med Phys Fitness* 2001; **41**:421–32

12. Newman MA, Daves H, van der Berg M, *et al.* Can aerobic treadmill training reduce the effort of walking and fatigue in people with multiple sclerosis? *Mult Scler* 2007;**13**:113–19

13. Suraka J, Romberg A, Ruutiainen J, *et al.* Effects of aerobic and strength exercise on motor fatigue in men and women with multiple sclerosis: a randomized controlled trial. *Clin Rehab* 2004;**18**:737–46

14. Storr LK, Sorensen PS, Ravnborg M. The efficacy of multidisciplinary rehabilitation in stable multiple sclerosis patients. *Mult Scler* 2006;**12**:235–42

15. Stuifbergen AK, Becker H, Blozis S, *et al.* A randomized clinical trial of a wellness intervention for women with multiple sclerosis. *Arch Phys Med Rehab* 2003;**84**:467–76

16. Langdon DW, Thompson AJ. Multiple sclerosis: a preliminary study of selected variables affecting rehabilitation outcome. *Mult Scler* 1999; 5:94–100

17. Grasso MG, Troisi E, Rizzi F, *et al.* Prognostic factors in multidisciplinary rehabilitation treatment in multiple sclerosis: an outcome study. *Mult Scler* 2005;**11**:719–24

Chapter 18

Clinical trials to test rehabilitation

Alessandra Solari

Randomized clinical trials (RCTs) are recognized as the gold-standard approach to assessing the efficacy of medical interventions. High-quality (rigorously designed, conducted, and analyzed) RCTs provide reliable evidence on which to base clinical practice. Rehabilitation interventions are widely used in the management of patients with multiple sclerosis (MS); however, relatively few interventions have been evaluated by RCTs.

Compared to drug trials, the design and conduct of RCTs to assess rehabilitation presents a number of major problems [1, 2]. This chapter examines sources of error in RCTs in general, discusses specific problems related to rehabilitation trials, and finally summarizes the available evidence regarding the methodological rigor of rehabilitation interventions in MS in three major areas: physiotherapy, cognitive retraining, and multidisciplinary rehabilitation. Clinical aspects of these interventions are discussed in other chapters of this volume.

Sources of error in RCTs

Randomized clinical trials are susceptible to two main types of error, those due to *chance* (random departure of results from the truth), and those due to *bias* (deviation of results from the truth) [3]. Many clinicians are familiar with errors due to chance, embodied in the concept of statistical significance or the *p* value, which estimates whether a difference between, say a treated and a control group, can reasonably be attributed to chance or considered real.

Bias is a much less familiar but equally important concept and the first step in reducing it is to use a rigorous randomization procedure. Randomization is the fundamental characteristic of an RCT that renders

it less susceptible to selection bias than other study designs for assessing therapeutic interventions. If assignment to the experimental vs. control intervention is random, any differences in characteristics between the two groups are due to chance alone. However, other types of bias can arise during the conduct of an RCT and the analysis of the results.

Two fundamental types of *chance* error can be distinguished:

(1) *Type 1 (alpha) error* At the basis of any RCT there are two possibilities: the experimental intervention has no effect: this is named the "null hypothesis"; the experimental intervention has an effect: this is named the "alternative hypothesis." A type 1 error is the chance to reject the null hypothesis (i.e., declaring that the experimental intervention has an effect) when it is not. This type of error is the most important error due to chance, and it is desirable that the probability of this error arising should be as low as possible (generally <0.05, or 5%).

(2) *Type 2 (beta) error* The other sort of error is the chance to miss the effect (i.e., declaring that the experimental intervention has no effect) when there is an effect. Usually the probability of this type of error is set a priori (before the study starts, when the "power analysis" is performed) at between 0.10 and 0.20 (10–20%). The *power* of a study corresponds to 1 minus the estimated type 2 error probability.

Bias is a systematic, non-random deviation of results and inferences from the truth. Any trend in the collection, analysis, interpretation, publication, or review of data that can lead to conclusions systematically different from the truth is a bias [3]. The main

Multiple Sclerosis: Recovery of Function and Neurorehabilitation, eds. J. Kesselring, G. Comi, and A. J. Thompson. Published by Cambridge University Press. © Cambridge University Press 2010.

types of bias encountered in RCTs are examined below, along with measures that can be taken to prevent or minimize them, considering for simplicity the example of a two-arm parallel group RCT.

(1) *Selection bias* Selection bias arises because of differences between the experimental and control group at the outset (e.g., differences in age, sex ratio, duration or severity of MS, presence of concomitant disease). Rigorous random allocation of participants to the experimental vs. control intervention prevents selection bias. If the trial is small (say fewer than 100 participants) differences between the two groups are still possible, but are due to chance.

(2) *Performance bias* Performance bias arises because of differences in care between the experimental and control groups, distinct from the intervention being studied. Such differences can take various forms, for example the treating physician may, unconsciously or otherwise, administer care, perform examinations, or elicit adverse events differently between experimental and control patients. Performance bias is prevented by masking the caring physician to the intervention received by the patient.

(3) *Detection bias* Detection bias arises because of differences in the *observation* of outcome measures. Detection bias is prevented by masking the outcome assessor to the intervention received by the patient.

(4) *Recall bias and social desirability bias* These biases arise because of differences in the reporting of *patient-reported* outcome measures. They are prevented by masking the patient to the intervention received.

(5) *Attrition bias* Attrition bias arises as a result of differences between the experimental and the control group in terms of the number of dropouts. Differences in patient commitment between the two groups may cause differential dropout, rendering the interpretation of the results problematic. Effective patient and physician blinding reduces attrition bias. However, differential attrition can also be due to poor acceptability or tolerability of the intervention. This differential attrition can be managed by including all randomized patients (including dropouts) in an intention-to-treat analysis, as well as performing an analysis of outcomes in patients who complete the study (per protocol analysis). If an intention-to-treat analysis is not performed, inferences from the per protocol analysis alone are likely to be biased.

From the above discussion it emerges that the procedures of randomization and blinding — essential characteristics of a well-designed and well-conducted RCT — achieve the greatest possible similarity between the experimental and control groups, so that the only difference between them is the intervention itself. Any differences in outcomes can then be reasonably attributed to the intervention. It should also be evident that the data must be analyzed according to the "intention-to-treat" principle.

Studies that manage to avoid, as far as possible, selection, performance, attrition, and detection bias, are considered to have *internal validity*. Scoring systems have been developed to quantify internal validity [4, 5]. Internal validity differs from *external validity* (or generalizability) which refers to the extent to which the study population of an RCT is comparable to the population of interest (in the present case whether participants with MS in an RCT correspond to people with MS in general or to the patients followed at a given center).

Methodological pitfalls in RCTs to assess rehabilitation

A number of pitfalls of rehabilitation RCTs are shared with those of drug RCTs, including those arising from variation in MS type and difficulties in choosing appropriate outcome measures. Other problems are specific to rehabilitation studies and arise because rehabilitation techniques are multifaceted, complex, and difficult to define and quantify; because the training and skills of clinicians administering the intervention can vary; and because patient blinding is difficult and often impossible. Furthermore, the resources necessary to conduct rehabilitation trials according to good clinical practice and high quality standards are generally lacking; well-powered multicenter studies are almost never performed. The pitfalls to be avoided in rehabilitation RCTs are considered under the headings experimental intervention, control intervention, blinding, and outcome measures.

Experimental intervention

The CONSORT statement on reporting clinical trials recommends that "precise details of the interventions intended for each group and how and when they were actually administered" should always be reported [5, 6]. Adherence to this recommendation is particularly important for RCTs on rehabilitation interventions because such interventions are complex. Factors contributing to this complexity are the specific rehabilitation technique or theory on which the intervention is based, the setting, intensity, and duration of the program, the patient's adherence to it, and above all the variability of the intervention in relation to experience and training of the therapist, and the way he/she interacts with the patient. By contrast there is much less variability in drug RCTs, where previous dose-finding trials have usually standardized the dose, and administration is uniform across studies.

Another reason why rehabilitation interventions should be described in detail is that their potential value can be appreciated: it must be clear whether the trial is pragmatic (with focus on whether the intervention has a beneficial effect that would be seen if introduced into clinical practice) or primarily explanatory (aiming to measure benefit under ideal conditions or determine which component of the intervention is efficacious) [7, 8].

Control intervention

In drug RCTs, the experimental intervention is compared to placebo or an established drug. The comparator in rehabilitation RCTs is much more problematic. An adequate sham intervention (equivalent to placebo) can be devised only in certain cases [9]. Waiting-list patients are not a good solution, since these patients know they are not receiving intervention, and this can result in bias [10]. (Bias can also arise because intervention patients know they are receiving the intervention.) Waiting-list patients should be used as controls only when no other solution is apparent. A more acceptable option is to use a low-intensity intervention as comparator [11], although this is likely to reduce the study power and require recruitment of more patients.

Blinding

As noted, patient masking is rarely possible in rehabilitation RCTs [9, 12]. However it is always possible to prevent detection bias by having an assessor who is different from the caring clinician, and from the treating clinician, and who is masked to the intervention assignment.

Outcome measures

To be clinically worthwhile an intervention must affect outcomes that are clinically meaningful, have a *clinically significant* effect, do more good than harm, and be cost-effective. Many RCTs conducted in the past had outcome measures of little direct relevance to people with MS [13]. Because of the complex nature of rehabilitation interventions, researchers often employ several outcome measures. However this increases the risk of type 1 errors (incorrectly concluding that the intervention has an effect) due to multiple significance testing. This type of error is also called the *cumulative Type 1 error rate*. The best way to minimize the impact of multiple testing is to specify one or two primary outcome measures a priori, on which the power analysis is based, and then select a limited number of other (secondary) outcome measures. Positive results for secondary measures must be considered preliminary and serve to suggest further exploration in specifically designed studies. Outcome measures (particularly primary outcome measures) should also be assessed on participants who drop out, to enable a genuine intention-to-treat analysis.

There is no real obstacle to designing rehabilitation RCTs with a limited number of outcome measures, all of which should be clinically relevant; nor is there any reason for not following all randomized patients, including dropouts, so as to allow a meaningful intention-to-treat analysis.

Quality of available evidence

The quality of an RCT has been defined as the likelihood of the trial design generating unbiased results [5], a definition that covers only the internal validity. A more comprehensive definition was given by Verhagen *et al.* [4] as the likelihood of the trial design generating unbiased results that are sufficiently precise and allow application in clinical practice.

The main findings of the available physiotherapy, cognitive retraining, and multidisciplinary rehabilitation RCTs in MS are summarized in Tables 18.1–18.3. When available, the score of the Physiotherapy Evidence Database (PEDro) scale (www.pedro.fhs.usyd. edu.au) is also reported [14]. The PEDro scale consists

Table 18.1 Published RCTs assessing the efficacy of physical rehabilitation

Study	Year	Primary outcome specified	Patient masking	Assessor masking	Intention-to-treat analysis	Pilot study	PEDro score
Petajan et al. [15]	1996	− [a]	−	+	−	−	5/10
Lord et al. [16]	1998	−	−	−	−	+	6/10
Jones et al. [17]	1999	−	−		−	−	N/A
Solari et al. [11]	1999	+	−	+	+	−	7/10
Armutlu et al. [18]	2001	−	−	+	−	+	6/10
Wiles et al. [19, 20]	2001 2003	+	−	+	−	−	7/10
Mostert and Kesselring [21]	2002	−	−	−	−	−	3/10
DeBolt and McCubbin [22]	2004	+	−	−	−	−	6/10
Romberg et al. [23]	2004	+	−	−	+	−	6/10
Romberg et al. [24]	2005	−	−	−	−	−	6/10
van den Berg et al. [25]	2006	+	−	+	−	+	6/10
McAuley et al. [26]	2007	+	−	−	+	−	N/A

Notes: [a] Bonferroni adjustment performed; − inadequate, not performed or not reported; + performed and adequate; N/A not available.

Table 18.2 Published RCTs assessing the efficacy of multidisciplinary rehabilitation

Study	Year	Primary outcome specified	Patient masking	Assessor masking	Intention-to-treat analysis	Pilot study	PEDro score
Francabandera et al. [27]	1988	−	−	−	−	−	4/10
Freeman et al. [10]	1997	−	−	−	−	−	N/A
Guagenti-Tax et al. [28]	2000	−	−	−	−	−	N/A
Craig et al. [29]	2003	+	−	−	−	−	5/10
Pozzilli et al. [30]	2002	−	−	−	−	−	N/A
Patti et al. [31, 32]	2002 2003	+	−	+	+	−	7/10
Stuifbergen et al. [33]	2003	−	−	−	−	−	N/A
Storr et al. [12]	2006	−	+	+	−	−	3/10

Notes: − inadequate, not performed or not reported; + performed and adequate; N/A not available.

of ten items, eight of which investigate internal validity (random allocation, concealed allocation, blind subjects, blind therapists, blind assessors, adequate follow-up, intention-to-treat analysis, and between-group comparisons), and two investigate the quality of the statistical information (baseline comparability, and reports of point estimates and measures of variability). Eight of the scale items are derived from the Delphi list [4]. The PEDro score is the number of items satisfied in the trial report, and ranges between 0 (no items satisfied) and 10 (all satisfied). The overall quality of the trials found was not particularly high (PEDro score, where available, in the range 3–7) (Tables 18.1 and 18.2).

Table 18.3 Published RCTs assessing the efficacy of cognitive retraining[a]

Study	Year	Primary outcome specified	Patient masking	Assessor masking	Intention-to-treat analysis	Pilot study
Jønsson et al. [36]	1993	−	−	−	−	−
Mendozzi et al. [37]	1998	−	−	−	−	+
Lincoln et al. [38]	2002	+	−	+	+	−
Solari et al. [9]	2004	+	+	+	+	−
Chiaravalloti et al. [39]	2005	−	−	−	−	−

Notes: [a] PEDro score not applicable to cognitive retraining; − inadequate, not performed or not reported; + performed and adequate.

Physiotherapy

There is mounting evidence that physical activity is associated with substantial health, economic, and societal benefits because it increases life expectancy, reduces risks of coronary heart disease, diabetes, colon cancer, hypertension, obesity, and osteoporosis, and also prolongs independent living in older adults [34]. Up to 1996, when the Petajan et al. study on aerobic training appeared [15], no RCT on physiotherapy in people with MS had been published. The Petajan study had the merit of providing evidence against the common belief that physical exercise increased the risk of exacerbation and clinical worsening in people with MS, and showed, conversely, that such people should not be discouraged from engaging in physical activity; it also proposed physical interventions suitable for MS patients [35]. The study inspired a series of further RCTs on physical rehabilitation in MS (12 RCTs, 13 publications; Table 18.1) [11, 15–26].

Cognitive retraining

Evidence for the effectiveness of rehabilitation interventions to help cognitively compromised MS people is scarce. Five RCTs [9, 36–39] have been published since 1993 (Table 18.3). Multiplicity of outcome measures and presence of a learning effect have heavily influenced the findings of these RCTs. In fact most studies assessing pharmacological and non-pharmacological interventions on cognitive functions in MS published over the last 10 years [9, 36, 38, 40–44], have found improvements in performance in all study arms, even over a 2-year follow-up [45] suggesting a learning effect. Similar improvements in cognitive performance are well documented for other diseases, including Alzheimer disease [46].

Multidisciplinary rehabilitation

Eight RCTs published between 1988 and 2006 [10, 12, 27–33] assessed the efficacy of interventions involving two or more rehabilitation areas among physical, occupational, and psychological therapy and cognitive retraining (Table 18.2). These RCTs are more heterogeneous than the others and are of variable quality [13].

Conclusions

Until 1988, no RCT assessing the efficacy of rehabilitation in MS patients had been published. In the 1990s and subsequently a series of studies appeared in a range of journals of clinical neurology and rehabilitation (Table 18.4) [47]. However, they were heterogeneous in terms of intervention type, outcome measures, and length of follow-up. As a consequence, systematic reviews attempting to summarize the results have been unable to perform meta-analyses and had to limit themselves to assessing study quality [13, 48]. A further limitation of most published studies is that details on components of the intervention were generally lacking.

There are in fact difficulties in defining, developing, documenting, and reproducing complex interventions that are not encountered in drug trials [1, 2]. The UK Medical Research Council framework (Fig. 18.1) produced a useful guide for developing and such interventions by RCTs [49]. It presents a phased approach to the process of development and evaluation as follows:

Pre-clinical phase In this phase the theoretical bases for the experimental intervention are considered in order to inform its choice.

Phase I The relevant components of the intervention and their interrelationships are defined by means of preliminary surveys, case studies, and qualitative studies (focus groups).

Table 18.4 Journals publishing RCTs on rehabilitation in MS

Journal	Number of studies	Publication year
Acta Neurologica Scandinavica	1	1993
Annals of Neurology	2	1996, 2000
Archives of Physical and Medical Rehabilitation	2	2003, 2004
Clinical Rehabilitation	1	1998
International Journal of MS Care	1	2000
Journal of the Neurological Sciences	1	2004
Journal of Neurology	3	2002, 2004
Journal of Neurology, Neurosurgery and Psychiatry	5	2002, 2003, 2006
Multiple Sclerosis	4	2002, 2005, 2006, 2007
Neurology	3	1994, 1999, 2004
Neurological Sciences	1	1998
Neurorehabilitation and Neural Repair	1	2001
Physiotherapy	1	1999
Rehabilitation Nursing	1	1988

Phase II The information gathered in Phase I is used to develop the optimum experimental intervention and study design, and the content of the control intervention (alternative treatment, or – if applicable –sham intervention). The use of a no-intervention control group may be unacceptable to patients, and a randomized waiting-list study in which all participants ultimately receive the intervention can produce biased results. Outcome measures for the succeeding RCT are also explored during this phase to allow assessment of effect size, and provide a basis for calculating sample sizes for the subsequent RCT.

Phase III The RCT is designed taking into account results of previous phases. The design must consider eligibility criteria, which should as far as possible match the characteristics of those to whom the intervention is likely to be offered. Outcomes relevant to people with MS and also encompassing economic measures (costs to patients, carers, and society) should also be considered in this phase.

Phase IV The results of the RCT are put into practice and their impact assessed, considering applicability of the intervention, the clinical characteristics of the patients, and adverse effects. Progression from one phase to the next may not be linear; instead an iterative procedure may prove useful leading to improved study design, execution, and results generalizability.

Theory	Modeling	Exploratory(R)CT	RCT	Long-term Implementation
Explore relevant theory to ensure best choice of intervention and hypothesis and to predict major confounders and strategic design issues	Identify the components of the intervention, and the underlying mechanisms by which they will influence outcomes to provide evidence that you can predict how they relate to and interact with each other	Describe the constant and variable components of a replicable intervention and a feasible protocol for comparing the intervention to an appropriate alternative	Compare a fully defined intervention to an appropriate alternative using a protocol that is theoretically defensible, reproducible and adequately controlled, in a study with appropriate statistical power	Determine whether others can reliably replicate your intervention and results in uncontrolled settings over the long term
Preclinical	Phase I	Phase II	Phase III	Phase IV

Continuum of increasing evidence

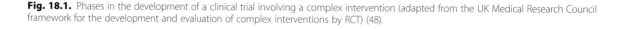

Fig. 18.1. Phases in the development of a clinical trial involving a complex intervention (adapted from the UK Medical Research Council framework for the development and evaluation of complex interventions by RCT) (48).

References

1. Plsek P E, Greenhalgh T. The challenge of complexity in health care. *BMJ* 2001;**323**:625–8

2. Campbell M, Fitzpatrick R, Haines A. Framework, design and evaluation of complex interventions to improve health. *BMJ* 2000;**321**:694–6

3. Last J M (ed). A dictionary of epidemiology. 4th ed. Oxford: Oxford University Press, 2001.

4. Verhagen A P, de-Vet H C W, de-Bie R A, *et al*. The Delphi list: a criteria list for quality assessment of randomized clinical trials for conducting systematic reviews developed by Delphi consensus. *J Clin Epidemiol* 1998;**51**:1235–41

5. Moher D, Jadad A R, Nichol G, *et al*. Assessing the quality of randomized controlled trials: an annotated bibliography of scales and checklists. *Control Clin Trials* 1995;**16**:62–73

6. Moher D, Schulz K F, Altman D G. The CONSORT statement: revised recommendations for improving the quality of reports of parallel-group randomized trials. *Lancet* 2001;**357**:1191–4

7. Hardeman W, Michie S, Prevost T, Fanshawe T, Kinmonth A L. Do trained intervention facilitators use theory-based behaviour change techniques? Results from the ProActive Fidelity Project. *Psychol Health* 2005;**20**(Suppl 1):107

8. Michie S, Hardeman W, Abraham C. Identifying effective techniques: the example of physical activity. *Psychol Health* 2005;**20**(Suppl 1):173–4

9. Solari A, Motta A, Mendozzi L, *et al*. Computer-aided retraining of memory and attention in people with multiple sclerosis: a randomized, double-blind controlled trial. *J Neurol Sci* 2004;**222**(1–2):99–104

10. Freeman J A, Langdon D W, Hobart J C, Thompson A J. The impact of inpatient rehabilitation on progressive multiple sclerosis. *Ann Neurol* 1997;**42**:236–44

11. Solari A, Filippini G, Gasco P, *et al*. Physical rehabilitation has a positive effect on disability in multiple sclerosis patients. *Neurology* 1999;**52**:57–62

12. Storr L K, Sørensen P S, Ravnborg M. The efficacy of multidisciplinary rehabilitation in stable multiple sclerosis patients. *Mult Scler* 2006;**12**:235–42

13. Khan F, Turner-Stokes L, Ng L, Kilpatrick T. Multidisciplinary rehabilitation for adults with multiple sclerosis. *Cochrane Database Syst Rev* 2007; CD006036

14. Physiotherapy Evidence Database. Available online at www.pedro.org.au

15. Petajan J H, Gappmaier E, White A T, *et al*. Impact of aerobic training on fitness and quality of life in multiple sclerosis. *Ann Neurol* 1996;**39**:432–41

16. Lord S E, Wade D T, Halligan P W. A comparison of two physiotherapy treatment approaches to improve walking in multiple sclerosis: a pilot randomized controlled study. *Clin Rehab* 1998;**2**:477–86

17. Jones R, Davies-Smith A, Harvey L. The effect of weighted leg raises and quadriceps strength, EMG and functional activities in people with multiple sclerosis. *Physiotherapy* 1999;**85**:154–61

18. Armutlu K, Karabudak R, Nurlu G. Physiotherapy approaches in the treatment of ataxic multiple sclerosis: a pilot study. *Neurorehab Neural Repair* 2001;**15**:203–11

19. Wiles C M, Newcombe R G, Fuller K J, *et al*. Controlled randomized crossover trial of the effects of physiotherapy on mobility in chronic multiple sclerosis. *J Neurol Neurosurg Psychiatry* 2001;**70**:174–9

20. Wiles C M, Newcombe R G, Fuller K J, Jones A, Price M. Use of videotape to assess mobility in a controlled randomized crossover trial of physiotherapy in chronic multiple sclerosis. *Clin Rehab* 2003; **17**:256–63

21. Mostert S, Kesselring J. Effects of a short-term exercise training program on aerobic fitness, fatigue, health perception and activity level of subjects with multiple sclerosis. *Mult Scler* 2002;**8**:161–8

22. DeBolt L S, McCubbin J A. The effects of home-based resistance exercise on balance, power, and mobility in adults with multiple sclerosis. *Arch Phys Med Rehab* 2004;**85**:290–7

23. Romberg A, Virtanen A, Ruutiainen J. Long-term exercise improves functional impairment but not quality of life in multiple sclerosis. *J Neurol* 2005;**252**:839–45

24. Romberg A, Virtanen A, Ruutiainen J, *et al*. Effects of a 6-month exercise program on patients with multiple sclerosis: a randomized study. *Neurology* 2004;**63**:2034–8

25. van den Berg M, Dawes H, Wade D T, *et al*. Treadmill training for individuals with multiple sclerosis: a pilot randomized trial. *J Neurol Neurosurg Psychiatry* 2006;**77**:531–3

26. McAuley E, Moti R W, Morris K S, *et al*. Enhancing physical activity adherence and well-being in multiple sclerosis: a randomized controlled trial. *Mult Scler* 2007;**13**:652–9

27. Francabandera F L, Holland N J, Wiesel-Levison P, Scheinberg L C. Multiple sclerosis rehabilitation: inpatient versus outpatients. *Rehab Nursing* 1988;**13**:251–3

28. Guagenti-Tax E M, DiLorenzo T A, Tenteromano L, LaRocca N G, Smith C R. Impact of a comprehensive

long-term care program on caregivers and persons with multiple sclerosis. *Int J MS Care* 2000;**2**:5–18

29. Craig J, Young C A, Ennis M, Baker G, Boggild M. A randomized controlled trial comparing rehabilitation against standard therapy in multiple sclerosis patients. *J Neurol Neurosurg Psychiatry* 2003;**74**:1225–30

30. Pozzilli C, Brunetti M, Amicosante A M W, *et al.* Home based management in multiple sclerosis: results of a randomised controlled trial. *J Neurol Neurosurg Psychiatry* 2002;**73**:250–5

31. Patti F, Ciancio M R, Reggio E, *et al.* The impact of outpatient rehabilitation on quality of life in multiple sclerosis. *J Neurol* 2002;**249**:1027–33

32. Patti F, Ciancio M R, Cacopardo M, *et al.* Effects of a short outpatient rehabilitation treatment on disability of multiple sclerosis patients: a randomized controlled trial. *J Neurol* 2003;**250**:861–6

33. Stuifbergen A K, Becker H, Blozis S, Timmerman G, Kulberg V. A randomized clinical trial of a wellness intervention for women with multiple sclerosis. *Arch Phys Med Rehab* 2003;**84**:467–76

34. Bo Andersen L. Physical activity and health. *BMJ* 2007;**334**:1173

35. Kahn E B, Ramsey L T, Brownson R C, *et al.* The effectiveness of interventions to increase physical activity: a systematic review. *Am J Prev Med* 2002;**22**(Suppl 4):73–107

36. Jønsson A, Korfitzen E M, Heltberg A, *et al.* Effect of neuropsychological treatment in patients with multiple sclerosis. *Acta Neurol Scand* 1993;**88**:394–400

37. Mendozzi L, Pugnetti L, Motta A, *et al.* Computer-assisted memory retraining of patients with multiple sclerosis. *Neurol Sci* 1998;**19**:S431–8

38. Lincoln N B, Dent A, Harding J, *et al.* Evaluation of cognitive assessment and cognitive intervention for people with multiple sclerosis. *J Neurol Neurosurg Psychiatry* 2002;**72**:93–8

39. Chiaravalloti N D, DeLuca J, Moore N B, Ricker J H. Treating learning impairments improves memory performance in multiple sclerosis: a randomized clinical trial. *Mult Scler* 2005;**11**:58–68

40. Beatty W W, Goodkin D E, Monson N, Beatty P A. Cognitive disturbances in patients with relapsing remitting multiple sclerosis. *Arch Neurol* 1989;**46**:1113–19

41. Weinstein A, Schwid S I L, Schiffer R B, *et al.* Neuropsychologic status in multiple sclerosis after treatment with Glatiramer. *Arch Neurol* 1999;**56**:319–24

42. Smits R C, Emmen H H, Bertlesmann F W, *et al.* The effects of 4-aminopyridine on cognitive function in patients with multiple sclerosis. *Neurology* 1994;**44**:1701–5

43. Greene Y M, Tariot P N, Wishart H, *et al.* A 12-week, open trial of donepezil hydrochloride in patients with multiple sclerosis and associated cognitive impairments. *J Clin Psychopharmacol* 2000;**20**:350–6

44. Barak Y, Achiron A. Effect of interferon-beta-1b on cognitive functions in multiple sclerosis. *Eur Neurol* 2002;**47**:11–14

45. Clare L, Woods R T, Moniz Cook E D, Orrell M, Spector A. Cognitive rehabilitation and cognitive training for early-stage Alzheimer's disease and vascular dementia (Cochrane Review). *Cochrane Library* 2003;**4**

46. Fischer J S, Priore R L, Jacobs L D, *et al.* Neuropsychological effects of interferon B-1a in relapsing multiple sclerosis. *Ann Neurol* 2000;**48**:885–92

47. Aisen M L. Justifying neurorehabilitation: a few steps forward. *Neurology* 1999;**52**:8

48. Rietberg M B, Brooks D, Uitdehaag B M J, Kwakkel G. Exercise therapy for multiple sclerosis. *Cochrane Database Syst Rev* 2004;CD003980

49. Medical Research Council. *A Framework for Development and Evaluation of RCTs for Complex Interventions to Improve Health.* London: Medical Research Council, 2000

Spasticity in multiple sclerosis

Mauro Zaffaroni

Definition and epidemiological aspects

Spasticity has become an equivocal term that includes several other symptoms related to positive components (rigidity, increased tendon reflexes, clonus, Babinski sign, contractures, and muscular spasms) and negative components (weakness, reduced skill, and fatigue) of the upper motor neuron syndrome (UMNS). Spasticity is most commonly defined as an inappropriate, velocity-dependent, increase in muscle tonic stretch reflexes, due to the amplified reactivity of motor segments to sensory input [1], but a more simple and useful definition for clinical purposes may be "an increased resistance, velocity-dependent to passive muscular stretching" [2].

Spasticity is a very common symptom in patients with multiple sclerosis (MS) and represents one main cause of disability, even more than strength loss. It is estimated that 40% to 84% of MS patients are affected and that 90% of patients present this symptom at some time during the course of the disease [3]. Impairments and disabilities associated with spasticity have also been reported in 40% to 70% of patients [4], contractures and sensory evoked muscle spasms being the most debilitating aspects of spasticity in MS [5].

Quality of life (QoL) is moderately or severely affected by spasticity in almost 78% of MS patients [6]. A survey study based on data from 20 380 MS patients [3] revealed that there is a direct relationship between spasticity scores and disease duration or disability and that one-third of patients modified or eliminated their daily activities as a result of spasticity. Six percent of the patients reported no spasticity, 31% minimal, 19% mild (occasional), 17% moderate (frequently affects activities), 13% severe (need to modify daily activities), and 4% total (prevents daily activities) [3].

Spasticity is more difficult to treat in MS in comparison to spinal trauma and cerebral palsy because of the disease progression that leads to an increasing neurological impairment. It means that, at different times, different sites of the central nervous system (CNS) are involved, that can modify the muscular tone in different ways.

The most typical pattern of spasticity in MS is represented by an increased tone of extensor muscles of lower limbs. As disease progresses, hip abductors are involved, causing extension spasms, mostly at night or on waking in the morning. Upper limbs are less frequently involved but give rise to higher disability. Later on, flexor spasticity and spasms appear, which are more frequently painful, and patients may fall over unexpectedly. In these phases, motor impairment is also aggravated by soft tissue contracture. In the latest phases, spasticity and contracture do not symmetrically affect agonist and antagonist muscles: this determines pathological postures and limb deformities that may become irreversible and associated with pressure sores in bedridden patients.

As only 78% of MS patients with severe/total spasticity report using medication for it, it appears that 22% are on no identifiable drug regimen [3]: these data stress that spasticity is underestimated and inadequately treated.

Pathophysiology of MS-related spasticity

Although spasticity is traditionally regarded as a "pyramidal" sign, both animal models and recent studies demonstrate that selective lesions of the

Multiple Sclerosis: Recovery of Function and Neurorehabilitation, eds. J. Kesselring, G. Comi, and A. J. Thompson.
Published by Cambridge University Press. © Cambridge University Press 2010.

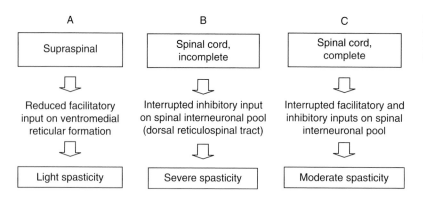

Fig. 19.1. Degrees of spasticity according to the three prototypic lesion levels, and the respective pathophysiological mechanisms.

corticospinal tract or of the primary motor cortex cause hyperreflexia but do not generate spasticity [7]. Consequently, these two clinical signs must be considered as distinct components of the UMNS.

Indeed, spinal spasticity is caused by damage to the inhibitory projections of the corticoreticulospinal fibers which originate from motor areas and reach the inhibitory medial bulbar reticular formation which, in turn, sends inhibitory projections to the spinal motor neurons through the dorsolateral reticulospinal tract running just anterior to the corticospinal tract in the lateral funiculus of the spinal cord as part of the so-called parapyramidal fibers. On the other hand, the lateral pontine reticular formation exerts an ipsilateral excitatory influence on the spinal cord through the anteromedial reticulospinal tract running in the ventral funiculus. A lesion involving the corticoreticulospinal fibers will release excitatory projections descending along the lateral pontine reticular formation, leading to a decreased inhibition (or to an increased facilitation) of the interneuronal pool in the spinal cord, and ultimately to spasticity.

These complex anatomical and functional relationships explain the different patterns of spasticity generated by different lesion levels: (a) supraspinal, (b) spinal cord, incomplete, (c) spinal cord, complete. According to the different excitatory or inhibitory pathways involved, these prototypic lesions cause different degrees of facilitation and remodeling of the spinal interneuronal network and, consequently, of spasticity (Fig. 19.1) [8]. For example, the different course of corticoreticular and corticospinal fibers in the internal capsule explains why selective lesions of the anterior limb or the genu of the internal capsule predominantly induce spasticity without a marked motor deficit and vice versa. Moreover, in the early phases of MS the lateral funiculus, the lateral corticospinal tract, and the dorsolateral reticulospinal tract are often involved, leading to severe spasticity. Conversely, in long-standing MS, with enlarging spinal cord lesions usually affecting both the dorsal and ventral reticulospinal tracts, as excitatory and inhibitory influences on the spinal circuits are in balance, the flexor reflex prevails and painful flexor spasms will appear [8].

Although spasticity is primarily generated by lesions located in the CNS, muscle paresis and immobilization, as well as muscle overactivity due to spasticity, induce secondary changes in the viscoelastic properties of muscle [9], leading to stiffness, contracture, atrophy, and fibrosis. The distinction between spastic hypertonia and stiffness due to rheological factors is relevant in that these two conditions are differently treated (see below).

From a neurochemical viewpoint, spasticity is a complex phenomenon not correlatable to any single reflex or synaptic neurotransmitter. However, at least in spasticity of spinal cord origin, a decrease was reported of the inhibitory neurotransmitters γ-aminobutyric acid (GABA) and glycine [10], which are involved in presynaptic inhibition of motoneurons. In turn, GABA and glycine receptors in the spinal cord are modulated by the inhibitory endocannabinoid neurotransmitter [11]. These concepts constitute the basis of pharmacological interventions in spasticity.

Measuring spasticity

These notions emphasize that scientifically sound and clinically meaningful spasticity measurement is indispensable to clinical practice and research in this area [12]. In clinical practice, the degree of spasticity

Table 19.1 Clinical scales for the assessment of muscle tone and spasm frequency

Scores
(a) Modified Ashworth Scale
0   No increase in muscle tone
1   Slight increase in muscle tone, manifested by a catch and release or by minimal resistance at the end of the range of motion when the affected part(s) is moved in flexion or extension
1⁺   Slight increase in muscle tone, manifested by a catch and release or by minimal resistance throughout the remainder (less than half) of the range of motion
2   More marked increase in muscle tone through most of the range of motion, but affected part(s) easily flexed
3   Considerable increase in muscle tone, passive movements difficult
4   Affected part(s) rigid in flexion or extension
(b) Penn Spasms Scale
0   No spasms
1   No spontaneous spasms/spasms induced by stimulation
2   Occasional spontaneous spasms and easily induced spasms
3   >1 but <10 spontaneous spasms/hr
4   >10 spontaneous spasms/hr

is measured by ordinal scales, the most validated and frequently used being the modified Ashworth scale [13], which is graduated in five steps (Table 19.1a). Usually the Ashworth scale is used in combination with the Penn scale [14] to evaluate spasm frequency per hour (Table 19.1b).

Recently, a patient-based, multi-item, interval-level measure of spasticity in MS patients was proposed [15]. This is an 88-item instrument made of eight subscales (muscle stiffness, pain and discomfort, muscle spasms and ADL, walking and body movements, emotional health, social functioning). In the author's opinion, the Multiple Sclerosis Spasticity Scale (MSSS-88) satisfies criteria for reliable and valid measurement of the impact of spasticity in MS and has the potential to advance measurement of outcomes in clinical trials and clinical practice, providing a new perspective in the clinical evaluation of spasticity.

Biomechanical techniques for dynamic registration of segmental mobility like the Wartenberg pendulum test or devices to measure the torque induced by passive mobilization like the isocinetic ergometer of Walsh provide objective measures but are applicable only to specific limb segments and are limited to research purposes.

Managing MS patients with spasticity

Unfortunately, there is no evidence-based model for spasticity management and all plans of action arise from experience-based practical approaches. Tentative algorithms derived from the experience of single groups [16] or from a board of experts [17] have been proposed only recently.

An effective treatment can not be apart from a methodologically correct approach, including an accurate clinical assessment with a clear definition of needs and problems, statement of goals, reassessment, and follow-up [18].

Spasticity needs to be treated when it is not useful for function and when symptoms give rise to disability or interfere with posture, motility, daily activities, and rehabilitation, in order to prevent muscular–skeletal deformities and other irreversible complications arising from immobility.

The treatment of spasticity in MS does not differ practically from that applied to other diseases of the CNS. However, it should be taken in mind that, in contrast to other diseases, MS will progress over time and, consequently, spasticity will increase or will be complicated (e.g., by pain), requiring therapy corrections or revision.

Before starting any treatment, we must always bear in mind that the main goal of the treatment is not reducing spasticity itself but minimizing the negative impact of spasticity on disability and quality of life.

Another important issue is to distinguish generalized spasticity from focal spasticity that involves few segments or body areas, since they need different therapeutic approaches.

In the early stage of MS, an increased tone of antigravity muscles may be helpful for standing, and may contribute to muscle trophism and prevent osteopenia: since antispastic drugs may increase weakness, aggravate fatigue, and limit deambulation, treatment would be detrimental. As the disease progresses over time, patients become unable to stand; at this stage spasticity is disadvantageous because it interferes with motor function and it would be rational to reduce muscle tone, even at the cost of increased weakness. Finally, in bedridden patients, severe spasticity leads to difficulties in nursing and hygiene, painful spasms, and sleep disturbances; in this phase the treatment is often mandatory to ameliorate quality of life and to prevent tertiary complications.

In all stages of MS it is very important to remove all noxious stimuli (e.g., urinary tract infections, constipation, dysmenorrhea, ingrown toenails, pressure ulcers, inadequate orthoses or wheelchair) that can increase the afferent input on the stretch reflex and thus can trigger or increase spasticity.

Treating spasticity

Several treatments are available for spasticity, including rehabilitation, oral medications, peripheral nerve blockage, intrathecal injections or infusions, and surgery. Severe spasticity usually requires a combination of such treatments [19], and should involve a patient-focused, coordinated, multidisciplinary team approach.

Physical therapy

Whereas these interventions have been more widely investigated in other diseases of the CNS, there are still very few studies on MS-related spasticity. They are usually safe and often low cost, but evidence-based results on their effectiveness are rather poor. Nevertheless, about 50% of MS patients with spasticity use physical therapy or a stretching regimen [3] and, even in the absence of evidence-based models, it is common opinion that physical therapy should always be the first choice and should become a real "lifestyle" for patients with spasticity. Among the several approaches proposed, facilitation techniques including cooling and muscular stretching are the most noteworthy [20].

Stretching may be useful to maintain the natural length of muscles and prevent fixed muscle contractures. Efficacy has been confirmed by electrophysiological evaluations, and in a blind cross-over study, it seemed to enhance the beneficial effects of baclofen [21]. Since muscle shortening is an early complication of spasticity [22], stretching should be introduced as soon as possible.

Many other physical therapy strategies have been reported [20]. Specifically, some authors have emphasized the role of cooling [23], hydrotherapy [24], reflexology [25], transcutaneous electrical nerve stimulation (TENS) [26], and functional neuromuscular stimulation (FNS) [27]. Casting may be indicated in the most advanced stage of the disease, when severe spasticity is complicated by stiffness due to rheological modifications and fibrosis [28].

Pharmacological therapy

The next step in treating spasticity after physical approaches is pharmacological therapy. Unfortunately, there are no well-documented studies that show the absolute and comparative efficacy and tolerability of antispasticity agents [29, 30], or their long-term effects [31]. However, a pragmatic approach allows one to outline post hoc the profile of most treatments, based on clinical practice. Mechanisms of action, doses, and main side effects of drugs approved for the treatment of spasticity are summarized in Table 19.2.

Baclofen is the most widely used oral antispastic drug. It acts by binding to $GABA_B$ receptors of spinal interneurons on which it exerts a presynaptic inhibitory effect on the release of the excitatory neurotransmitters glutamate and aspartate. Postsynaptically it decreases the firing of motor neurons. This results in inhibition of monosynaptic and polysynaptic spinal reflexes. Since baclofen also acts non-selectively on $GABA_B$ receptors on brain neurons, its main adverse effects include sedation or somnolence, excessive weakness, vertigo, and psychological disturbances. Fortunately, the majority of adverse effects are not severe and most are dose-related, transient, and/or reversible. The only severe, although rare, adverse effect is a withdrawal syndrome characterized by seizures, psychic symptoms, and hyperthermia. The syndrome improves after the reintroduction of baclofen, usually without sequelae. When not related to withdrawal, these symptoms occur mainly in patients with brain damage and in the elderly [32].

Tizanidine is the second most used oral antispastic drug. Its α_2-adrenergic action strengthens inhibitory projections descending from the locus coeruleus, acting both at spinal and supraspinal level. Tizanidine seems to be no more effective than baclofen but has a slightly different side effects profile. Despite claims that it causes less muscle weakness, there is very little evidence that tizanidine performs better than other drugs in this respect, although it is more expensive.

Table 19.2 Drugs approved for the treatment of spasticity

Drugs	Mode of action	Doses	Side effects
Baclofen	Agonistic action on GABA receptors in the spinal cord inhibits stretch reflex by reducing the release of excitatory neurotransmitters glutamate and aspartate	10–75 mg/day per os	Sedation, dizziness, weakness, fatigue, addiction
Tizanidine	Agonistic action on α2- adrenergic receptors in CNS	6–32 mg/day per os	Drowsiness, dry mouth, hypotension, bradycardia
Diazepam	Increases presynaptic inhibition by stimulating agonistic action on $GABA_A$ receptors in the brainstem and spinal cord	4–10 mg/day per os	Sedation, dizziness, weakness, fatigue, ataxia, constipation, hypotension, bladder dysfunction
Dantrolene	Blocks voltage-dependent Ca^{2+} channels; inhibits Ca^{2+} release from the sarcoplasmic reticulum	25–200 mg/day per os	Liver toxicity, muscle weakness, diarrhea, heart failure
Gabapentin	Agonistic action on $GABA_B$ receptors	900–3600 mg/day per os	Sedation, dizziness, weakness, fatigue, headache, hypotension
Eperisone		300 mg/day per os	Weakness
Clonidine	Agonistic action on α2- adrenergic receptors in CNS	100–150 mg/day per os	Dry mouth, sedation, nocturnal akathisia, dizziness, nausea, depression
Botulinum toxin	Inhibits presynaptical cholinergic transmission by preventing acetylcholine release	Botox® 50–200 U Dysport® 250–1000 U Intramuscular	Bruising at the injection site, muscular weakness
Botox®		250–1000 U	Muscular weakness
Dysport®	Inhibits presynaptic cholinergic transmission by preventing acetylcholine release	intramuscular	
Phenol	Blocks peripheral nerves or motor points by chemical neurolysis	5%–7% aqueous solution intramuscular	Bruising at the injection site, muscular weakness, vascular lesions, sensory loss
Intrathecal baclofen	Agonistic action on GABA receptors in the spinal cord inhibits stretch reflex by reducing the release of excitatory neurotransmitters glutamate and aspartate	25–1200 µg/day	Bladder and sexual dysfunction Overdosage: nausea, vomiting, respiratory depression, coma Withdrawal: hypertension, hyperthermia, hallucinations, seizures

Benzodiazepines increase presynaptic inhibition by an agonist action on $GABA_A$ receptors in the CNS. In patients with MS, diazepam was found to reduce spasticity but causes significantly more side effects, including asthenia, dizziness, ataxia, somnolence, and addiction, in comparison to baclofen, dantrolene, and tizanidine [29]. Diazepam is very commonly used in combination with other antispastic drugs or procedures and extemporarily to treat spasms because of its rapid action.

Dantrolene is the only drug acting at muscular level, blocking voltage-dependent calcium channels, thus inhibiting calcium release from sarcoplasmic reticulum. Despite this unique profile which makes it suitable for combination therapy, its use is much limited by liver toxicity and the risk of heart failure.

Gabapentin is structurally similar to the GABA neurotransmitter. However, it does not seem to act on GABA receptors. Therefore, its exact mechanism of action is unknown. A statistically significant reduction of spasticity was found in gabapentin-treated subjects as measured by the physician-administered Ashworth scale and plantar stimulation response and by the self-report scales of spasm severity, interference with function, and painful spasms [33].

Cannabinoids, in the form of natural (cannabidiol) or synthetic (delta9-tetrahydrocannabinol, Δ9-THC) derivatives of cannabis, are still under investigation after several anecdotal reports indicated their efficacy in relieving some symptoms of MS, including spasticity. Results are not conclusive since one double-blind, placebo-controlled trial showed a statistically and clinically significant reduction in spasticity [34] while another one provided positive effects only in patients' opinions [35]. Side effects are generally mild, such as dry mouth, dizziness, somnolence, and nausea. However, longer-term studies are needed to evaluate the risk of lung cancer and other respiratory dysfunction. Hence, at present, results from clinical trials do not support recommendation for the use of cannabinoids in MS.

Eperisone hydrochloride is a recently developed central muscle relaxant, active on both spinal and supraspinal structures, reducing alpha- and gamma-efferent activities. In an explorative report it was found to be as effective and as tolerable as baclofen but with some additional clinical benefits as found by clinical and instrumental measures [36].

Other molecules have been proposed to treat MS-related spasticity, including carbamazepine, vigabatrin, progabide, and clonidine. Although they all have different mechanisms of action and safety profiles that make them suitable for combination therapy, their efficacy is not sufficiently supported by adequate clinical studies.

Side effects from antispastic drugs are more likely to occur with dose escalation and the use of multi-drug regimens. These adverse effects include sedation, fatigue, cognitive impairment, weakness, and imbalance.

Intrathecal baclofen (ITB)

Direct spinal intrathecal administration of baclofen is a major step forward in treatment of severe spasticity.

This method, first proposed in 1985 [37], is now well established in many centres. Baclofen can be administered intrathecally via a subcutaneously implanted electronic pump with a reservoir and a catheter (Synchromed® Infusion System, Medtronic Ltd.) with the tip placed at dorsal level. This system is completely programmable by external telemetry, allowing different dose regimes to be delivered [37, 38].

Due to its poor lipid solubility, oral baclofen crosses the blood–brain barrier poorly and very high plasma concentrations are needed to reach CNS neurons. Moreover, its action is not selective for spinal cord [39] and high plasma concentrations are often required to obtain clinical efficacy. Delivering baclofen intrathecally accentuates its antispasticity effect while minimizing the systemic side effects associated with oral intake. It has been calculated that intrathecal doses 100-fold lower than oral ones can lead to elevated and stable intrathecal concentrations 50-fold higher [40] with almost no side effects.

It has been proposed that the antispastic effects of ITB might be a direct result of depression of motor neuron excitability [39]. Other authors speculate that ITB might have a selective effect on certain spinal cord receptors which are receiving supraspinal input that is modified by cerebral disease [41, 42].

Intrathecal baclofen is indicated for use in patients with severe spasticity of spinal origin, grade 4–5 on the Ashworth scale, who are unresponsive to maximal doses of oral baclofen and other oral myorelaxants, or developed unacceptable side effects at maximal effective dosages. Limited data suggest that also ambulatory MS patients are good candidates for ITB [43].

Daily doses are extremely variable, depending on the degree of spasticity. In contrast to patients with other diseases, MS patients often need an increase in the ITB daily dose to control spasticity. The steady increase in the daily dose in the first years indicates that tolerance to baclofen can occur [44]. On the other hand, in some patients with longer follow-up a decreased daily requirement of baclofen can be observed, probably due to structural changes of $GABA_B$ receptors, with phenomena of adaptation and consequent remodeling of myotatic circuits [45].

In the majority of published papers, the results concerning MS are scattered in miscellaneous series of patients. Although randomized, double-blind clinical trials with ITB are impracticable, the efficacy is well demonstrated. Benefits are maximal on spasticity and spasms [46] since more than 80% and 65% of patients respectively have improvement in tone and spasms [47], and also sleep quality, pain, and other symptoms are positively affected. In a limited number of patients, slight functional improvements can be observed [48–52]. Efficacy was also demonstrated by reduced amplitude of the short-latency stretch reflex [51]. In comparison to patients assuming oral medications, ITB-treated patients report lower levels of spasticity, less stiffness in the legs, less pain, and fewer spasms at any time [3]. Another benefit is that ITB also decreases caregiver burden [5, 43, 47].

Specific benefits of ITB therapy depend upon the patient, his/her functional status, and personal goals. In a review of MS patients treated with ITB, 87% showed sustained improvements, from the clinician's perspective, in at least one treatment goal that had been identified prior to ITB implant, and 79% showed sustained improvements in at least one treatment goal from the patient's perspective [53]. Despite higher levels of disability among the ITB-treated patients, satisfaction with therapy appears most favorable with ITB compared to the oral treatments [3]. In addition, higher satisfaction with oral drugs was reported by patients already under ITB treatment: it may be inferred that ITB facilitates an additive effect from oral medications [3]. Some studies report also improvements in quality of life [3, 45, 50, 54] and fatigue [3], and favorable results in pharmacoeconomic evaluations. Although expensive, the use of ITB may be associated with significant savings in hospitalization costs in relation to bedbound patients who are at risk of developing pressure sores, thus enhancing its cost-effectiveness [46, 55, 56].

The two unwanted events that clinicians are most concerned with are drug overdose and withdrawal. Overdose primarily arises from drug test doses or human error during refill and programming of the pump. Initial symptoms include nausea and vomiting, thereafter, progressive loss of muscle tone, respiratory depression, and drowsiness until coma may develop. Withdrawal most commonly occurs as a result of delivery system dysfunction [49]. It starts insidiously with itching or tingling, then a marked rebound of hypertonia, hallucinations, hyperthermia, hypertension, and restriction of consciousness develop. However, the most alarming symptoms are incoming seizures leading to status epilepticus. If this condition is not adequately treated, within a few days a rapid and life-threatening evolution may be seen with rhabdomyolysis, renal or liver failure, and intravascular disseminated coagulation [57]. Withdrawal syndrome must be distinguished from malignant hyperthermia and malignant neuroleptic syndrome. Out of 16 cases described to date, six patients have died because this condition was not adequately treated with intrathecal or oral administration of baclofen [58].

Peripheral nerve blockage

These procedures lead to functional or physical neurolysis and can effectively treat localized and loco-regional spasticity.

Botulin toxin is injected at small doses intramuscularly, producing a local paralysis of the involved muscle. Although it is not approved for spasticity in MS, it is often used for the treatment of adductor hypertonia, equinus spastic foot, flex elbow, or flex wrist. It may be used to treat loco-regional or severely asymmetric spasticity or, in combination with ITB, to treat upper limb spasticity. These conditions, however, are not frequent in MS. The high cost of this biological product prevents its diffusion in the treatment of large muscle masses.

Phenol can be used to block peripheral nerves or motor points by chemical neurolysis. Only case series have been published in MS-related spasticity. Unfortunately, despite the low cost and the long duration of effects which last for some months, chemical denervation is irreversible. Moreover, vascular and sensory structures can also be damaged [59].

Phenol may be also injected intrathecally; this procedure might be recommended for those patients with generalized and severe spasticity who do not respond to or tolerate ITB.

Palliative surgical procedures

These are indicated only for those spastic limbs with no more functional voluntary movements. Open ablative procedures include tenotomy, neurotomy, selective posterior rhizotomy (DREZotomy), or lumbar myelotomy. Since these procedures are irreversible, they represent the extreme therapeutic options in the treatment of MS-related spasticity. In very rare cases, they may be indicated in severe regional spasticity associated with intractable pain [60].

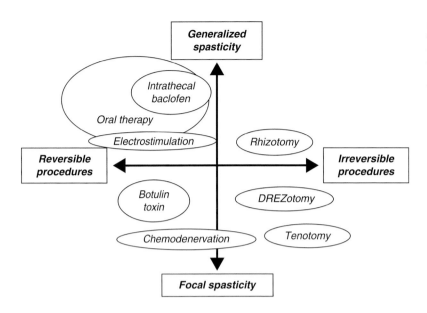

Fig. 19.2. Different approaches to treating spasticity according to the distinction between focal or generalized distribution and reversible or irreversible procedures. DREZotomy, ablation of the dorsal root entry zone.

Conclusions

A helpful approach in the management of spasticity is to treat it according to the level of severity and to distinguish generalized from focal spasticity since they require different treatments, with the possibility of choosing between reversible and irreversible procedures (Fig. 19.2).

Although we do not discard evidence-based therapeutic strategies, a rational approach suggests that a monotherapy should be started first, then a multi-drug regimen could be set out and, finally, more invasive treatments should be introduced after previous steps have failed.

Physical therapy plays the main role in the initial phases of the disease, when spasticity is mild. At this stage, exercise and stretching may be sufficient to manage symptoms. As the disease progresses and spasticity becomes more severe, physical therapy will be useful in combination with other strategies (oral drugs, neuromuscular blocks, intrathecal infusions).

There is limited evidence of the effectiveness of four oral drugs: baclofen, tizanidine, diazepam, and dantrolene. Oral baclofen is the most commonly prescribed drug for spasticity but is often suboptimally managed being usually underdosed for fear of side effects [54]. Utilization of other treatments, including benzodiazepines, dantrolene, anti-convulsants, and tizanidine, appears to be non-standardized and practitioner-dependent, but forthcoming data regarding the potential use of cannabinoids are encouraging. It will be interesting to carry out double-blind randomized controlled trials of interventions used in current practice, where outcomes could include functional benefit and impact on quality of life.

There is also good evidence that both botulinum toxin and intrathecal baclofen are effective in reducing focal and generalized spasticity respectively and both are associated with functional benefit. For patients who do not respond to combined oral therapy at maximal doses or do not tolerate side effects, a device for ITB becomes the elective option. Although invasive and substantially more expensive, this procedure showed elevated efficacy, tolerability, and safety. Moreover, ITB demonstrated the highest satisfaction rating among patients compared to all oral treatments [3].

Finally, to obtain best results and reach established therapeutic goals in the treatment of spasticity, a key component is to form a multidisciplinary team which should include a neurologist, a neurosurgeon, physiatrist, a rehabilitation therapist, and a dedicated nurse, and, not least, the patient with his/her caregiver and family.

References

1. Lance J W. Symposium synopsis. In: Feldman R G, Young R R, Koella W P, eds. *Spasticity: Disordered Motor Control*. Chicago, IL: Year Book Medical Publishers, 1980:485–95

2. Burke D, Gillies J D, Lance J W. An objective assessment of a gamma aminobutyric acid derivative in the control of spasticity. *Proc Austr Assoc Neurol* 1971;**8**:131–4

3. Rizzo M A, Hadjimichael O C, Preiningerova J, Vollmer T L. Prevalence and treatment of spasticity reported by multiple sclerosis patients. *Mult Scler* 2004;**10**:589–95

4. Avourou K J, Goldenberg E, Cleghon G. Sociodemographic and health status characteristics of persons with MS and their caregivers. *Mult Scler Management* 1996;**3**:6–17

5. Vender J R, Huges M, Hughes B D, *et al.* Intrathecal baclofen therapy and multiple sclerosis: outcomes and patient satisfaction. *Neurosurg Focus* 2006;**2**:E6–9

6. MS Society. *MS symptom management survey*. London: MS Society, 1999

7. Sherman S J, Koshland G F, Laguna J F. Hyper-reflexia without spasticity after unilateral infarct of the medullary pyramid. *J Neurol Sci* 2000;**175**:145–55

8. Sheean G. The pathophysiology of spasticity. *Eur J Neurol* 2002;**1**:3–9

9. Lieber R L, Steinman S, Barash I A, *et al.* Structural and functional changes in spastic skeletal muscle. *Muscle Nerve* 2004;**29**:615–27

10. Maertens de Noordhout A, Delvaux V, Delwaide P J. Muscular tone and its disturbances. *Encycl Méd-Chir, Neurology* 2001;17–007–A–20

11. Baker D, Pryce G, Giovannoni G, *et al.* The therapeutic potential of cannabis. *Lancet Neurol* 2003;**2**:291–8

12. Voerman G E, Gregoric M, Hermens H J. Neurophysiological methods for the assessment of spasticity: the Hoffmann reflex, the tendon reflex, and the stretch reflex. *Disabil Rehab* 2005;**27**:33–68

13. Ashworth B. Preliminary trial of carisoprodol in multiple sclerosis. *Practitioner* 1964;**192**:540–2

14. Penn R D, Savoy S M, Corcos D, *et al.* Intrathecal baclofen for severe spinal spasticity. *N Engl J Med* 1989;**320**:1517–21

15. Hobart J C, Riazi A, Thompson A J, *et al.* Getting the measure of spasticity in multiple sclerosis: the Multiple Sclerosis Spasticity Scale (MSSS-88). *Brain* 2006;**129**:224–34

16. Thompson A J, Jarrett L, Lockley L, Marsden J, Stevenson V. Clinical management of spasticity. *J Neurol Neurosurg Psychiatry* 2005;**76**:459–63

17. Haselkorn J K, Richer C B, Fry-Welch D, *et al.* Spasticity management in multiple sclerosis: evidence-based strategies for spasticity treatment in multiple sclerosis. *J Spinal Cord Med* 2005; **28**:167–99

18. Kesselring J, Beer S. Symptomatic therapy and neurorehabilitation in multiple sclerosis. *Lancet Neurol* 2005;**4**:643–52

19. Crayton H, Heyman R, Rossman H. A multimodal approach to managing the symptoms of multiple sclerosis. *Neurology* 2004;**63**:S12–18

20. Richardson D. Physical therapy in spasticity. *Eur J Neurol* 2002;**9**(Suppl 1):17–22

21. Brar S P, Smith M B, Nelson L M, *et al.* Evaluation of treatment protocols on minimal to moderate spasticity in multiple sclerosis. *Arch Phys Med Rehab* 1991;**72**:186–9

22. Gracies J M. Pathophysiology of spastic paresis. II: Emergence of muscle overactivity. *Muscle Nerve* 2005;**31**:552–71

23. Petrilli S, Durufle A, Nicolas B, *et al.* Influence of temperature changes on clinical symptoms in multiple sclerosis: an epidemiologic study. *Ann Readapt Med Phys* 2004;**47**:204–8

24. Kesiktas N, Paker N, Erdogan N, *et al.* The use of hydrotherapy for the management of spasticity. *Neurorehab Neural Repair* 2004;**18**:268–73

25. Siev-Ner I, Gamus D, Lerner-Geva L, Achiron A. Reflexology treatment relieves symptoms of multiple sclerosis: a randomized controlled study. *Mult Scler* 2003;**9**:356–61

26. Armutlu K, Meric A, Kirdi N, *et al.* The effect of transcutaneous electrical nerve stimulation on spasticity in multiple sclerosis patients: a pilot study. *Neurorehab Neural Repair* 2003;**17**:79–82

27. Ring H, Rosenthal N. Controlled study of neuroprosthetic functional electrical stimulation in sub-acute poststroke rehabilitation. *J Rehab Med* 2005;**37**:32–6

28. Lannin N A, Herbert R D. Is hand splinting effective for adults following stroke? A systematic review and methodologic critique of published research. *Clin Rehab* 2003;**17**:807–16

29. Shakespeare D T, Boggild M, Young C. Anti-spasticity agents in multiple sclerosis. *Cochrane Database Syst Rev* 2001;CD001332

30. Beard S, Hunn A, Wight J. Treatments for spasticity and pain in multiple sclerosis: a systematic review. *Health Technol Assess* 2003;**7**:1–111

31. Paisley S, Beard S, Hunn A, Wight J. Clinical effectiveness of oral treatments for spasticity in multiple sclerosis: a systematic review. *Mult Scler* 2002;**8**:319–29

32. Dario A, Tomei G. A benefit–risk assessment of baclofen in severe spinal spasticity. *Drug Saf* 2004;**27**:799–818

33. Cutter N C, Scott D D, Johnson J C, Whiteneck G. Gabapentin effect on spasticity in multiple sclerosis: a. placebo-controlled, randomized trial. *Arch Phys Med Rehab* 2000;**81**:164–9

34. Vaney C, Heinzel-Gutenbrunner M, Jobin P, *et al.* Efficacy, safety and tolerability of an orally administered cannabis extract in the treatment of spasticity in patients with multiple sclerosis: a randomized, double-blind, placebo-controlled, crossover study. *Mult Scler* 2004;**10**:339–40

35. Zajicek J P, Sanders H P, Wright D E, *et al.* Cannabinoids in multiple sclerosis (CAMS) study: safety and efficacy data for 12 months follow-up. *J Neurol Neurosurg Psychiatry* 2005;**76**:1664–6

36. Bresolin N, Zucca C, Pecori A. Efficacy and tolerability of eperisone and baclofen in spastic palsy: a double-blind randomized trial. *Adv Ther* 2009; **26**:563–73

37. Penn R D, Kroin J S. Continuous intrathecal baclofen for severe spasticity. *Lancet* 1985; **1**:215–17

38. Penn R D. Intrathecal baclofen for spasticity of spinal origin: seven years of experience. *J Neurosurg* 1992;**77**:236–40

39. Ørsnes G, Crone C, Krarup C, Petersen N, Nielsen J. The effect of baclofen on the transmission in spinal pathways in spastic multiple sclerosis patients. *Clin Neurophysiol* 2000;**111**:1372–9

40. Kroin J S, Penn R D Cerebrospinal fluid pharmacokinetics of lumbar intrathecal baclofen. In: Lakke JPWF, Delhaas E M, Rutgers AWF, eds. Parenteral drug therapy in spasticity and Parkinson's disease. Carnforth, UK: Parthenon, 1991:67–77

41. Kofler M, Quirbach E, Schauer R, Singer M, Saltuari L. Limitations of intrathecal baclofen for spastic hemiparesis following stroke. *Neurorehabil Neural Repair* 2009; **23**:26–31

42. Meythaler J M, Guin-Renfroe S, Brunner R C, Hadley M N. Intrathecal baclofen for spastic hypertonia from stroke. *Stroke* 2001;**32**:2099–109

43. Sadiq S A, Wang G C. Long-term intrathecal baclofen therapy in ambulatory patients with spasticity. *J Neurol* 2006; **253**:563–9

44. Nielsen J F, Hansen H J, Sunde N, Christensen J J. Evidence of tolerance to baclofen in treatment of severe spasticity with intrathecal baclofen. *Clin Neurol Neurosurg* 2002;**104**:142–5

45. Middel B, Kuipers-Upmeijer H, *et al.* Effect of intrathecal baclofen delivered by an implanted programmable pump on health related quality of life in patients with severe spasticity. *J Neurol Neurosurg Psychiatry* 1997;**63**:204–9

46. Ordia J I, Fischer E, Adamski E, Spatz E L. Chronic intrathecal delivery of baclofen by a programmable pump for the treatment of severe spasticity. *J Neurosurg* 1996;**85**: 452–457

47. Ben Smail D, Peskine A, Roche N, Mailhan L, Thiebaut I, Bussel B. Intrathecal baclofen for treatment of spasticity of multiple sclerosis patients. *Mult Scler.* 2006;**12**:101–3

48. Azouvi P, Mane M, Thiebaut J-B, *et al.* Intrathecal administration for control of severe spinal spasticity: functional improvement and long-term follow-up. *Arch Phys Med Rehabil* 1996;**7**:35–39

49. Dario A, Scamoni C, Bono G, Ghezzi A, Zaffaroni M. Functional improvement in patients with severe spinal spasticity treated with chronic intrathecal baclofen infusion. *Funct Neurol* 2001;**16**:311–5

50. Dressnandt J, Conrad B. Lasting reduction of severe spasticity after ending chronic treatment with intrathecal baclofen. *J Neurol Neurosurg Psychiatry* 1996;**60**:168–173

51. Nielsen J F, Sinkjaer T. Guided intrathecal baclofen administration by using soleus stretch reflex in moderate-severe spastic multiple sclerosis patients with implanted pump. *Mult Scler* 2004;**10**:521–5

52. Boviatsis E J, Kouyialis A T, Korfias S, Sakas D E. Functional outcome of intrathecal baclofen administration for severe spasticity. *Clin Neurol and Neurosurg* 2005;**107**:289–295

53. Jarrett L, S M Leary, B Porter, D Richardson, T Rosso, M Powell, *et al.* Managing spasticity in people with multiple sclerosis: a goal-oriented approach to intrathecal baclofen therapy. *Int J MS Care* 2001;**3**:1–11

54. Gianino J M, York M M, Paice J A, *et al.* Quality of life: effect of reduced spasticity from intrathecal baclofen. *J Neurosci Nurs* 1999;**30**:47–54

55. Nance P, Schryvers O, Schmidt B, *et al.* Intrathecal baclofen therapy for adults with spinal cord spasticity: therapeutic efficacy and effect on hospital admissions. *Can J Neurol Sci* 1995;**22**:22–9

56. Postma TJB, Oenema D, Terpstra S, *et al.* Cost analysis of the treatment of severe spinal spasticity with a continuous intrathecal baclofen infusion system. *Pharmacoeconomics* 1999;**4**:395–404

57. Green L B, Nelson V S. Death after acute withdrawal of intrathecal baclofen: case report and literature review. *Arch Phys Med Rehab* 1999;**80**:1600–4

58. Coffey R J, Ridgely P. Abrupt intrathecal baclofen withdrawal: management of potentially life-threatening sequelae. *Neuromodulation* 2001;**4**:142–5

59. Carda S, Molteni F. Selective neuromuscular blocks and chemoneurolysis in the localized treatment of spasticity. *Eur Med Phys* 2004;**40**:123–30

60. Lazorthes Y, Sol J-C, Sallerin B, Verdié J. The surgical treatment of spasticity. *Eur J Neurol* 2002;**9** (Suppl 1):35–41

Chapter 20

Cognitive rehabilitation in multiple sclerosis

Dawn W. Langdon

Cognitive impairment adversely affects the lives of people with multiple sclerosis (MS) in far-reaching ways [1]. Perhaps most pertinent for this volume is the evidence that cognitive deficits are associated with a worse outcome in physical rehabilitation [2, 3]. Motor learning in virtual reality is compromised in MS, when tasks require more complex integration of information [4]. There is good evidence that cognitive impairments reduce everyday functional status in MS [5, 6]. Cognitive impairment, defined by neuropsychology test results, is usually demonstrated in just under half of people with MS in community samples and a little over half in clinic samples. Generalized dementia is rare in MS [7]. Processing speed is the aspect of cognition most often affected. Other particularly vulnerable functions include complex attention, memory, and executive functions. Typically, language functions are preserved, which can make cognitive impairments in MS difficult to detect at interview. No clear trajectory of cognitive change over time has been described, although the few longitudinal studies spanning a decade or more have shown increased risk over time of both worsening cognitive impairment, and new cognitive impairment for those who were previously unaffected [8].

The different MS subtypes do not have very distinct cognitive profiles, although large studies have tended to show that secondary progressive patients have the most marked cognitive impairments, with perhaps primary progressive patients being slightly less affected and relapsing–remitting patients usually demonstrating the least impairment. Most rehabilitation studies tend to include a range of MS subtypes and do not report outcomes separately for the different subtypes. Disease and magnetic resonance imaging (MRI) variables correlate moderately well with cognitive performance, especially in cross-sectional studies [8]. Although some medications have been shown to slow the progression of cognitive impairment, they are as yet not a complete solution [9].

There are fierce methodological challenges for those seeking to evaluate a cognitive rehabilitation intervention in MS. Patients with MS experience a varying, progressive disease that is often clinically silent and virtually unpredictable on a short-term, individual basis, in both the physical and cognitive domains. This may in part account for the paucity of evidence for cognitive rehabilitation. A recent review identified only 16 articles that addressed cognitive rehabilitation in MS, of which only four were rated as the most convincing, Class I evidence [10]. The *Cochrane Review* on psychological interventions for MS stated that the available evidence did not allow any conclusions about cognitive rehabilitation to be drawn [11]. It is not yet established what should be targeted in rehabilitation, what form training should take, what the length and spacing of sessions should be, or what level or profile of cognitive impairment is best addressed. The field of cognitive rehabilitation as a whole has no one shared methodology or evaluation model. Wilson [12] identified four main approaches, which are still apparent:

Type 1 – cognitive retraining through drills and exercises;

Type 2 – neuropsychology-model-based interventions;

Type 3 – eclectic approaches, drawing on neuropsychology, cognitive psychology, and behavioral psychology;

Type 4 – the holistic approach, addressing motivation, emotion, and other psychological needs, in addition to specific cognitive skill training.

Multiple Sclerosis: Recovery of Function and Neurorehabilitation, eds. J. Kesselring, G. Comi, and A. J. Thompson. Published by Cambridge University Press. © Cambridge University Press 2010.

This typology will be used to categorize interventions throughout this chapter. Delivering and describing some of these interventions in a controlled, reliable, and replicable way is not easy. Quite clearly, the appropriate outcomes also differ.

Wilson recommended that disability should be the focus of rehabilitation, rather than impairment [12]. She has argued that performance and competence in everyday tasks should be the measured change, not neuropsychology test scores. However, if a person's memory function improves after training, and if the skill generalizes to all memory tasks, neuropsychology memory test performance may also improve. Other methodological dilemmas include the difficulty of "blinding" patients and therapists to the active intervention and there has been strong advocacy for designs other than randomized controlled trials (RCTs) [13]. Over time the production of Class I evidence with acquired brain injury and stroke populations is increasing [14]. However, there remains a strong feeling among experts that clinical judgment and acknowledgement of the patients' values and beliefs remain essential [15]. It is likely that cognitive rehabilitation in MS will follow the path of that taken in head injury and stroke research, with growing numbers of randomized controlled trials building an increasingly convincing evidence base. For the moment, the few studies available require caution in appraisal and application to clinical settings.

Cognitive assessment for rehabilitation

A number of specialized cognitive batteries have been validated in MS [16]. Cognitive test performance can be affected by changes in sensory and motor function, which may confound measurement [17]. However, performance on a pen-and-paper cognitive test has been shown to be independent of motor speed [18]. The standardized batteries are designed to minimize the impact of sensory and motor deficits on test performance; however, this is harder to achieve when longitudinal assessments are required and change over time is being assessed. Whilst many traditional neuropsychology tests measure cognitive impairment fairly well, they cannot explain all cognitive disability in everyday life. Rather than repeating lists of words to be recalled, for example, which is a rather artificial behavior, more

"ecologically valid" tests have been developed that involve quasi-everyday activities, such as remembering to post a letter albeit in the clinic room. Interestingly, whilst both traditional neuropsychology tests and the more "ecologically valid" tests correlate with functional status, the two types of test do not always correlate with each other [19]. It may be that the two types of tests are measuring different things and that both should be included in an assessment for rehabilitation. Understanding the patient's experience is crucial in identifying the main problem area and designing an acceptable, effective rehabilitation program. However, it should be borne in mind that patient self-report does not relate closely to objective test performance, and this is particularly true when high levels of cognitive problems are reported [20]. It is accepted in the general neuropsychological rehabilitation literature that neurological impairments, emotional and psycho-social problems, and behavioral problems should be identified and explored as part of an assessment [13]. This is also a requirement in the context of the complex disability that MS brings.

The evidence base for cognitive rehabilitation in MS

Effects of cognitive rehabilitation on attention in MS

Several studies have evaluated the effects of computerized attention training packages, which have the advantages of a being a reliably administered and reproducible intervention. One of the earliest studies [21] used a computerized assessment of the MS patients' attention skills at baseline. Only those with attention deficits on computer assessment were recruited to the study. A computerized training package was then selected for each patient, to target one of their two weakest attention domains (Type 1). The results showed that specific training of particular impaired domains of attention (alertness, divided attention, vigilance, or selective attention) uniquely improved the target domain and not other aspects of attention [21]. A small RCT [22] allocated half the MS patients to computer-based treatment targeting their two most impaired cognitive areas (Type 1), being taught everyday compensation strategies (Type 2), and self-control techniques (Type 3), and they also received outpatient multidisciplinary rehabilitation that did not address cognition, structured according to individual needs. The MS control group only received the multidisciplinary rehabilitation. The authors do not report results separately for those patients who received training in attention; however, overall the treated group did not do better than the control group on tests of attention [22].

The largest and best-designed study of attention training in MS was a randomized, double-blind, controlled trial (Type 1) [23]. The MS patients were selected to have both self-reported impairments in attention and to have impairments on neuropsychological tests. Participants were randomized to either memory and attention computer retraining (treatment group), or to visual construction and visual–motor coordination computer training (control group). Both groups received 16 training sessions across 8 weeks. About 45% of patients improved in both groups, with no treatment effect on tests of attention [23]. One small study [24] utilized non-specific cognitive training tasks on paper, that were handed out weekly for 6 weeks, for participants to complete at home several times a day (Type 1). The MS patients were compared with healthy control participants. At baseline the patients were significantly worse than the control group on some computer assessments of attentional skills (but not on memory or executive tests), and both groups showed significant improvements on some parts of the computerized assessment of attention; but there was no group effect of treatment. Both groups improved equally [24]. This makes the benefit to MS patients hard to judge.

Overall the studies of fairly intensive attention training are rather contradictory. In addition, access to and individual suitability of retraining programs restricts their usefulness. It seems safe to conclude that they are unlikely to cause harm and, if sufficiently precisely targeted, may bring improvement.

Experimental studies of memory

Laboratory studies of learning and memory with MS patients offer some insights into which cognitive processes are most vulnerable to MS pathology and the strategies most likely to facilitate improvement. The simplest characterization of memory impairment in MS is that recall (i.e., unprompted remembering) is more affected than recognition (i.e., prompted

remembering) [25]. However, a study that first trained participants to specific learning criteria on a range of verbal and non-verbal memory tasks showed no difference between the MS group's and the healthy control group's recall at 30 minutes, 60 minutes, or even 1 week follow-up [26]. Although the MS group required more learning trials to reach criterion, once they had learnt the material they could recall it as efficiently as the healthy control group. The authors suggested that the MS patients' primary difficulty was with acquisition, rather than recall per se [26].

There are several strands of evidence that suggest that the way information is presented to MS patients, and the extent to which they process it at first encounter, can significantly affect how well they remember it later. For example, simple repetition is much less helpful at improving later recall performance for MS patients than for healthy controls [27]. It seems that repetition in isolation is not enough to support memory functions in MS, but rather more processing ("encoding") and more organization of information is required. Those MS patients who were able to recall a list of target words entirely normally were significantly disadvantaged when the target words were presented along with "distracter" items [28]. Apparently, paring down presented information to the essential items facilitates remembering, whereas unnecessary or unrelated information alongside important items impairs memory performance. Grouping words together that are related may also be helpful [29]. Although the provision of cues and prompts is often helpful, it is a fairly robust finding that if the MS patients generate their own cue (rather than having it given to them by another person), they are more likely to remember the target word. This holds for both minimal and more severe memory impairment, for both recall and recognition, and for both laboratory and everyday tasks [30, 31].

In summary, there seem to be many ways of presenting information to people with MS that can improve their remembering. The constraint of valid and reliable experimental designs, aiming to identify the effects of individual components, leaves us without knowledge of the efficacy of combining these strategies in rehabilitation settings or everyday life. It would seem a sensible course of action to discuss these possibilities with patients with memory problems and advise health professionals and family members to routinely employ these procedures. They can be fine-tuned and amended as appropriate with patient feedback.

Effects of cognitive rehabilitation on memory

The Brenk *et al.* study [24] compared MS patients with healthy control participants, who all completed paper-based non-specific cognitive training tasks that also targeted memory (Type 1). The MS patients had improved short-term and working memory after treatment, but their verbal long-term memory deteriorated (assessed on standardized tests). There were no significant group differences with the normal control participants, making interpretation of the findings difficult in terms of usefulness for MS patients [24]. The large RCT conducted by Solari *et al.* [23] also trained memory skills using a computerized battery (Type 1). There was no treatment effect on memory test scores immediately after treatment, or at 2 months follow-up, when the treated and control MS group were compared [23].

A single-blind controlled study of computer-based memory rehabilitation [32] used higher intensity training at home (Type 1). The MS patients in the treatment group were given a disk with memory and working memory tasks. They were required to spend 30 minutes a day, 5 days a week on training. The program gave feedback and adjusted to patients' performance levels, repeating lists and reducing item numbers if the patient failed, and conversely increasing task difficulty if the patient succeeded. The control group received no treatment. At baseline, almost half of participants in both groups scored below 1 SD of the published mean on at least one standardized test, the criterion for cognitive impairment adopted by this study. The treated MS group showed significant improvement on verbal memory and working memory tests. These occurred in the context of small improvements in the treated group and small decrements in the control group, leading the authors to conclude that the treatment partly improved performance and partly counteracted functional loss [32]. The Tesar *et al.* study [22] also evaluated the effects of cognitive training on memory function (Type 1, 2, and 3). The authors do not report results separately for those patients receiving the targeted memory training. However, although the entire treated MS group showed significant improvement in verbal and spatial learning over time, there were no significant differences between the treated and control group on standardized memory tests after treatment [22].

Research highlighting how the acquisition phase of information contributes to poor memory function in MS has shaped memory rehabilitation programs. Typically, quality of acquisition is enhanced by context, organization, and imagery. A small uncontrolled study [33] used the Ridiculously Imaged Story technique (RIS, "ridiculous" meaning salient; Type 2). Baseline testing indicated at most mild impairments for the group on memory and other cognitive tests. Fifteen computer-assisted training sessions took place over 5 weeks. After the training period, there was no increase in correct free verbal recall responses, compared to baseline performance [33]. The Story Memory Technique (SMT), which uses context and imagery, was utilized in an RCT [34] where all participants had impaired verbal learning (defined as scoring at least 1 SD below published means on a standardized test [Type 2]). The SMT training comprised eight sessions over 4 weeks, in a group led by a therapist. The MS treatment group was taught the application of imagery (visualization) and context (a story) in a structured, graded program. Those MS patients in the treated group who had moderate to severe learning impairment showed significant improvement in verbal learning, on standardized tests, compared to MS participants in the control group. However, those treated MS patients with mild learning impairments did not improve significantly on standardized tests.

An RCT [35] compared specific cognitive treatment (Type 1), and neuropsychotherapy (Type 4) in a treated MS group, with non-specific mental stimulation for the control MS group. Both groups performed below matched healthy control levels on all seven cognitive tests in a battery at baseline, except for the non-treated group being within normal limits on visual perception. There were no significant differences immediately after treatment between the two MS groups on the battery. There was a significant improvement in visuo-spatial memory for the treated group at 6 months follow-up [35].

It appears that the computerized program that was individually tailored to each patient's performance was effective at improving memory function [32], and it may be that individually tailored training is most likely to be effective. The use of stories as context also appears to be a way of improving memory function [34]. The successful study used fairly intensive training in therapist-led groups, which requires considerable expertise and other resources.

However, once again, within the group the therapist may have been able to tailor exercises to individual needs, which may have increased the likelihood of improving memory function.

Effect of rehabilitation on executive skills in MS

Executive skills are involved in planning, judgment, reasoning, and organization. When asked to choose and complete several simple cognitive tasks from an array, to maximize points scored within a given time, MS patients reliably do significantly worse than healthy control participants [17]. Because of their superordinate, supervisory role, executive skills are involved in many aspects of everyday life, especially those that are not routine. Executive skills could in principle be improved by direct training and, because of their involvement in all novel and challenging tasks, could also be improved by cognitive training of other skills. The Tesar *et al.* study [22] did not separately report the outcomes of patients who received computer-based executive skill training, but overall the MS treated group showed improvement on a test of executive functioning, compared to the MS control group, and the advantage was maintained at 3 months follow-up (Type 1, 2, and 3). It is worth noting that the general compensatory strategy package that all the treatment group received included building up routines of behavior and "problem-solving and planning," which could explain the improvement in executive test scores [22]. The Solari *et al.* RCT [23] utilized a computer program designed to train attention and memory skills (Type 1). However, the one test that showed superior performance after training was a test of executive skills. The authors suggest that this may be explicable by regression to the mean (the control arm was significantly better at baseline) [23].

There are fewer retraining programs that have targeted executive skills. Overall, it seems that the study that involved direct training of executive skills by a therapist was the most successful [22].

Use of technology and other aids in cognitive rehabilitation

In the general field of neuropsychological rehabilitation, some promising results have been achieved with technological aids, such as paging systems [13]. There is some evidence that electronic personal organizers can improve daily function in MS [36]. A number of gadgets available commercially on the general market can help support everyday function and they have the advantage of normality. These include pens that dispense post-it notes, voice recorders, and devices to locate keys and other small items. Whilst many people with MS may well be able to select suitable items and incorporate them into their everyday life, for those with more subtle or severe cognitive deficits, the health professional will need to support the patient learning to use the gadget and evaluate its usefulness.

Patient evaluation of cognitive rehabilitation programs

The patient must feel that the cognitive rehabilitation program is congenial and worthwhile. In experimental studies, good feedback is often obtained. After receiving computerized training for their two weakest attentional domains, the patients in the Plohmann *et al.* study [21] reported decreased distractibility and increased speed of mental processing. The patients in the Tesar *et al.* study [22] also reported benefit, after receiving computer training addressing their two weakest areas and being taught compensation strategies; 60% reported average or above average benefit from training, and 80% assessed the compensation strategies as above average. For comparison, 90% rated the relaxation exercises as very helpful. The MS treated group in the SMT study [34] reported more memory improvement than the untreated MS control group.

A large single-blind RCT relied entirely on self-report outcome measures [37]. Patients were screened for cognitive impairment, but its presence or absence was not used to select study participants. The study compared no intervention (control), with brief cognitive assessment and information (assessment), and an outpatient cognitive rehabilitation program designed for each patient individually (intervention), according to current practice (Type 2). There were no significant group effects on subjective cognitive impairment or independence, save for a few favoring the control group. It is of note that a standardized questionnaire of self-reported cognitive status in MS was significantly correlated with some neuropsychology tests, but was not correlated with self-report of daily functioning or objectively measured daily function [38].

For most evaluation purposes, patient self-perception and evaluation forms an essential part of a larger picture that includes objective measures of cognition and functional status. If the target activity is not a concern of the patient, the assessment has failed and the patient is unlikely to be motivated. MS patients and treating teams do not necessarily agree on specific gaols of general rehabilitation, at least [39]. If the training is uncomfortable or difficult to access, attendance is likely to suffer. If there is not sufficient progress discernible to the patient, the enterprise will not seem worthwhile. In a general rehabilitation setting, MS patients reported requiring a higher average improvement to achieve a meaningful benefit, compared to the health professionals treating them [39]. Some of these potential problems can be overcome by regular meetings to monitor progress and systematic goal-setting. Individualized and incremental goal-setting for MS patients has proven efficacy in a general rehabilitation setting [40]. Although no evidence exists for MS patients and cognition goals, Goal Attainment Setting has been shown to be reliable in another population with progressive cognitive disorders [41].

Cognitive rehabilitation and MRI findings

There are few studies that investigate the link between cognitive rehabilitation and MRI parameters. Brain parenchymal fraction (BPF, a measure of tissue volume and therefore brain atrophy) was reported by Hildebrandt *et al.* [32], in the study utilizing a home-based computer training program that adjusted to each participants' performance level (Type 1). In this study BPF was highly correlated with disease duration and duration of symptoms, which is a typical finding. Baseline BPF was linked to improvement on a test of complex attention (only patients with low BPF at baseline profited from treatment). However, baseline BPF was not related to the significant improvement demonstrated on a test of verbal memory [32]. Perhaps of more interest is the suggestion that computer-based training of attention skills led to additional activation of regions in the cingulate gyrus, precuneus, and frontal cortex, a network that has been functionally related to attentional processing (Type 1) [42]. This finding points towards targeted cognitive rehabilitation creating a measurable increase in specific cortical network activation. It may be that in the future MRI can be used to identify suitable candidates for rehabilitation, indicate appropriate rehabilitation programs, and monitor efficacy of

rehabilitation. However, it is unlikely that the clinical skills of communication, assessment, problem-solving, evaluation, and empathy will ever become entirely redundant in cognitive rehabilitation.

References

1. Pierson S H, Griffith N. Treatment of cognitive impairment in multiple sclerosis. *Behav Neurol* 2006;**17**:53–67

2. Langdon D W, Thompson A J. Multiple sclerosis: a preliminary study of selected variables affecting rehabilitation outcome. *Mult Scler* 1999;**5**:94–100

3. Grasso M G, Troisi E, Rizzi F, Morelli D, Paolucci S. Prognostic factors in multidisciplinary rehabilitation treatment in multiple sclerosis: an outcome study. *Mult Scler* 2005;**11**:719–24

4. Leocani L, Comi E, Annovazzi P, *et al.* Impaired short-term motor learning in multiple sclerosis: evidence from virtual reality. *Neurorehab Neural Repair* 2007;**21**:273–8

5. Goverover Y, Genova H M, Hillary F G, DeLuca J. The relationship between neuropsychological measures and the Timed Instrumental Activities of Daily Living task in multiple sclerosis. *Mult Scler* 2007;**13**:636–44

6. Kalmar J H, Gaudino E A, Moore N B, Halper J, DeLuca J. The relationship between cognitive deficits and everyday functional activities in multiple sclerosis. *Neuropsychology* 2008;**22**:442–9

7. Rogers J M, Panegyres P K. Cognitive impairment in multiple sclerosis: evidence-based analysis and recommendations. *J Clin Neurosci* 2007;**14**:919–27

8. Hoffman S, Tittgemeyer M, von Cramon D Y. Cognitive impairment in multiple sclerosis. *Curr Opin Neurol* 2007;**20**:275–80

9. Amato M P, Zipoli V, Portaccio E. Multiple sclerosis-related cognitive changes: a review of cross-sectional and longitudinal studies. *J Neurol Sci* 2006;**245**:41–6

10. O'Brien A R, Chiaravalloti N, Goverover Y, DeLuca J. Evidence-based cognitive rehabilitation for persons with multiple sclerosis: a review of the literature. *Arch Phys Med Rehab* 2008;**89**:761–9

11. Thomas P W, Thomas S, Hillier C, Galvin K, Baker R. Psychological interventions for multiple sclerosis. *Cochrane Database Syst Rev* 2006;CD004431

12. Wilson B A. Cognitive rehabilitation: how it is and how it might be. *J Int Neuropsychol Soc* 1997;**3**:487–96

13. Wilson B A. Neuropsychological rehabilitation. *Annu Rev Clin Psychol* 2008;**4**:141–62

14. Cicerone K D, Dahlberg C, Malec J F, *et al.* Evidence-based cognitive rehabilitation: updated review of the literature from 1998 through 2002. *Arch Phys Med Rehab* 2005;**86**:1681–92

15. Cicerone K D. Evidence-based practice and the limits of rational rehabilitation. *Arch Phys Med Rehab* 2005;**86**:1073–4

16. Benedict R H, Fischer J S, Archibald C J, *et al.* Minimal neuropsychological assessment of MS patients: a consensus approach. *Clin Neuropsychol* 2002;**16**:381–97

17. Birnboim S, Miller A. Cognitive strategies application to multiple sclerosis patients. *Mult Scler* 2004;**10**:67–73

18. Arnett P A, Smith M M, Barwick F H, Benedict R H, Ahlstrom B P. Oralmotor slowing in multiple sclerosis: relationship to neuropsychological tasks requiring oral response. *J Int Neuropsychol Soc* 2008;**14**:454–62

19. Higginson C I. Arnett P A, Voss W D. The ecological validity of clinical tests of memory and attention in multiple sclerosis. *Arch Clin Neuropsychol* 2000;**15**:185–204

20. Schwartz C E, Kozora E, Zeng Q. Towards patient collaboration in cognitive assessment: specificity, sensitivity, and incremental validity of self-report. *Ann Behav Med* 1996;**18**:177–84

21. Plohmann A M, Kappos L, Ammann W, *et al.* Computer assisted retraining of attentional impairments in patients with multiple sclerosis. *J Neurol Neurosurg Psychiatry* 1998;**64**:455–62

22. Tesar N, Bandion K, Baumhackl U. Efficacy of a neuropsychological training programme for patients with mutiple sclerosis: a randomised controlled trial. *Wien Klin Wochenschr* 2005;**117**:747–54

23. Solari A, Motta A, Mendozzi L, *et al.* Computer-aided retraining of memory and attention in people with multiple sclerosis: a randomized, double-blind controlled trial. *J Neurol Sci* 2004;**222**:99–104

24. Brenk A, Laun K, Haase C G. Short-term cognitive training improves mental efficacy and mood in patients with multiple sclerosis. *Eur Neurol* 2008;**60**:304–9

25. Seinela A, Hamalainen P, Koivisto M, Ruutiainen J. Conscious and unconscious uses of memory in multiple sclerosis. *J Neurol Sci* 2002;**198**:79–85

26. Demaree H A, Gaudino E A, DeLuca J, Ricker J H. Learning impairment is associated with recall ability in multiple sclerosis. *J Clin Exp Neuropsychol* 2000;**6**:865–73

27. Chiaravalloti N D, Demaree H, Gaudino E A. Can the repetition effect maximize learning in multiple sclerosis? *Clin Rehab* 2003;**17**:58–68

28. Coolidge F L, Middleton P A, Griego J A, Schmidt M M. The effects of interference on verbal learning in multiple scelrosis. *Arch Clin Neuropsychol* 1996;**11**:605–11

29. Andrade V M, Oliveira M G, Miranda M C, *et al.* Semantic relations and repetitions of items enhance the free recall of words by multiple sclerosis patients. *J Clin Exp Neuropsychol* 2003;**25**:1070–8

30. Basso M R, Lowery N, Ghormley C, Combs D, Johnson J. Self-generated learning in people with multiple sclerosis. *J Int Neuropsychol Soc* 2006;**12**:640–8

31. Goverover Y, Chiaravalloti N, DeLuca J. Self-generation to improve learning and memory of functional activities in persons with multiple sclerosis: meal preparation and managing finances. *Arch Phys Med Rehab* 2008;**89**:1514–21

32. Hildebrandt H, Lanz M, Hahn H K, *et al.* Cognitive training in MS: effects and relation to brain atrophy. *Res Neurol Neurosci* 2007;**25**:33–43

33. Allen D A, Goldstein G, Heyman R A, Rondinelli T. Teaching memory strategies to persons with multiple sclerosis. *J Rehab Res Dev* 1998;**35**:405–10

34. Chiaravalloti N D, DeLuca J, Moore N B, Ricker J H. Treating learning impairments improves memory performance in multiple sclerosis: a randomized clinical trial. *Mult Scler* 2005;**11**:58–68

35. Jonsson A, Korfitzen E M, Heltberg A, Ravnborg M H, Byskov-Ottosen E. Effects of neuropsychological treatment in patients with multiple sclerosis. *Acta Neurol Scand* 1993;**88**:394–400

36. Gentry T. PDAs as cognitive aids for people with multiple sclerosis. *Am J Occup Ther* 2008;**62**:18–27

37. Lincoln N B, Dent A, Harding J, *et al.* Evaluation of cognitive assessment and cognitive intervention for people with multiple sclerosis. *J Neurol Neurosurg Psychiatry* 2002;**72**:93–8

38. O'Brien A, Gaudino-Goering E, Shawaryn M, *et al.* Relationship of the Multiple Sclerosis Neuropsychological Questionnaire (MSNQ) to functional, emotional, and neuropsychological outcomes. *Arch Clin Neuropsychol* 2007;**22**:933–48

39. Bloom L F, Lapierre N M, Wilson K G, *et al.* Concordance in goal setting between patients with multiple sclerosis and their rehabilitation team. *Am J Phys Med Rehab* 2006;**85**:807–13

40. Stuifbergen A K, Becker H, Timmerman G M, Kullberg V. The use of individual goal setting to facilitate behaviour change in women with multiple sclerosis. *J Neurosci Nurs* 2003;**35**:94–9

41. Bouwens S F, van Heugten C M, Verhey F R. Review of goal attainment scaling as a useful outcome measure in psychogeriatric patients with cognitive disorders. *Dement Geriatr Cogn Disord* 2008;**26**:528–40

42. Penner I K, Kappos L. Retraining attention in MS. *J Neurol Sci* 2006;**245**:147–51

Disorders of mood and affect in multiple sclerosis

Anthony Feinstein and Omar Ghaffar

Introduction

Disorders of mood and affect in multiple sclerosis (MS) may be separated into four main categories: depression, bipolar disorder, euphoria, and pseudo-bulbar affect. Depression may be further subdivided according to the taxonomy followed. For the purposes of this chapter, only two subdivisions will be discussed, namely major depression and subsyndromal depression. This chapter will outline the clinical characteristics of each disorder, discuss possible mechanisms underlying etiology, and provide recommendations for treatment. As the data will make clear, some of these disorders have been well studied while others have remained in relative obscurity. What all the disorders have in common, however, is the deleterious effect they exert on quality of life, not only for the individual with MS but also for family members and caregivers.

Definitions

The term "mood" refers to an individual's subjective sense of emotional well being. "Affect," on the other hand, is an objective rating of a person's mood. Usually, mood and affect are congruent, but in the disorder of pseudobulbar affect, this is not the case.

Depression
Major depression

Major depression has been defined in the *Diagnostic and Statistical Manual* (DSM-IV) [1] as a syndrome consisting of five or more symptoms that have been present during the same 2-week period and that represents a change from previous functioning. At least one of the symptoms is either depressed mood

or loss of interest or pleasure. Additional features consist of significant weight loss when not dieting or weight gain (a change of more than 5% of body weight in a month); insomnia or hypersomnia; psychomotor agitation or retardation (observable by others); fatigue or loss of energy; feelings of worthlessness or excessive or inappropriate guilt; diminished ability to think or concentrate or indecisiveness; and recurrent thoughts of death. These symptoms by definition cause clinically significant distress or impairment in social, occupational, or other important areas of functioning.

Subsyndromal depression

Subsyndromal depression refers to patients who have fewer than the five symptoms required for a diagnosis of major depression. By definition, at least three symptoms are required. In MS, the most common are irritability, sadness, and discouragement. Subsyndromal depression should not be ignored by clinicians. It exerts a negative effect on quality of life, is often the harbinger for the development of the full syndrome of major depression, and has a negative impact on the lives of relatives and other family members [2]. It should therefore be treated as aggressively as major depression.

Prevalence

Major depression is common in multiple sclerosis. Lifetime prevalence rates approach 50% [3–5]. Of note is that the studies cited here contain data derived from tertiary referral MS clinics, introducing a potential bias. This possible confounder has, however, been laid to rest by the Canadian Community Health Survey of 115 071 subjects [6]. A self-report

Multiple Sclerosis: Recovery of Function and Neurorehabilitation, eds. J. Kesselring, G. Comi, and A. J. Thompson. Published by Cambridge University Press. © Cambridge University Press 2010.

questionnaire followed by a brief interview to detect the 12-month prevalence of major depression was used. The results confirmed an elevated prevalence rate which exceeded not only that found in individuals without MS but also in those with other long-term medical illnesses. The 12-month prevalence rate in MS patients aged 18–45 years was 25.7%, a figure that declined with increasing age.

Symptoms

Reviewing the symptom checklist for major depression, it is apparent that some symptoms may not represent a mood disorder at all but could rather reflect a direct consequence of the neurological disorder. The most prominent symptom in this regard is fatigue, but other symptoms such as sleep disturbance, appetite change, and poor concentration may also be viewed in this light. It is therefore important to note that research using detailed clinical inquiry to take this symptom overlap into account has still shown significantly elevated rates of depression in MS [3]. The importance of teasing out the correct attribution of symptoms has been acknowledged in the development of screening instruments for depression in the medically ill. The Hospital and Anxiety Depression Scale [7] and the Beck Fast Screen for Depression in Medically Ill Patients [8] are two examples of scales developed for this purpose. The latter has also been validated for MS patients [9], with cut-off scores provided to stratify the severity of depression (0–3, minimal; 4–6, mild; 7–9, moderate; 10–21, severe).

Anxiety

Little attention has been paid to anxiety as a symptom of MS, despite the fact that patients endorse anxiety more often than depression [10]. The evidence also suggests that anxiety exerts a strongly negative effect on a patient's quality of life. Anxiety comorbid with depression, rather than anxiety or depression alone, is associated with heightened thoughts of self-harm, more somatic complaints, and greater social dysfunction. Anxiety has also been linked to MS patients' excessive consumption of alcohol [11]. Research that has focused on discrete anxiety disorders has shown that the lifetime prevalence rates for generalized anxiety disorder, panic disorder, and obsessive–compulsive disorder in MS patients are three times those in the general population [12].

Suicide

A Scandinavian epidemiological investigation of 5525 MS patients reported significantly elevated suicide rates in MS patients. Males and those diagnosed with MS before the age of 30 years were most at risk [13]. Confirmatory evidence has come from a study of 3126 MS patients followed over 16 years, demonstrating that suicide accounted for 15% of all ascertained deaths. This was 7.5 times that for the age-matched, but not sex-matched, general population. With these figures in mind, it is not surprising that MS patients also show increased rates of suicidal intent. In a sample of 140 consecutive clinic attendees, 28.6% endorsed harboring suicidal intent over the course of their illness with 6.4% of the sample actually attempting to harm themselves at some point [14]. The study also revealed that over a third of patients with suicidal intent had received no psychological help for their stress. Factors that predicted suicidal thinking were the presence of major depression, the severity of depression, social isolation, and alcohol abuse. These four predictors are not difficult to elicit in patients and should be part of routine clinical inquiry.

Etiology

Findings with respect to a genetic link between MS and depression are equivocal, with some [15] but not others [3, 16] reporting an association. The data are, however, clearer with respect to brain imaging correlates of low mood. Depression has been linked to the presence of T2-weighted lesions in the arcuate fasciculus [17] and temporal lobe [18]. Others have highlighted T1-weighted lesion volume and atrophy as the more relevant cerebral correlations [19]. In a detailed magnetic resonance imaging (MRI) study incorporating whole brain and regional measures of T1- and T2-weighted lesions together with atrophy, a composite picture emerged with depression clearly linked to both lesions and atrophy affecting medial inferior frontal and anterior temporal regions [20]. In this study, brain pathology accounted for 40% of the depression variance. While informative, this suggests that the search for etiological factors needs to be widened to incorporate additional indices of brain pathology together with selected psycho-social variables. With respect to the former, modest albeit significant correlations have been found between depression and fractional anisotropy measurements obtained from inferomedial frontal regions [21].

The brain imaging data are complemented by a large literature looking at psycho-social correlates of depression. A number of factors have emerged as potentially significant, namely the presence of uncertainty [22], inadequate coping strategies [23, 24], helplessness [25], social relationships [26], loss of recreational activities [27], and high levels of stress [15]. A limitation of all these findings, however, is the problem of retrospective bias. Depressed patients, looking back over their lives in a search for potential etiological clues, are likely to view things in a negative light. This in turn could affect how they rate the quality of relationships and levels of support. To date, psycho-social inquiry has failed adequately to address this conundrum. While the MS patient cannot be viewed in isolation from their environment and social milieu, the etiological significance of the many psycho-social factors mentioned above should be viewed with this in mind.

Treatment

The treatment of major depression and subsyndromal depression may be divided into two broad categories: psychotropic medication and psychotherapy. The two treatment modalities are not mutually exclusive and combination therapy can be tried in more intractable cases. With respect to antidepressant medication, MS-related depression responds well to tricyclic drugs [28], selective serotonin reuptake inhibitors (SSRIs) [29], and the reversible monoamine oxidase A inhibitor moclobemide [30]. Generally, the SSRI drugs are better tolerated than the tricyclic preparations where anticholinergic side effects such as dry mouth and constipation are more troublesome. One side effect that may hinder compliance with SSRI medications is sexual dysfunction. It is therefore not uncommon for a patient's depression to respond to treatment at the cost of aggravating or inducing sexual difficulties, leaving the individual with an uncomfortable choice of continuing or stopping treatment. Two antidepressant drugs, bupropion and mirtazapine, have fewer sexual difficulties as a side effect. There are, however, no treatment studies with either medication, and both are not without their own potential complications; in the case of bupropion it is seizures while mirtazapine is associated with fatigue and weight gain.

A form of psychotherapy, namely cognitive behavioral therapy (CBT), has been shown to be effective in treating MS patients with mild to moderately severe major depression. In a 16-week trial, CBT was as effective as the SSRI sertraline in alleviating low mood [31]. Data also revealed that CBT given over the telephone is effective, a finding of particular relevance to patients with MS given their difficulties with mobility and the challenges of getting in to see a therapist [32].

Finally, in cases of treatment-resistant depression, particularly when a patient is acutely suicidal, electroconvulsive therapy (ECT) can be tried. This is an effective and safe choice although should the patient have active disease as shown by gadolinium-enhancing lesions on brain MRI, treatment with ECT may precipitate a relapse in the MS [33]. In these circumstances, clinicians have to weigh carefully the potential benefits and risks before proceeding with treatment.

Bipolar disorder

Bipolar disorder was formerly called manic–depressive psychosis. There is a paucity of research related to this topic in patients with MS.

Mania is characterized by the following triad: elevated or irritable mood, grandiose or persecutory thoughts, and overactivity. The latter takes the form of a decreased need for sleep, a marked increase in goal-directed activity either at work or socially, excessive involvement in pleasurable activities that have a high potential for painful consequences, hyper-talkativeness or a pressure to keep talking, and distractibility. By definition [1], symptoms have to be present for at least 1 week or be associated with psychosis or hospitalization to be called mania. Lesser variants with symptoms present for at least 4 days are considered hypomania.

Prevalence

An epidemiologic inquiry from Monroe County, New York revealed that the prevalence rate of bipolar disorder in MS patients was double that in the general population [34]. This was confirmed in a Canadian study [4].

Etiology

The etiological basis for the increased rates of mania in MS remains unclear. Treatment with steroids cannot account for it [35]. Of note is that patients who do go "high" on steroid medication are more likely to have a history of major depression, or a family history of depression, alcoholism, or both.

Too few brain imaging studies have been undertaken to ascertain whether there is a link between elevated mood and cerebral indices in MS. Associations between mania and the presence of hyperintense lesions in frontal white matter [36] and the regions surrounding the temporal horns of the lateral ventricles [37] have been noted but sample sizes were small and the imaging data were compromised by methodological limitations.

Treatment

There are no published treatment trials of mania associated with MS. Data are limited to case reports and anecdotal evidence. The basic treatment principles are as follows: hypomanic patients may respond to a mood-stabilizing drug such as lithium carbonate or valproic acid. A benzodiazepine may need to be introduced to help with sedation and insomnia. For the patient who is floridly manic and who may have lost touch with reality because of persecutory and grandiose delusions, additional drugs are required. The newer antipsychotic agents such as olanzapine, risperidone, and quetiapine are preferred to the older ones such as chlorpromazine and haloperidol because of fewer side effects. Benzodiazepines can be used on an as-needed basis for sedation. At times, in the presence of a floridly manic patient, it is difficult to follow the treatment maxim of "start low and go slow" with respect to drug dosing. Grossly disinhibited behavior, outbursts of verbal and physical aggression, reluctance to take treatment, and lack of insight make this one of the most challenging clinical conditions to treat. Patients may need to be detained against their will in hospital, adding a further layer of difficulty to the treatment plan. However, it is important to remember that this is a treatable disorder and that mania invariably gets better and in the majority of cases resolves completely. Maintenance treatment with a mood-stabilizing agent is then advisable. In this regard, while lithium carbonate is a useful agent, some MS patients with a neurogenic bladder have difficulty tolerating the treatment because it promotes a diuresis. In these cases, valproic acid or carbamazepine is a useful alternative.

Euphoria

Euphoria may bear some superficial similarities to hypomania as individuals show signs of an elevated mood and affect. However, euphoric patients lack the motor activity and increased energy characteristic of the manic individual. Euphoria may be best defined as a fixed state of mental well-being in patients who invariably have significant levels of neurological impairment.

An influential early paper defined four particular states: mental well-being or "euphoria sclerotica," characterized by a persistently cheerful mood; physical well-being or "eutonia," distinguished by lack of concern over physical disability; "pes scleroticus," an incongruous optimism for the future; and emotional lability [38]. The validity of the subdivision has never been proven but the clinical descriptors contained therein summarize succinctly the syndrome of euphoria characteristic of certain MS patients.

Prevalence

Given that euphoria is linked to MS patients with marked neurological disability, some researchers consider a median rather than a mean prevalence rate to be more appropriate. Depending on the approach adopted, a median rate of 25% [39] or a mean rate of 9–13% [40, 41] has been reported.

Correlates

Euphoria is a feature of advanced MS. Associations have been reported with increased physical disability and cognitive impairment [40, 42], progressive disease course [42], large cerebral ventricles on computed tomography (CT) brain scan [42], frontal lesions on MRI [36, 41], and more widespread lesions in general on MRI [43].

Treatment

There are no treatment studies for euphoria in MS and indeed the question has been asked, why treat patients with marked physical disability who are not distressed by impairments? This, however, does not take into account the distress experienced by family members of euphoric MS patients. Saddled with the burden of care for a relative with marked physical disability, it is often confusing and distressing to the relative when the patient expresses a relative lack of concern for their disability coupled with a failure to appreciate the consequences of this disability for all concerned. At the very least, robust psycho-education for the family of the euphoric patient is warranted, though the effect on caregiver burden has not been systematically studied.

Pseudobulbar affect

Pseudobulbar affect (PBA) goes by a number of different synonyms including pathological laughing and crying, emotional incontinence, and excessive emotionalism. Recently, the term, "involuntary emotional expression disorder" was put forward and a set of diagnostic criteria defined [44]. This plethora of names reflects dissatisfaction with "pseudobulbar affect" as a term of choice given that many patients with this syndrome do not display other pseudobulbar signs. Be that as it may, for the purposes of this chapter and with an eye on history, the term pseudobulbar affect is retained.

The syndrome may be defined as tears without sadness and/or laughter without mirth. Patients with PBA cry involuntarily without feeling depressed or laugh without feeling happy. It represents a disconnection of mood and affect and is considered involuntary, unwanted, and distressing. In some patients, tears and laughter may occur together as part of the same clinical picture.

Prevalence

Pseudobulbar affect may occur in up to 10% of MS patients [45]. Like all the syndromes described in this chapter, severity lies along a continuum. While the more florid manifestations of inappropriate laughter and crying are difficult to miss, subtle changes may be easily overlooked. However, when these are teased out as part of the mental state assessment, the prevalence rate increases and helps explain why one in ten MS patients can show evidence of abnormal affect.

Clinical correlates

Pseudobulbar affect is associated with disease of long-standing duration and progressive, significant physical disability not necessarily of brainstem origin. There is no gender predilection. The abnormal affect is associated with greater cognitive impairment, particularly in those aspects of cognition mediated by frontal–subcortical circuits. Thus, MS patients with PBA have been shown to perform poorly on tasks such as the Stroop and the Controlled Oral Word Association Test [46].

Etiology

Unlike major depression where causation is linked to cerebral and psycho-social factors, PBA is quite clearly a product of brain dysfunction. In an MRI study comparing MS patients with and without PBA, the former were found to have significantly more hyperintense lesions in bilateral inferior parietal and bilateral inferior frontal regions. In addition, PBA patients had a higher hypointense lesion volume in the brainstem [47]. The brain findings could account for upward of 75% of the PBA variance, a figure almost double that reported for brain pathology causally implicated in the pathogenesis of major depression. The more robust variance statistic confirms that PBA is a "hard-wired" brain disorder arising from a disconnection of widely dispersed neural networks. The imaging data suggest that PBA is more likely to arise if there is bilateral brain involvement, an observation shared by other researchers [48].

Treatment

Pseudobulbar affect can be effectively and quickly treated by a number of different medications. A low dose of the tricyclic drug amitriptyline is helpful [49] as are SSRIs [50], levodopa [51], and amantadine [51]. More recently, a serendipitous discovery revealed that dextromethorphan combined with quinidine was singularly effective in reducing the frequency and severity of abnormal displays of affect [52]. This preparation, still undergoing clinical trials, has not yet received approval by the Food and Drug Administration. The medication was, however, well tolerated by MS patients, with dizziness emerging as the most troubling side effect affecting 26.3% of those treated.

Summary

This chapter has reviewed the four main disorders affecting mood and affect in patients with MS. All are clinically significant. Three of the four, namely depression, bipolar affective disorder, and pseudobulbar affect, can be effectively treated. Not only will treatment enhance the quality of life for MS patients, it will reduce the possibility of suicide in the case of major depression and bipolar disorder. Timely diagnosis and treatment is therefore essential. As such, when confronted by a depressed MS patient, neurologists should not necessarily wait for a psychiatric opinion should that entail a delay. Rather, as a consensus statement makes clear, early intervention with medication and supportive psychotherapy is warranted [53].

References

1. American Psychiatric Association. Diagnostic and statistical manual. 4th ed. Washington, DC: American Psychiatric Press, 1994

2. Feinstein A, Feinstein K J. Depression associated with multiple sclerosis: looking beyond diagnosis to symptom expression. *J Affect Disord* 2001;**66**:193–8

3. Minden S L, Orav J, Reich P. Depression in multiple sclerosis. *Gen Hosp Psychiatry* 1987;**9**:426–34

4. Joffe R T, Lippert G P, Gray T A, Sawa G, Horvath Z. Mood disorder and multiple sclerosis. *Arch Neurol* 1987;**44**:376–8

5. Sadovnik A N, Remick R A, Allen J, *et al.* Depression and multiple sclerosis. *Neurology* 1996;**46**:628–32

6. Patten S B, Beck C A, Williams J V A, Barbui C, Metz L M. Major depression in multiple sclerosis: a population-based perspective. *Neurology* 2003;**61**:1524–7

7. Zigmond A S, Snaith R P. The Hospital and Anxiety Depression Scale. *Acta Psychiatr Scand* 1983;**67**:361–70

8. Beck A T, Steer R A, Brown G K. BDI-Fast Screen for Medical Patients manual. San Antonio, TX: The Psychological Corporation, 2000.

9. Benedict R H, Fishman I, McClellan M M, Bakshi R, Weinstock-Guttman B. Validity of the Beck Depression Inventory-Fast Screen in multiple sclerosis. *Mult Scler* 2003;**9**:393–6

10. Feinstein A, O'Connor P, Gray T, Feinstein K. The effects of anxiety on psychiatric morbidity in patients with multiple sclerosis. *Mult Scler* 1999;**5**:323–6

11. Quesnel S, Feinstein A. Multiple sclerosis and alcohol: a study of problem drinking. *Mult Scler* 2004;**10**:197–201

12. Korostil M, Feinstein A. Anxiety disorders and their clinical correlates in multiple sclerosis patients. *Mult Scler* 2007;**13**:67–72

13. Stenager E N, Stenager E, Koch-Hendrikson N, *et al.* Suicide and multiple sclerosis: an epidemiological investigation. *J Neurol Neurosurg Psychiatry* 1992;**55**:542–5

14. Feinstein A. An examination of suicidal intent in patients with multiple sclerosis. *Neurology* 2002;**59**:674–8

15. Patten S B, Metz L M, Reimer M A. Biopsychosocial correlates of lifetime major depression in a multiple sclerosis population. *Mult Scler* 2000;**6**:115–20

16. Schiffer R B, Caine E D, Bamford K A, Levy S. Depressive episodes in patients with multiple sclerosis. *Am J Psychiatry* 1983;**140**:1498–500

17. Pujol J, Bello J, Deus J, Marti-Vilalta J L, Capdevila A. Lesions in the left arcuate fasciculus region and depressive symptoms in multiple sclerosis. *Neurology* 1997;**49**:1105–10

18. Berg D, Supprian T, Thomae J, *et al.* Lesion pattern in patients with multiple sclerosis and depression. *Mult Scler* 2000;**6**:156–62

19. Bakshi R, Czarnecki D, Shaikh Z A, *et al.* Brain MRI lesions and atrophy are related to depression in multiple sclerosis. *NeuroReport* 2000;**11**:1153–8

20. Feinstein A, Roy P, Lobaugh N, Feinstein K J, O'Connor P. Structural brain abnormalities in multiple sclerosis patients with major depression. *Neurology* 2004;**62**:586–90

21. Moradzadeh L, Feinstein A, Lobaugh N, Ramirez J. Multiple sclerosis and depression: a diffusion MRI study. (Abstract.) *J Neuropsychiatry Clin Neurosci* 2007;**19**:232

22. Lynch S G, Kroencke D C, Denney D R. The relationship between disability and depression in multiple sclerosis: the role of uncertainty, coping and hope. *Mult Scler* 2001;**7**:411–16

23. Mohr D C, Goodkin D E, Gatto N, van der Wende J. Depression, coping and level of neurological impairment in multiple sclerosis. *Mult Scler* 1997;**3**:254–8

24. Pakenham K I. Adjustment to multiple sclerosis: application of a stress coping model. *Health Psychol* 1999;**18**:383–92

25. Shnek Z M, Foley F W, LaRocca N G, *et al.* Helplessness, self-efficacy, cognitive distortions, and depression in multiple sclerosis and spinal cord injury. *Ann Behav Med* 1997;**19**:287–94

26. Maybury C P, Brewin C R. Social relationships, knowledge and adjustment to multiple sclerosis. *J Neurol Neurosurg Psychiatry* 1984;**47**:372–6

27. Voss W D, Arnett P A, Higginson C I, *et al.* Contributing factors to depressed mood in multiple sclerosis. *Arch Clin Neuropsychol* 2002;**17**:103–15

28. Schiffer R B, Wineman N M. Antidepressant pharmacotherapy of depression associated with multiple sclerosis. *Am J Psychiatry* 1990;**147**:1493–7

29. Scott T F, Nussbaum P, McConnell H, Brill P. Measurement of treatment response to sertraline in depressed multiple sclerosis patients using the Carroll scale. *Neurol Res* 1995;**17**:421–2

30. Barak Y, Ur E, Archiron A. Moclobemide treatment in multiple sclerosis patients with co-morbid depression: an open label safety trial. *J Neuropsychiatry Clin Neurosci* 1999;**11**:271–3

31. Mohr D C, Boudewyn A C, Goodkin D, Bostrom A, Epstein L. Comparative outcomes for individual

cognitive-behavior therapy, supportive-expressive group therapy, and sertraline for the treatment of depression in multiple sclerosis. *J Consult Clin Psychol* 2001;**69**:942–9

32. Mohr D C, Likosky W, Bertagnoli A, *et al.* Telephone-administered cognitive-behavioral therapy for the treatment of depressive symptoms in multiple sclerosis. *J Consult Clin Psychol* 2000;**68**:356–61

33. Mattingley G, Baker K, Zorumski C F, Figiel G S. Multiple sclerosis and ECT: possible value of gadolinium enhanced magnetic resonance scans for identifying high risk patients. *J Neuropsychiatry Clin Neurosci* 1992;**4**:145–51

34. Schiffer R B, Wineman M, Weitkamp L R. Association between bipolar affective disorder and multiple sclerosis. *Am J Psychiatry* 1986;**143**:94–5

35. Minden S L, Orav J, Schildkraut J J. Hypomanic reactions to ACTH and prednisone treatment for multiple sclerosis. *Neurology* 1988;**38**:1631–4

36. Reischies F M, Baum K, Bräu H, Hedde J P, Schwindt G. Cerebral magnetic resonance imaging findings in multiple sclerosis: relation to disturbance of affect, drive and cognition. *Arch Neurol* 1988;**45**:1114–16

37. Feinstein A, du Boulay G, Ron M A. Psychotic illness in multiple sclerosis: a clinical and magnetic resonance imaging study. *Br J Psychiatry* 1992;**161**:680–5

38. Cottrell S S, Wilson S A K. The affective symptomatology of disseminated sclerosis. *J Neurol Psychopath* 1926;**7**:1–30

39. Rabins P V. Euphoria in multiple sclerosis. In: Rao S M, ed. Neurobehavioral aspects of multiple sclerosis. New York: Oxford University Press, 1990:180–5

40. Fishman I, Benedict R H B, Bakshi R, Priore R, Weinstock-Guttman B. Construct validity and frequency of euphoria sclerotica in multiple sclerosis. *J Neuropsychiatry Clin Neurosci* 2004;**16**:350–6

41. Diaz-Olavarrieta C, Cummings J L, Velasquez J, Garcia de la Cadena C. Neuropsychiatric manifestations of multiple sclerosis. *J Neuropsychiatry Clin Neurosci* 1999;**11**:51–7

42. Rabins P V, Brooks B R, O'Donnell O P, *et al.* Structural brain correlates of emotional disorder in multiple sclerosis. *Brain* 1986;**109**:585–97

43. Ron M A, Logsdail S J. Psychiatric morbidity in multiple sclerosis: a clinical and MRI study. *Psychol Med* 1989;**19**:887–95

44. Cummings J L, Arcinegas D B, Brooks B R, *et al.* Defining and diagnosing involuntary emotional expression disorder. *CNS Specr* 2006;**11**:1–7

45. Feinstein A, Feinstein K J, Gray T, O'Connor P. The prevalence and neurobehavioral correlates of pathological laughter and crying in multiple sclerosis. *Arch Neurol* 1997;**54**:1116–21

46. Feinstein A, O'Connor P, Gray T, Feinstein K. Pathological laughing and crying in multiple sclerosis: a preliminary report suggesting a role for the prefrontal cortex. *Mult Scler* 1999;**5**:69–73

47. Ghaffar O, Chamelian L, Feinstein A. Neuroanatomy of pseudobulbar affect: a quantitative MRI study in multiple sclerosis. *J Neurol* 2008;**255**:406–12

48. Sakheim H A, Greenberg M S, Weinman A L, *et al.* Hemisphere asymmetry in the expression of positive and negative emotions. *Arch Neurol* 1982;**39**:210–18

49. Schiffer R B, Herndon R M, Rudick R A. Treatment of pathologic laughing and weeping with amitriptyline. *New Engl J Med* 1985;**312**:1480–2

50. Seliger G M, Hornstein A, Flax J, Herbert J, Schroder K. Fluoxetine improves emotional incontinence. *Brain Inj* 1992;**6**:267–70

51. Udaka F, Yamao S, Nagata H, Nakamura S, Kameyama M. Pathologic laughing and crying treated with levodopa. *Arch Neurol* 1984;**41**:1095–6

52. Panitch H S, Thisted R A, Smith R A, *et al.* Randomized controlled trial of dextromethorphan/quinidine for pseudobulbar effect in multiple sclerosis. *Ann Neurol* 2006;**59**:780–7

53. **Goldman Consensus Group**. The Goldman Consensus statement on depression in multiple sclerosis. *Mult Scler* 2005;**11**:328–37

Chapter 22

Bladder dysfunction in multiple sclerosis

Clare J. Fowler and Gustav Kiss

Prevalence

Since bladder dysfunction in multiple sclerosis (MS) depends to a large extent on the severity of spinal cord involvement, estimates of its prevalence have varied depending on the severity of disability of the population studied. A recent questionnaire survey of an unselected group of patients with MS studied over a 5-year period showed that half reported significant symptoms due to bladder dysfunction [1]. Other population studies have given estimates of between 58% [2] and 75% [3], the problem becoming increasingly common with a longer duration of illness and an increasing level of disability.

Nature of the problem
Underlying pathophysiology

Figure 22.1 shows the location of the micturition center in the pons (PMC), and whilst various higher cortical functions are known to effect its ultimate control and activation, "switching" it on for voiding, connections between the pons and the sacral segments of the spinal cord are critical for coordinated, physiological bladder function. It is known that there are direct connections between the PMC and the parasympathetic outflow to the detrusor muscle and innervation within the spinal cord which sends reciprocal inhibition of the striated urethral sphincter muscle so that when the detrusor contracts for voiding the sphincter relaxes [4]. These activation processes are reversed during the storage phase. If the integrity of the spinal connections is compromised the coordinated detrusor sphincter behavior is lost and "detrusor–sphincter dyssynergia" (DSD) [5] occurs. This may impair bladder emptying and contribute to

pathologically raised detrusor contraction pressures as the bladder contracts against a closed sphincter. Such abnormal activity can lead to upper tract damage, ureteric reflux, hydronephrosis, and renal damage.

A further pathophysiological consequence of disconnection of the sacral cord from the upper brainstem is detrusor overactivity (DO). It is now known that an important relay center for the bladder's afferent activity is in the periaqueductal gray (PAG) [6] and interruption of this afferent pathway leads to the emergence of a new sacral segmental reflex: formerly quiescent unmyelinated afferents become functionally active and drive detrusor contractions in response to low bladder volumes [7]. It is DO that causes urinary urgency, the sensation experienced as an involuntary bladder contraction occurs, if sufficient afferent activity reaches consciousness.

Less commonly and for reasons as yet unknown, the detrusor muscle loses its effective emptying properties. This appears to be a problem that is particularly pronounced in the bladder pathophysiology of MS and somewhat different from the situation of patients following spinal cord injury. Urodynamic studies have shown a median of 17% of patients with MS have a "hypocontractile detrusor" [8, 9]; lower detrusor contraction pressures have been demonstrated in women with MS [10]; and other studies have found that injection of the sphincter to treat DSD does not improve bladder emptying [11]. It may be because of this that the incidence of upper tract damage in MS is so low. A speculative explanation for this phenomenon is that whereas the disconnected spinal cord distal to a level of traumatic injury is likely to be healthy and serve as a synaptic relay center for aberrant reflex activity such as that causing DO or even autonomic dysreflexia, the same is not the case in MS, a disease

Multiple Sclerosis: Recovery of Function and Neurorehabilitation, eds. J. Kesselring, G. Comi, and A. J. Thompson. Published by Cambridge University Press. © Cambridge University Press 2010.

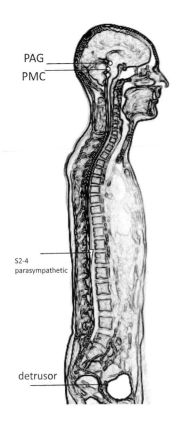

Fig. 22.1. Illustration of the pathways involved in micturition. PAG, periaqueductal gray; PMC, pontine micturition center.

PAG

PMC

S2-4
parasympathetic

detrusor

that can affect the entire spinal cord leading to atrophy in advanced cases.

An individual patient may have a combination of all three problems: DO, DSD, and inefficient emptying.

Symptoms

The effect of these pathophysiologies in producing symptoms is shown in Figure 22.2. Urgency, urgency incontinence, and frequency reflect the underlying DO and have been universally demonstrated to be the commonest problems in MS [8]. A particular characteristic of urgency resulting from spinal cord disease is that the patient may describe that they are able to remain continent whilst sitting in the same position but that rising to stand or walk precipitates urgency and urgency incontinence.

Urinary frequency can result either from a reduced bladder capacity or incomplete bladder emptying.

The symptoms of abnormal voiding due to DSD and inefficient detrusor contractions are hesitancy, an interrupted flow pattern, and possibly a complaint of incomplete emptying. Difficulty in emptying is much less commonly volunteered as a complaint by patients but may be admitted to on direct questioning when the patient reports that they can void twice at a short interval, rather than because they have a positive sensation of incomplete emptying. In a study of patients' bladder

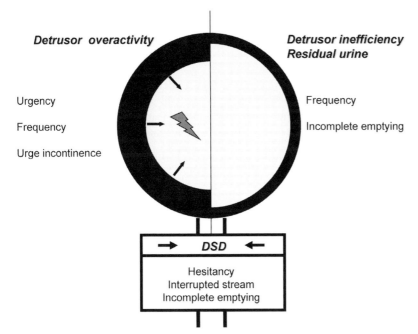

Fig. 22.2. The relationship between pathophysiology and symptoms.

Detrusor overactivity

Detrusor inefficiency
Residual urine

Urgency

Frequency

Urge incontinence

Frequency

Incomplete emptying

→ *DSD* ←

Hesitancy
Interrupted stream
Incomplete emptying

191

symptoms it was demonstrated that the majority (83%) of those who thought they were not emptying their bladders were correct whereas the converse was untrue: of those demonstrated to have a raised post-micturition residual volume only 47% were aware of it [12].

Management of bladder symptoms in MS: first-line treatments

Antimuscarinic medication

Antimuscarinic medications have long been known to improve bladder control. Until relatively recently it was supposed that the medication was effective through blockade of the parasympathetic neurotransmission to the detrusor muscle. However, the medication results in a demonstrable increase in bladder capacity and reduction in urgency incontinence in patients with DO treated with antimuscarinics, suggesting that there is a more complex mechanism of action, possibly through an effect on the afferent innervation of the bladder [13].

There are now a number of antimuscarinic medications available (Table 22.1). The detrusor muscle expresses mostly M2 muscarinic receptors [14], although M3 are the functionally important ones in the detrusor muscle, in conditions of health. The benefits of selective blockade of M2 or M3 muscarinic receptors have yet to be translated into clinical effect. The formulation of these medications to give a long-acting preparation (extended life, "XL") is a significant advantage for patients, who need only take the tablet once a day to provide 24-hour cover for symptoms. Both tolterodine and trospium chloride have a chemical structure which renders them less lipophilic and therefore theoretically less likely to cross the blood–brain barrier, possibly conferring the advantage of lesser central side effects. Darifenacin is a selective M3 antagonist, which it is claimed reduces adverse effects on memory, a function dependent on M1 central receptors [15]. Probably the cautions about prescribing antimuscarinics to elderly patients because of their central effects should be extended to those with cognitive impairment due to MS.

Recent studies of patients with neurogenic DO found that doubling the dose of antimuscarinics increased effectiveness in controlling incontinence without excessive side effects [16, 17]: a daily dosage of trospium chloride up to 135 mg appears to be effective and safe in patients [18]. Alternative means of administering antimuscarinics include intravesical atropine [19] or dermal patches of slow-release oxybutynin [20].

Management of incomplete emptying

Although immediate treatment of the symptoms of DO (see Fig. 22.2) by an antimuscarinic might at first glance seem desirable, it is important first to measure the post-micturition residual volume (PRV). This can be conveniently done using a small, easily operated portable ultrasound device. The importance of recognizing incomplete emptying is that any residual volume in the bladder can trigger volume-determined reflex detrusor contractions, and thus exacerbate the clinical situation. As already explained, many patients are not aware of the extent to which they have incomplete emptying, and bladder emptying efficiency may be further compromised by antimuscarinics. Figure 22.3 shows a simple algorithm for managing the common early symptoms of bladder dysfunction in MS [21]. Although some authorities prefer to use one-third of capacity as a significant PRV, for ease and simplicity a figure in excess of 100 ml is generally agreed to be an indicator of significant incomplete emptying. This can be demonstrated either by "in/out catheterization" or by use of a small portable ultrasound machine. The latter, although by no means inexpensive, have been developed to be reliable and easy to use. Many of these devices simply display a figure rather than an image of the residual volume and since precision is not required, this is a satisfactory means of monitoring the situation.

If a raised PRV is demonstrated, the patient, or possibly their carer, will need to be taught clean intermittent self-catheterization (CISC). This is best done by a nurse who is knowledgeable about the use of catheters, etc., such as a specially trained continence advisor nurse. The technique can be taught to the patient as an outpatient procedure in approximately an hour. They can be provided with supportive literature and a telephone number to call if further advice is needed.

The requirements for success with CISC include the ability to comprehend the principle of the technique and adequate motivation. The patient needs to be able to get into a position to access their urethra with the catheter, clearly more difficult in women than men, and severe lower limb spasticity may be a

Table 22.1 Oral antimuscarinic agents used to treat symptoms of detrusor overactivity

Generic name	UK trade name	Dose (mg)	Frequency of administration	Receptor subtype selectivity	Molecule type	Elimination half-life of parent drug (hrs)
Propantheline	Pro-Banthine	15	tds	Non-selective	Quaternary amine	<2
Tolterodine tartrate	Detrusitol	2	bd	Non-selective	Tertiary amine	2.4
Tolterodine tartrate	Detrusitol XL	4	od	Non-selective	Tertiary amine	8.4
Trospium chloride	Regurin	20	bd	Non-selective	Quaternary amine	20
Oxybutynin chloride	Ditropan	2.5–5	bd–qds	Non-selective	Tertiary amine	2.3
Oxybutynin chloride XL	Lyrinel XL	5–30	od	Non-selective	Tertiary amine (R and S isomers)	13.2
Propiverine hydrochloride	Detrunorm	15	od–qds	Non-selective	Ester	4.1
Darifenacin	Emselex	7.5–15	od	Selective muscarinic M3 receptor antagonist	Tertiary amine	13–18
Solifenacin	Vesicare	5–10	od	Selective muscarinic M2 and M3 receptor antagonist	Tertiary amine	40–68

Notes: od, once daily; bd, twice daily; tds, three times daily; qds, four times daily; XL, extended life.

limiting factor. Manual dexterity sufficient to do up buttons of clothes is needed and, although some blind patients do manage the technique, good eyesight makes things easier. There are now a range of catheters, most of them single-use disposable ones, and some which come pre-wetted with a hydrophilic coating so that they are ready lubricated. Patients' concerns are often around the risk of infection, and infections may be a problem particularly in the early stages of learning the technique. The patient should be given advice on how to collect a specimen and obtain antibiotics at the early onset of symptoms of infection, but long-term prophylactic antibiotics are rarely indicated.

The only other means of improving bladder emptying, which may benefit some patients, is the application of a suprapubic vibrating stimulus. It was shown many years ago that vibration applied to this region can induce bladder contraction [22]. Although this may have no effect in healthy individuals, in those with DO, the vibrating stimulus may trigger a detrusor contraction and thus help initiate micturition and possibly improve bladder emptying. Various devices including a small hand-held battery-operated vibrator are commercially available and some patients find these helpful [23, 24].

Although CISC is undoubtedly the best and most effective means of improving bladder emptying, some alternative is much needed for those patients who are unwilling or unable to carry this out on a regular basis. It has been claimed that alpha blockers, which are used to treat prostatic hypertrophy and outflow obstruction, can reduce PRV [25] but the evidence is poor and clinical experience rarely shows them to be effective [11]. This, of course, is not surprising since the abnormality causing incomplete emptying is poor

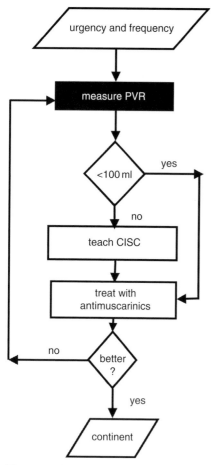

Fig. 22.3. Algorithm for the management of neurogenic incontinence. CISC, clean intermittent self-catheterization. (Reproduced with permission from "Investigation of the neurogenic bladder" by Clare J Fowler in *Neurological Investigations*, ed. RAC Hughes, 1997, published by Blackwell Publishing.)

coordination of the detrusor contraction and detrusor sphincter dyssynergia, a disorder of the striated musculature.

Desmopressin (DDAVP)

The synthetic antidiuretic hormone desmopression (DDAVP) was originally licensed to treat the polyuria of diabetes insipidus. Subsequently it became an established treatment for nocturnal enuresis and studies were then carried out to look at its efficacy in women with MS and night-time frequency [26]. If used at night, normal sleep patterns may be restored which results in a significant improvement in quality of life [27]. A number of small placebo-controlled trials have shown that it is effective if taken during

the day in providing the patients with a period up to 6 hours during which they are not troubled by urinary frequency, without any rebound night-time frequency [27]. Patients must, however, be cautioned to use it only once in 24 hours despite the convenience of the effect it has. It should be given with extreme caution to patients over the age of 65 and not be used by those with dependent leg edema through immobility who have night-time frequency when recumbent. Measurements of serum sodium should be made if it is used in the elderly.

Point of controversy

Clean intermittent self-catheterization in combination with an antimuscarinic provides the best chance of improving urinary incontinence in a patient with DO and incomplete emptying. Both these management options are included in the simple algorithm shown in Fig. 22.3, although this has been viewed as contentious for more than 15 years because it does not include cystometry as part of routine investigations [28]. The additional information that may be obtained from cystometry includes the severity of DO and the extent of DSD. However, it can be argued that both those pathophysiologies are optimally treated with the combination of CISC and antimuscarinics and in circumstances where cost-effective use of personel is a driving force, time spent teaching the patient CISC is probably most valuable.

Thus the algorithm in Fig. 22.3 is recommended as a first-line management for patients presenting initially with urinary symptoms. Undoubtedly as the disease progresses and bladder symptoms may become worse, complications can arise requiring further investigations and urological interventions, as shown in Fig. 22.4. Table 22.2 stresses the symptoms that warrant immediate urological referral.

Risk of urological damage in MS

Some 20–30 years ago when the importance of bladder dysfunction in patients with MS started to be acknowledged as the problem it is, urologists were concerned that the upper tract disorders that can follow traumatic spinal cord injury and may result in renal damage, renal failure, and death were going to be complications of other neurogenic bladder disorders, including those of MS. For unknown reasons but possibly related to the already highlighted phenomenon of poor detrusor contractility in MS, this

Table 22.2 Indications for referral to a urologist

1. Recurrent urinary tract infections

2. Hematuria

3. Evidence of impaired renal function

4. Pain thought to be arising from the upper or lower urinary tract

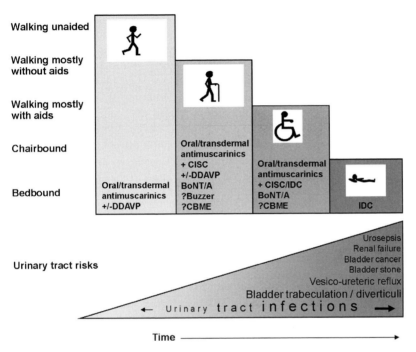

Fig. 22.4. The bladder symptoms in MS becoming increasingly difficult to manage with progression of spinal cord disease. The diagram summarizes the various measures that may be effective at each stage. DDAVP, desmopressin; CBME, cannabis-based medical extract; CISC, clean intermittent self-catheterization; BoNT/A, botulinum neurotoxin type A; IDC, indwelling catheter. The figure also illustrates the increasing risk of development of urological problems.

does not appear to be the case. A study has shown that there is no increased risk of death from renal failure in MS, compared with the general UK population [29], in contrast to the situation following spinal cord injury. However urinary tract damage such as urinary tract infections, bladder diverticulae and trabeculation, dilatation of upper tracts, vesico-ureteric reflux, bladder cancer, stone formation, and renal failure may all occur in patients with MS and a recent systematic study has identified a number of factors shown in Table 22.3 [8] and these data are illustrated in Fig. 22.4.

It is, however, important to note that patients with the typical at-risk profile will necessarily be highly symptomatic from their bladder disorder, and having become non-responsive to simple first-line measures will already have needed urological intervention.

Further urological efforts to improve their symptomatology will also be appropriate to manage their underlying urinary tract disease, be it severe DO, the consequences of DSD, or recurrent infection.

Second-line treatments for overactive bladder

Although not absolute, there is a clinically observable correlation between increasing disability and difficulty controlling bladder symptoms, as shown in Fig. 22.4. As mobility deteriorates first-line measures become insufficient to prevent troublesome incontinence; the patient is not in a robust state of health and yet does not want to have a long-term indwelling catheter. Major continence surgery is not therefore appropriate and furthermore may be unsuitable for a

Table 22.3 Risk factors for developing urological complications

Definite risk factors	Probable risk factors
Duration of MS >15 years	Detrusor–sphincter dyssynergia
Indwelling urinary catheter	Age > 50
Urodynamically demonstrated frequent detrusor contractions and high detrusor pressure	Male

patient who is likely to experience further neurological deterioration. Various new non-operative treatments have recently become available and some of these second-line treatments are proving highly effective.

Cannabinoids

The use of cannabis by patients with MS is common in European countries, and a diagnosis of MS is sometimes argued as extenuating circumstances by people found growing the plant *Cannabis sativa* in Member States where its possession is illegal. In 1998 a high-level UK government report argued that the medicinal properties of cannabis should be further explored, giving rise to a number of open-label studies. These included a small, open-label study in patients with advanced MS in whom first-line conventional available treatments were ineffective and who were therefore facing the prospect of having a long-term indwelling catheter. The results of this pilot study showed there were no serious adverse effects but a significant decrease in urinary urgency and reduction in the number and volume of incontinence episodes, frequency, and nocturia, and reduction in spasticity and improvement in quality of sleep [30]. Encouraged by this finding a larger multi-center randomized placebo-controlled study was undertaken to look at the effect of sublingual sprays of medicinal cannabis extracts on bladder function. So far reported on only in abstract, the findings are that although improvements in incontinence were not statistically significant, there was a significant reduction in night-time frequency and patients rated their bladder control much improved.

The UK Medical Research Council funded a large multi-center placebo-controlled trial to look at the effect of oral Nabilone and THC (Δ-tetrahydrocannabinol) in patients with MS (the "CAMS study" – Cannabis in Multiple Sclerosis). The primary focus was to look at the effect of cannabinoids on spasticity and although no change was demonstrated on the Ashworth Scale, the patients did report subjective improvements [31]. In a substudy patients' incontinence was assessed by diaries and a significant difference in the groups treated with cannabis extract and THC compared to the placebo group were shown. Whereas medicinal cannabis extract is now a licensed treatment for pain in Canada, its use has not been approved for any indication in the UK as yet.

Intravesical vanilloids

That the afferent fibers of the sacral segmental reflex that emerge following spinal cord damage are sensitive to capsaicin [7] led to the use of intravesical capsaicin in patients with MS [32] in an attempt to de-afferent the bladder. Although further work demonstrated that this could have a significant therapeutic effect [33, 34], its use was generally abandoned both because of the discomfort of the instillations and its non-licensed status. However work continued in Bordeaux where it was found that by using glucidic acid as the solvent, irritant effects were reduced, and such a formulation has continued to be used ever since [35].

Other molecules with the same selective neurotoxic effect by virtue of a vanilloid chemical ring, the so called "vanilloids," include resiniferatoxin. Resiniferatoxin (RTX) is an ultra potent capsaicinoid but with much less pungency than capsaicin. It was hoped that this could have the same selective neurotoxin effect on the bladder afferents without the irritant effect [36]. Clinical trials with RTX were unfortunately marred by an unrecognized effect of the compound's tendency to adhere to plastic and for this reason the number of patients in whom it was effective in treatment trials was small [37, 38]. However one of the authors (GK) has found continuing beneficial effects in a small group of patients with MS. Also, at the time of writing there has been renewed interest in this molecule and a pharmaceutical preparation may become available again.

De-afferentation of the bladder using other vanilloids remains the aim of other pharmaceutical companies attempting to develop agents to treat the pathologically overactive bladder.

Detrusor injections of botulinum toxin type A

Botulinum toxin A (BoNT/A) was injected into the detrusor muscle of patients with spinal cord injury with the intention of blocking parasympathetic release of acetylcholine, paralyzing the detrusor muscle, and so reducing involuntary detrusor contractions. However, the findings of the first systematic study of this treatment far exceeded expectations [39], with a marked reduction in incontinence episodes without complete retention. A subsequent placebo-controlled study showed highly significant efficacy [40] and subsequently studies from all over the world have reported the benefits in both neurogenic and idiopathic DO [41, 42]. In fact the clinical findings have been so exceptional that a hypothesis was proposed suggesting that BoNT/A acts on afferent mechanisms that are involved in the pathogenesis of DO [43].

The original description of the method for injection used a rigid cystoscope so that a general anesthetic was necessary, particularly in men, if sensation was intact. Thirty equally spaced injection points in the bladder, sparing the trigone, are given, each injection consisting of 10 mouse units of BOTOX® (1 ml). The use of a flexible cystoscope through which to inject has meant that it is possible to reduce the intervention to a minimally invasive outpatient procedure, taking on average up to 15 minutes, with a mean level of discomfort of 3, rated on a 1–10 scale [44, 45].

Although some of the many reports of using BoNT/A in neurogenic DO have included patients with MS, the larger proportion of patients in each series have had spinal cord injury. A recent study, which included 43 patients exclusively with MS, demonstrated highly significant improvements in incontinence episiodes, urinary urgency, daytime frequency, and nocturia when the patients were assessed at 4 and at 16 weeks [46]. An important observation arising from this study that will affect clinical practice was that 98% of patients needed to perform CISC following the treatment, even the 28% who had not

done so previously, but that this did not affect their quality of life. Highly significant improvements in quality of life were found (Fig. 22.5). The duration of effect in most studies has been found to be about 10 months and in the MS study the mean duration following the first injection was 9.7 months and 11.7 months following the second [46]. Figure 22.6 shows the duration of benefit in six patients from that study who have had four repeated injections and suggests that the response duration is fairly consistent and individual for each patient.

Such a remarkably effective minimally invasive treatment, with few side effects, is obviously going to have a major impact on the future management of bladder dysfunction in MS. It is currently still undergoing the trials to obtain licensing in the EU and USA but it is hoped that it will then become widely available as a treatment.

Injection of BoNT/A in the external urethral sphincter to treat DSD

The first use of BoNT/A in urology was to inject the striated urethral sphincter in patients with DSD following spinal cord injury. It was with this same aim and the expectation that PVR might be reduced, that sphincter injections were used in a group of patients with MS [47]. Interestingly, a placebo-controlled study which examined this carefully found no reduction in PVR in the patients injected with BoNT/A [11]. This suggests incomplete emptying is due more to inefficient detrusor contractions than DSD.

Long-term indwelling catheter

If the level of disability increases such that the patient is chair- or bedbound, has severe lower limb spasticity, loss of manual dexterity, and possibly also cognitive impairment, intermittent self-catheterization or even intermittent catheterization by their caregiver becomes impossible. At this stage a permanent indwelling catheter or some other measure becomes necessary.

A suprapubic catheter is recommended in preference to a long-term urethral catheter in both men and women since urethral catheters in men are likely to cause splitting of the distal urethra and in women, damage to the urethra and bladder neck [48]. Their use should be considered as a temporary measure

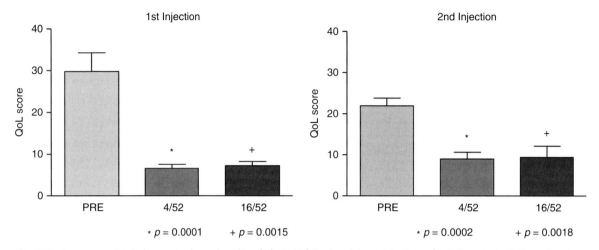

Fig. 22.5. Improvement in leakage episodes and quality of life (QoL) following detrusor injections of botulinum toxin A. (Reproduced with permission from [47].)

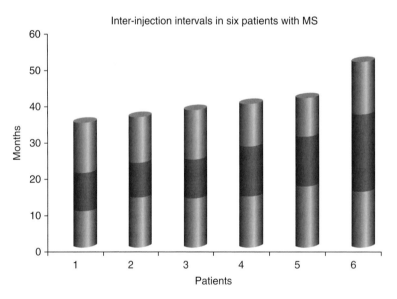

Fig. 22.6. The duration of efficacy of repeated detrusor injections of BoNT/A in six patients with MS.

only – possibly to familiarize the patient and their caregiver with the collecting bag system. As soon as possible the patient should be referred to a urologist for insertion of a suprapubic catheter.

Most urologists, anxious about the risk of bowel perforation when inserting a trochar into a small, shrunken bladder, prefer to carry out the procedure under cystoscopic control and general anesthetic. The suprapubic catheter tract must be left to epithelialize for 6–8 weeks before the first catheter change which should ideally be performed by the team who

performed the operation. Subsequent changes of the catheter will be at intervals of about 3 months, and may be done in the clinic or even in the community.

Once a suprapubic catheter has been inserted the patient should remain under urological supervision so that catheter blockages, infection, and the possible increased risk of bladder cancer can be monitored [48]. Those with an indwelling catheter who have formerly received cytotoxic treatment, cyclophosphamide in particular, have been shown to be at increased risk of developing bladder cancer.

Summarizing conclusion

In the early stages of MS, symptoms of bladder dysfunction can be effectively managed by oral antimuscarinic agents and the addition of CISC if incomplete bladder emptying is demonstrated. With accumulating disability, bladder symptoms may become more difficult to treat and urological complications more likely. Fortunately, a new and highly effective treatment in the form of detrusor injections of BoNT/A is becoming available to reduce the symptoms and urological consequences of DO, although incomplete bladder emptying remains a problem requiring intermittent catheterization.

At each stage of the disease there is much that can be done to improve bladder control and there are few patients with MS who cannot be offered effective treatment for incontinence.

References

1. Nortvedt M W, Riise T, Frugard J, *et al*. Prevalence of bladder, bowel and sexual problems among multiple sclerosis patients two to five years after diagnosis. *Mult Scler* 2007;**13**:106–12

2. Hennessey A, Robertson N P, Swingler R, Compston D A. Urinary, faecal and sexual dysfunction in patients with multiple sclerosis. *J Neurol* 1999;**246**:1027–32

3. Miller H, Simpson C A, Yeates W K. Bladder dysfunction in multiple sclerosis. *BMJ* 1965;**1** (5445):1265–9

4. Blok B F, de Weerd H, Holstege G. The pontine micturition center projects to sacral cord GABA immunoreactive neurons in the cat. *Neurosci Lett* 1997;**233**:109–12

5. Blaivas J G, Sinha H P, Zayed A A H, Labib K B. Detrusor–external sphincter dyssynergia: a detailed electromyography study. *J Urol* 1981;**125**:545–8

6. Blok B F, Holstege G. Direct projections from the periaqueductal grey to the pontine micturition centre (M-region): an antegrade and retrograde tracing study in the cat. *Neurosci Lett* 1994;**166**:93–6

7. de Groat W, Kawatani T, Hisamitsu T, *et al*. Mechanisims underlying the recovery of urinary bladder function following spinal cord injury. *J Auton Nerv Syst* 1990;**30**:S71–8

8. de Seze M, Ruffion A, Denys P, Joseph P A, Perrouin-Verbe B. The neurogenic bladder in multiple sclerosis: review of the literature and proposal of management guidelines. *Mult Scler* 2007;**13**:915–28

9. Mayo M E, Chetner M P. Lower urinary tract dysfunction in multiple sclerosis. *Urology* 1992;**39**:67–70

10. Lemack G E, Frohman E, Ramnarayan P. Women with voiding dysfunction secondary to bladder outlet dyssynergia in the setting of multiple sclerosis do not demonstrate significantly elevated intravesical pressures. *Urology* 2007;**69**:893–7

11. Gallien P, Reymann J M, Amarenco G, *et al*. Placebo controlled, randomised, double blind study of the effects of botulinum A toxin on detrusor sphincter dyssynergia in multiple sclerosis patients. *J Neurol Neurosurg Psychiatry* 2005;**76**:1670–6

12. Betts C D, D'Mellow M T, Fowler C J. Urinary symptoms and the neurological features of bladder dysfunction in multiple sclerosis. *J Neurol Neurosurg Psychiatry* 1993;**56**:245–50

13. Andersson K E. Antimuscarinics for treatment of overactive bladder. *Lancet Neurol* 2004;**3**:46–53

14. Chess-Williams R. Muscarinic receptors of the urinary bladder: detrusor, urothelial and prejunctional. *Auton Autacoid Pharmacol* 2002;**22**:133–45

15. Kay G G, Wesnes K A. Pharmacodynamic effects of darifenacin, a muscarinic M selective receptor antagonist for the treatment of overactive bladder, in healthy volunteers. *BJU Int* 2005;**96**:1055–62

16. Horstmann M, Schaefer T, Aguilar Y, Stenzl A, Sievert K D. Neurogenic bladder treatment by doubling the recommended antimuscarinic dosage. *Neurourol Urodyn* 2006;**25**:441–5

17. Bennett N, O'Leary M, Patel A S, *et al*. Can higher doses of oxybutynin improve efficacy in neurogenic bladder? *J Urol* 2004;**171**:749–51

18. Menarini M, Del Popolo G, Di Benedetto P, *et al*. Trospium chloride in patients with neurogenic detrusor overactivity: is dose titration of benefit to the patients? *Int J Clin Pharmacol Ther* 2006;**44**:623–32

19. Fader M, Glickman S, Haggar V, *et al*. Intravesical atropine compared to oral oxybutynin for neurogenic detrusor overactivity: a double-blind, randomized crossover trial. *J Urol* 2007;**177**:208–13; discussion 13

20. Dmochowski R R, Nitti V, Staskin D, *et al*. Transdermal oxybutynin in the treatment of adults with overactive bladder: combined results of two randomized clinical trials. *World J Urol* 2005;**23**:263–70

21. Fowler C J. Investigation of the neurogenic bladder. *J Neurol Neurosurg Psychiatry* 1996;**60**:6–13

22. Nathan P. Emptying the paralysed bladder. *Lancet* 1977;**1**(8007):377

23. Dasgupta P, Haslam C, Goodwin R, Fowler C. The Queen Square bladder stimulator: a device for assisting emptying of the neurogenic bladder. *Br J Urol* 1997;**80**:234–7

24. Prasad R S, Smith S J, Wright H. Lower abdominal pressure versus external bladder stimulation to aid

bladder emptying in multiple sclerosis: a randomized controlled study. *Clin Rehabil* 2003;**17**:42–7

25. O'Riordan J, Doherty C, Javed M, *et al.* Do alpha-blockers have a role in lower urinary tract dysfunction in multiple sclerosis? *J Urol* 1995;**153**:1114–16

26. Hilton P, Hertogs K, Stanton S. The use of desmopressin (DDAVP) for nocturia in women with multiple sclerosis. *J Neurol Neurosurg Psychiatry* 1983;**46**:854–5

27. Bosma R, Wynia K, Havlikova E, De Keyser J, Middel B. Efficacy of desmopressin in patients with multiple sclerosis suffering from bladder dysfunction: a meta-analysis. *Acta Neurol Scand* 2005;**112**:1–5

28. Fowler C J, van Kerrebroeck P E V, Nordenbo A, Van Poppel H. Treatment of lower urinary tract dysfunction in patients with multiple sclerosis. *J Neurol Neurosurg Psychiatry* 1992;**55**:986–9

29. Lawrenson R, Wyndaele J J, Vlachonikolis I, Farmer C, Glickman S. Renal failure in patients with neurogenic lower urinary tract dysfunction. *Neuroepidemiology* 2001;**20**:138–43

30. Brady C M, DasGupta R, Dalton C, *et al.* An open-label pilot study of cannabis-based extracts for bladder dysfunction in advanced multiple sclerosis. *Mult Scler* 2004;**10**:425–33

31. Zajicek J, Fox P, Sanders H, *et al.* Cannabinoids for treatment of spasticity and other symptoms related to multiple sclerosis (CAMS study): multicentre randomised placebo-controlled trial. *Lancet* 2003;**362**:1517–26

32. Fowler C, Beck R, Gerrard S, Betts C, Fowler C. Intravesical capsaicin for treatment of detrusor hyperreflexia. *J Neurol Neurosurg Psychiatry* 1994;**57**:169–73

33. De Ridder D, Chandiramani V, Dasgupta P, *et al.* Intravesical capsaicin as a treatment for refractory detrusor hyperreflexia: a dual center study with long-term follow-up. *J Urol* 1997;**158**:2087–92

34. de Seze M, Wiart L, Ferriere J, *et al.* Intravesical instillation of capsaicin in urology: a review of the literature. *Eur Urol* 1999;**36**:267–77

35. de Seze M, Wiart L, de Seze M P, *et al.* Intravesical capsaicin versus resiniferatoxin for the treatment of detrusor hyperreflexia in spinal cord injured patients: a double-blind, randomized, controlled study. *J Urol* 2004;**171**:251–5

36. Cruz F, Guimaraes M, Silva C, Reis M. Suppression of bladder hyperreflexia by intravesical resiniferatoxin. (Letter). *Lancet* 1997;**350**:640–1

37. Brady C M, Apostolidis A N, Harper M, *et al.* Parallel changes in bladder suburothelial vanilloid receptor TRPV1 and pan-neuronal marker PGP9.5 immunoreactivity in patients with neurogenic detrusor overactivity after intravesical resiniferatoxin treatment. *BJU Int* 2004;**93**:770–6

38. Kim J H, Rivas D A, Shenot P J, *et al.* Intravesical resiniferatoxin for refractory detrusor hyperreflexia: a multicenter, blinded, randomized, placebo-controlled trial. *J Spinal Cord Med* 2003;**26**:358–63

39. Schurch B, Stohrer M, Kramer G, *et al.* Botulinum-A toxin for treating detrusor hyperreflexia in spinal cord injured patients: a new alternative to anticholinergic drugs? Preliminary results. *J Urol* 2000;**164**:692–7

40. Schurch B, de Seze M, Denys P, *et al.* Botulinum toxin type a is a safe and effective treatment for neurogenic urinary incontinence: results of a single treatment, randomized, placebo controlled 6-month study. *J Urol* 2005;**174**:196–200

41. Dmochowski R, Sand P K. Botulinum toxin A in the overactive bladder: current status and future directions. *BJU Int* 2007;**99**:247–62

42. Patel A K, Patterson J M, Chapple C R. Botulinum toxin injections for neurogenic and idiopathic detrusor overactivity: a critical analysis of results. *Eur Urol* 2006;**50**:684–709; discussion 710

43. Apostolidis A, Dasgupta P, Fowler C J. Proposed mechanism for the efficacy of injected botulinum toxin in the treatment of human detrusor overactivity. *Eur Urol* 2006;**49**:644–50

44. Harper M, Popat R, Dasgupta R, Fowler C J, Dasgupta P. A minimally invasive technique for outpatient local anaesthetic administration of intradetrusor botulinum toxin in intractable detrusor overactivity. *BJU Int* 2003;**92**:325–6

45. Sahai A, Kalsi V, Khan M S, Fowler C J. Techniques for the intradetrusor administration of botulinum toxin. *BJU Int* 2006;**97**:675–8

46. Kalsi V, Gonzales G, Popat R, *et al.* Botulinum injections for the treatment of bladder symptoms of multiple sclerosis. *Ann Neurol* 2007;**62**:452–7

47. Schulte-Baukloh H, Schobert J, Stolze T, *et al.* Efficacy of botulinum-A toxin bladder injections for the treatment of neurogenic detrusor overactivity in multiple sclerosis patients: an objective and subjective analysis. *Neurourol Urodyn* 2006;**25**:110–15

48. De Ridder D, Ost D, Van der Aa F, *et al.* Conservative bladder management in advanced multiple sclerosis. *Mult Scler* 2005;**11**:694–9

Chapter 23

Ataxia and imbalance in multiple sclerosis

Luigi Tesio

What is ataxia?

More than 80% of patients with multiple sclerosis (MS) experience deficits of balance and/or coordination during the course of their disease [1]. Impaired balance is often one of their earliest complaints. Hence, "ataxia" is a major target of their treatment. But what does this term really mean?

Ataxia is a word of Greek origin meaning disorder or confusion. In clinical language it broadly denotes motor incoordination. During most movements, either voluntary or involuntary, our muscles are recruited following a precise spatial–temporal chain. Ataxia may stem from weakness, spasm, or wrong timing (early or late onset) of contraction across the linked muscles [2]. With any of these mechanisms, ataxia can affect movement of the limbs as well as speech, swallowing, respiration, and bowel or bladder voiding.

Balance deficits can also be ascribed to the family of ataxic symptoms, although balance disturbances may accompany many other motor disorders. Given the higher prevalence and disabling impact of balance disturbance in MS patients, compared to limb ataxia, most of this chapter will focus upon the balance issue. Also, the words ataxia and imbalance will sometimes be used interchangeably.

Intention tremor is also an ataxic symptom. In MS it may be absent, mild, or indeed devastating. As a sign of ataxia, it may be interpreted simply as a series of hypermetric corrections of misdirected voluntary motions (frequently detected in the classic finger-to-nose test). A discussion of the classification of tremor [3] is beyond the scope of this chapter.

Pathophysiology: a sensorimotor perspective

Ataxia is roughly classified as cerebellar and/or sensory. This rules out "disordering" caused by purely efferent mechanisms such as central paresis and muscular–skeletal deficits. The cerebellum–sensation dichotomy highlights that in the former type of ataxia the control of motor output is primarily affected, whereas the latter type is a consequence of lacking or misleading sensory information. The two forms of ataxia may coexist. Whether vestibular disorders should be included or not is a matter of convention: in this chapter, they will be.

Things are not as simple as that. The cerebellum requires good sensory information. The sensory flow requires good cerebellar performance.

The cerebellum performs on-line tracking of a welter of visual, vestibular, and somatosensory information, and creates complex spatial–temporal patterns of muscle recruitment ("synergisms") in response to both voluntary commands and external perturbations. In fact these patterns must include both the chaining of the so-called "focal" muscles, i.e., those acting on the body segments one is thinking of, and the "postural" muscles, i.e., the muscles (usually very many) acting on other, often very remote segments in order to stabilize the uninvolved motor segments and/or the center of mass of the body with respect to the base of support [4]. The distinction between focal and postural movements dates back to the nineteenth century and can be accredited to Joseph Babinski who highlighted that leaning backwards with the trunk whilst standing requires the

Multiple Sclerosis: Recovery of Function and Neurorehabilitation, eds. J. Kesselring, G. Comi, and A. J. Thompson.
Published by Cambridge University Press. © Cambridge University Press 2010.

previous flexion of the knees, otherwise the center of mass (CM) will go beyond the base of support and the subject will fall, which is often the case after cerebellar damage [5].

The cerebellum is also involved in learning, based on previous experience, either voluntary or involuntary movements. This holds for both slow movements as well as fast "ballistic" movements that can only rely upon previous experience and predictions. In the former case, sensory feedback helps to guide the movement on-line. In the latter case, memory of previous movements helps the prediction of the best muscle output, while an updated "sensory" upgrade provides the initial body coordinates (mass distribution and position of all body segments) before the movement is "launched."

"Reflex" actions in response to perturbations may also improve with practice. Both the selection of a given response and its time-course must be adapted to: (a) the environmental context and (b) the expectations. Box 23.1 gives a classic example taken from the literature.

Box 23.1 Anticipatory postural actions: the dark side of will

"Rising on tiptoes" in free stance is mostly based on the work done by the plantar–flexor muscles. Yet the anterior leg muscles must be activated first, thus pulling the body forwards to counteract the tendency towards a backward push implied by the relative motion of the leg with respect to the foot, were the latter kept flat on the ground. If one stands with one's back leaning against a wall, however, the early activation of the anterior leg muscles must be suppressed.

During free stance on a wide surface, a forward push from the back will evoke a stretch reflex by the plantar–flexors (which, in this case, "pull" the lower limb backwards with respect to the feet), nearly synchronous with the contraction of a chain of extensor muscles, such as the hamstrings, the glutei, etc. (the so-called ankle strategy). If the feet are on a thin support (e.g., the edge of a pool) the stretch reflex is suppressed and the reaction will initiate with knee and hip flexion, the leg muscles staying relaxed. The center of mass will be lowered, thus undergoing a shorter oscillation forward, while plantar flexion is avoided (the so-called hip strategy). This strategy prevents the subject from slipping and falling into the water.

Sensory feedback is not a passive picture of the external stimuli. The main sources of information needed for motor control come through the visual, the vestibular, and the kinesthetic (somatosensory) systems. Each of the three systems may be more or less informative depending on the contexts, so that full efficiency of all of them is not required in most instances. Cerebellar learning is involved in "weighting" the type of sensory information, thus privileging the most relevant in any given context [6], and in scaling the motor responses accordingly [7]. For instance, in a subject standing blindfolded just touching the ground with a walking stick may improve stability. This is more evident in the elderly than in the young, perhaps due to lower efficiency of the proprioceptive channel caused by subclinical neuropathies [8]. Sometimes the different systems convey conflicting information. Seasickness in the cabin of a rolling ship arises, perhaps as an alarm signal, from a conflict between the visual system signaling stability and the vestibular system signaling oscillations. The cerebellum is engaged in the process of sensory weighting [9]. Recently, it has been revealed to participate in cognitive performances such as motor learning of either conscious or reflex movements [10, 11].

Specificity of ataxia in MS patients

Demyelinating lesions can be found in any of the aforementioned central circuits, and they may also affect the vestibular nerve, which is provided with central-type myelin in its proximal segment. Persons with MS can also suffer from weakness and/or spasticity, adding to their overall disability. For this reason, the prescription of exercise is a major challenge, given the need for it to be tailored accurately to the individual patient.

Most traditional exercise approaches focus on drawing attention to voluntary movements and/or smoothing the distal oscillations through inertial (e.g., by applying heavy armbands or by adopting heavy tools for writing or eating) or viscous reactions [12]. None of these approaches is satisfactory, however, given that they may only provide a mild adaptive, not intrinsic, functional recovery in a very limited set of activities.

A basic conceptual framework for rehabilitation of ataxia

It must be emphasized that sensation and movement are inextricably linked, and that sensory–motor integration is almost entirely unconscious. The therapeutic approach should be based on three milestones:

(1) diagnosing the functional sensorimotor alterations affecting each patient;
(2) prescribing an individual set of exercises based on the diagnosis and according to decision-tree rules;
(3) privileging "implicit" learning.

Diagnosis: sensory–motor disturbances underlie dysmetria and/or imbalance

Patients with ataxia usually complain of balance deficits and/or intentional tremor and dysmetria, which impair mostly manual activities. Upper limb dysmetria is the topic of a number of studies investigating the neural–mechanical characteristics of reaching trajectories [13]. Unfortunately, evidence for effective treatments is still scarce, if not entirely lacking [14]. This conclusion should be attenuated by considering that the detection of functional recovery is hindered by the poor metric quality of the available scales [15]. In the author's experience, distal tremor and dysmetria, reflecting a disorder in spatio-temporal muscular recruitment, are but signs of a more general loss of coordination rooted in a disorder of the postural, unconscious control of movement (see below). From the clinical standpoint, impaired balance is often found without concurrent evidence of tremor or dysmetria, whereas the opposite is not true. This is not to say that dysmetria is rare. This symptom may appear mild or absent because of the low forces involved in conventional clinical testing. Traditionally this focuses on displacements of distal segments (e.g., the finger-to-nose and heel-to-knee tests). Instability of the maximal isometric force output, for which the term dystenia is proposed here, appears to be a more sensitive test. Very often dystenia affects trunk and girdle muscles. These undergo moderate shortening while sustaining heavy forces because they are acting against long lever arms amplifying the displacements and de-amplifying the forces (this is the case for the humeral and the femoral rotators). For instance, if the examiner resists arm flexion, oscillations of the force provided by the scapular muscles may pass undetected, yet they cause an appreciable "tremor" of the hands (actually, revealing whole-arm rotations). If the patient is supine with hip and knee flexed, and extension is resisted at the foot, oscillations of the force provided by muscles acting on hip rotations will cause the leg to visibly oscillate in the right–left direction (the author's "wobbly hip" sign [16]). Scapular and pelvic muscles are fundamental for postural control and walking, so this kind of test provides more functional information compared to conventional tests. Also, they confirm that the alteration of postural control may subtend both loss of balance and dysmetria and some form of tremor, by causing proximal dystenia.

A unified view of dysmetria and loss of balance as a single postural disorder

Most human actions require the chaining of several muscles linking the body segments to provide countless degrees of freedom and even extraordinarily precise movements. The issue of the control of "multi-joint" movements, both in voluntary and involuntary actions, is a continuous challenge for scientists [17].

Voluntary movements
Will and consciousness

Ataxia is a disorder of voluntary movement. In recent years a new vision of "will," as far as movements are concerned, has emerged. There is converging evidence from clinical, biomechanical, neurophysiological, and imaging studies, that:

(a) some brain activity time-locked with the voluntary movement anticipates consciousness of the will itself [18]. When a person is able to state "I want to move" his/her brain has already been at work for at least 100 ms;
(b) unconscious movements, allowing within-body and body–ground stabilization, are time-locked (and again in advance) with respect to the "willed" movement [19]. In other words, "willed movement" is not synonymous with "conscious movement." To avoid confusion, a small glossary can be proposed linking the psychological and the mechanical viewpoints of the voluntary

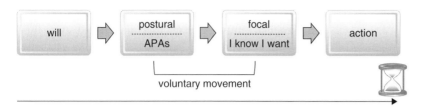

Fig. 23.1. The sequence of events subtending an intended action, from "will" to action. The timescale is arbitrary, but each arrow may represent an interval in the order of 30 to 300 ms, reflecting both neural processing and mechanical delays.

movement. At a psychological level, one should speak of conscious and unconscious action components, both contributing to the intended action. At a mechanical level, the conscious component translates into a "focal-intended" movement, while the unconscious component translates into the so-called "anticipatory postural actions" (APAs) [19]. The neural hardware and software provides the machine allowing translation of the intangible "will" into a tangible "action." The temporal sequence of events underlying this translation is shown in Fig. 23.1.

Targets of studies on ataxia

The most varied hand-reaching tasks represent perhaps the most popular paradigms for studies on ataxia. In this approach a privileged perspective is the optimization of the "smoothness" of the trajectories. This goal is usually formalized as the minimization of hand-jerking (the first derivative of acceleration) although in actual fact this requires a complex chaining of all of the proximal segments. Given the high performance of the neural machine, it is unsurprising that upper limb movements can be "optimal" according to several criteria simultaneously, in addition to that of smoothness [13, 20].

A less emphasized research target, as far as ataxia is concerned, is the way focal and postural movements interact during intended actions. In cases of lesions of the central nervous system, the planning and performing of the correct APAs may be selectively affected, with respect to the planning and performing of the focal component of a movement [21]. In rhythmic movements of the hands and feet, respecting the sequence of recruitment of muscles foreseen by the APAs may make hand–foot coupling easier (i.e., faster and less fatiguing), or else [22] very much more difficult. When overt APAs are not detectable, subliminal excitation of the proper motoneurons (wherever they may be) occurs nonetheless [23]. The rules of recruitment of muscles within a

given postural chain are not yet fully understood, but it is reasonable to assume that they comply with the need to stabilize body segments with respect to each other, and the CM of the body with respect to the ground. An empirical rule to predict the muscles participating in the postural chaining has been proposed by the author as the "fan rule" [24]. In Fig. 23.2 it can be seen that the action of "lifting a bag" by abducting one's arm triggers the recruitment of a chain of muscles along the same plane (in this case frontal). This linking of muscles (a) prevents the proximal segments (the homolateral scapula first) from moving towards the arm, and (b) ultimately provides a compact mass allowing the proper inertial reactions against the forces generating the focal movement. If the ground provides the proper resistance (i.e., it is sufficiently hard and rough), the chain can be interrupted at the level of the contralateral foot. The length and the timing of the chain may be highly variable, yet in accordance with the mechanical needs imposed by the weight of the object lifted, the acceleration of the movement, and the mass distribution of the chained segments. The sketch in Fig. 23.2 should clarify that weakness of any relevant "link" of the chain may ultimately lead to apparent weakness and dysmetria of the "focal" movement, to which hypermetric corrections may follow. The same holds true for inappropriate timing across muscles leading to fractioning of the stabilizing mass. If wrong linking entails an excessive displacement of the body's CM, the balance of the body as a whole may be seriously challenged.

For this reason, during the neuromotor examination of an ataxic patient the clinician should give importance, once again, to tests of isometric force. While one of the examiner's hands provides resistance, the other should palpate distant "postural" muscles. In the case depicted in Fig. 23.2, for instance, the examiner may resist maximal voluntary arm abduction while palpating the contralateral trapezius. The faster and greater the subject's effort, the earlier and stronger the contraction of the trapezius and

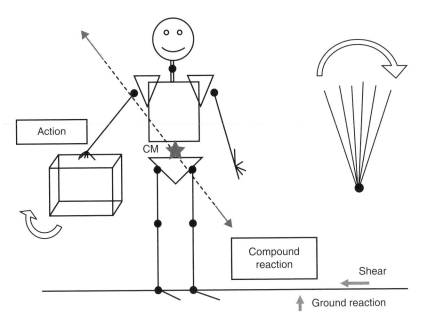

Fig. 23.2. The "fan rule." Within an intended action (lifting a weight on a frontal plane) the focal movement is associated with anticipatory postural actions (APAs), entailing the unconscious recruitment of several "chained" muscles. This provides the necessary reaction to "focal" forces either by adding up the mass of the chained segments or ultimately by stabilizing the body system (i.e., its center of mass, CM) against the ground. The length and timing of the chain can vary, depending on the mechanical needs; however, the active muscles must be located along the plane of action, which can be imagined as an opening fan (see the right sketch). The "fan" may be open in any plane, depending on the plane of action. (From Tesio 2009 [24], modified; reprinted with permission.)

other postural muscles should be. Incidentally, in the case of weakness, the lack of postural fixation may indicate decreased or missing voluntary effort. For instance, this may be the case for central fatigue, conversion disorders, or malingering [25].

Once a deficit in either the timing or the strength of the APAs has been detected, an attempt can be made to diagnose its sensory and/or motor origin. Conventional neurological examination may reveal sensory deficits. These are a source of ineffective "sensory upgrade." On-line knowledge of the mechanical context (including joint positions and forces) is a requisite for the correct programming of ballistic movements. The sensory deficit may not necessarily affect the segments engaged in the focal movement. For instance, again referring to Fig. 23.2, it can be forecasted that decreased sensation in the lower limbs leads to a less precise estimation of the forces and the joint rotations subtending the action. In clinical testing, weakness and dysmetria may appear at any level along the chain (e.g., arm, head, shoulder) whenever the lower limb is involved in the corresponding APAs. If the postural alteration is not associated with sensory deficits, it may stem from a primitive disorder of motor programming. This is often the case in cerebellar lesions. Usually, in this case, all movements are affected, including speech, swallowing, and eye movements. Cerebellar lesions may lead to

distinct motor impairments (e.g., truncal instability in case of vermian lesions, and distal dysmetria and dysarthria in case of hemispheric lesions). This seems not to be the rule in MS patients, given that demyelination may simultaneously affect various cerebellar structures. In the author's experience, the high prevalence and/or severity of balance disorders in MS patients stems from the frequent coexistence of lesions scattered within the cerebellum, the brainstem, and the spinal sensory pathways.

Involuntary movements

Muscle chaining is required also in most responses to external perturbations. Again, there is evidence that normal responses consist in preset patterns of recruitment which require sensory updating and can be foreseen in the light of optimization of balance. Not surprisingly, normal patterns may be disrupted in ataxia and other neural disorders [4, 8, 26].

Decomposing the sensory–motor disturbance

In MS patients impaired balance is often seen without concurrent dysmetria, the most frequent cause being a sensory deficit and/or a deficit of sensory–motor integration. It is now acknowledged that the three

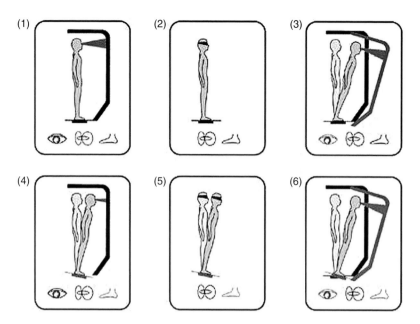

Fig. 23.3. The six conditions of testing standing balance, according to the Sensory Organization Test (SOT) on the EquiTest™ force platform. It is assumed that three sensory streams are critical for balance in quiet stance. These are provided by three functional systems: eyes–vision, vestibulum–head orientation, and kinesthesia–ankle motion (see the corresponding symbols below the outline of the human form). The subject stands quietly for 20 s on a force plate recording the oscillations of the center of pressure (CP), either with eyes open or blindfolded. The visual surround and/or the support surface can be made to tilt "tuned" with the spontaneous oscillations of the subject. "Tuning" makes one or two of the corresponding sensory system (vision in condition 3, kinesthesia in conditions 4 and 5, both of them in condition 6) unreliable: they signal stability, whereas the body is actually oscillating. The remaining reliable systems must be able to compensate for the sensory loss, and must be properly "up-weighted". A frequent problem is vision remaining the dominant system when it is actually misleading (visual "preference"). (After http://www.onbalance.com; reproduced with permission, courtesy of Neurocom Inc., Clackamas, OR, USA.)

main sensory systems contributing to balance are, in order of decreasing clinical relevance, the somatosensory, the vestibular, and the visual systems. Actually, vision seems to be the most sensitive to whole body inclinations, but the other two systems have much faster responses and, most importantly, are more directly nested within the circuitries of postural control. Blind people do not fall, ataxic people do. The EquiTest™ designed by L. Nashner [27] perhaps provides the best diagnostics of the performances of the above sensory systems. Figure 23.3 shows the basic principles of the test. The subject stands with each foot on a force platform, which provides the displacement of the body center of pressure (CP). The basic idea underlying this ingenious device is creating a conflict between the three controlling systems.

Vision can be removed through blindfolding, and either vision or (ankle) kinesthesia, or both, can be neutralized through the "tuning" of the visual surround or of the support surface with the subject's spontaneous oscillations. One or two systems always remain reliable but three requirements must be met for a successful performance: (a) the reliable systems must be "healthy" enough to compensate for the missing information; (b) they must undergo a proper "re-weighting"; and (c) the misleading information must be detected and suppressed. The latter point deserves special attention. Condition 6 (kinesthesia and vision unreliable) is more difficult than condition 5 (kinesthesia unreliable and vision removed), due to the so-called "visual preference." The process of re-weighting and/or suppression across sensory systems is still the object of intense biomedical research: yet it is certain that it requires the integrity of brain areas where sensory flows converge. In the author's experience, imbalance or a feeling of "unsteadiness" due to an excess of "visual preference" is very frequent in MS patients. This may reflect the scatter of lesions across the somatosensory and the vestibular circuits. However, the fact that instability and visual preference are often associated in patients with an otherwise low burden of disease and disability may reflect significant, though minimal, demyelination within "multisensory" areas of the cerebellum and brainstem [28].

Designing rational treatments: some examples

Postural training in ataxia: basic principles

How can proper postural chaining be restored? The onset delays between the contractions of the muscles involved are in the order of 10–100 ms. Furthermore, within any given voluntary movement the postural chains may involve tenths of muscles and must continuously adapt to even the smallest changes in the features of the focal movement itself, in the arrangement of body segments, or in the environmental context. For this reason, explicit/declarative teaching is both inappropriate and doomed to failure [29]. During motor learning, help can come from some feedback on the success or failure of the action. However, if problems arise from faulty APAs, feedback on the hidden postural performance should be provided [30]. Take the example of "rising on toes," shown in Fig. 23.4. Due to mechanical reasons (see legend of Fig. 23.5) a fast sequence of recruitment of focal and postural muscles is necessary for a successful completion of the task. Ataxic patients may "rise on toes" indeed. However, they are unable to produce the proper APAs, and tend to lean their trunk precariously forward until passive elevation of the heels occurs. Implicit learning [31] becomes possible, if knowledge of the delay between the onset of contraction of a key focal and a key postural muscle is offered to the patient while the action is attempted. Figure 23.4 illustrates an application of the "dynamic electromyogram (EMG) biofeedback" proposed by the author [32].

Figure 23.5 gives the EMG tracings recorded during the "rise on toes" action, and made to generate an acoustic feedback. A tone from each of two muscles is sent to each ear. The high temporal acuity of human hearing [33] makes it very easy to identify the recruitment order. Awareness of even a handful of successful actions is a reward triggering motor learning and priming long-term retention [34]. Learning from motor errors requires intervals, across subsequent trials, of between 4 and 10 seconds to allow for optimal consolidation [35]. In case of ataxia, three to eight half-hour sessions per week are advisable, and an improvement should be detected within ten sessions. This form of EMG biofeedback may help either to diagnose or to treat difficulties in focal–postural timing in any other

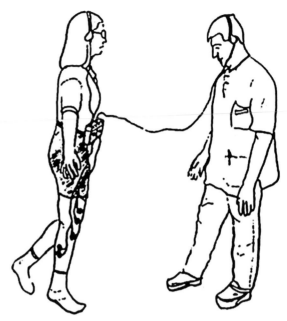

Fig. 23.4. The "dynamic electromyogram biofeedback" for postural training: task of "rising on toes". Information about the timing of recruitment of two muscles involved in the same action (here, gastrocnemius lateralis – focal, and vastus lateralis – postural) is obtained during exercise. The surface electromyogram (EMG) signal from each muscle is captured and transformed into a tone sent to one ear. Through dichotic listening, the onset time of both muscles can be easily recognized. A couple of stereo earphones allow the patient (right) and the therapist (left) to share the information. (From Tesio *et al.* [31], modified. Reprinted with permission.)

action. The key point is identifying the proper focal muscle and one representative postural muscle: the optimal pair can be identified with the help of the "fan rule" depicted in Fig. 23.2.

Rationale for "postural" exercises

One should ask whether the improvement in the APAs, if any, could be transferable to other movements beyond the trained one, and to patients with postural disturbances caused by different lesions. It has been known for decades that for any motor skills:

- some transfer to other movements occurs
- it is unavoidable
- it never reaches 100%
- it may differ very much across movement types and training contexts
- it is long-lasting [35, 36, 37].

The underlying neural mechanisms are being increasingly elucidated. For instance, in one-handed tasks a

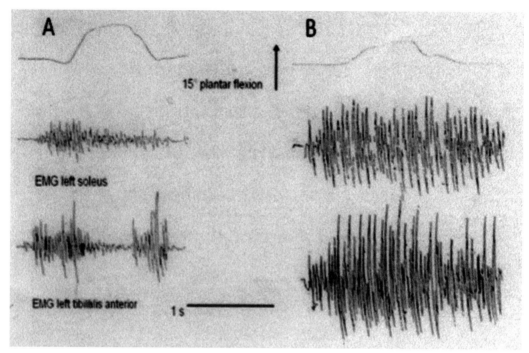

Fig. 23.5. The action of "rising on toes on the left foot" requires (among others) the soleus as a focal muscle, and the tibialis anterior. In this case, the latter is not working as an antagonist but as a postural agonist instead. Panel A shows, from top to bottom, the sagittal rotation of the ankle and the surface EMG recorded from the soleus and the tibialis anterior, respectively. The latter muscle is activated in advance, with respect to the "focal" muscle, thus realizing an APA. This APA allows the leg and the body system to start leaning forward, thus providing the proper inertial reaction to the backward pull of the leg exerted by the "focal" muscles, including the soleus. The net result of the plantar flexion thus becomes the body lift. Panel B refers to an ataxic patient unable to provide the correct sequence of muscle recruitment: both the "focal" and the "postural" muscles are co-activated synchronously. "Rise on toes" is transformed into a heel-rise action following the forward leaning of the trunk, entailing the risk of falling (personal results).

substantial disinhibition of the "untrained" hemisphere from the (usually inhibiting) "trained" hemisphere has been proven for skill transfer between hands [37]. What about the specific family of "postural" skills? There is now growing evidence that transfer of motor learning is higher the more the requested task can rely upon hard-wired sets of high-order neurons. Some of these sets are inherited through the genetic evolution of the control of general aspects of movements: e.g., plane of action, synergisms between focal and postural muscles [38], synergisms across muscles engaged in reactions to various perturbations [26, 39]. It can be speculated that postural adaptations during standing and locomotion were privileged during the evolution of vertebrates. Neuroplasticity when novel voluntary actions are required would thus imply the re-weighting of synaptic efficiency across a limited number of preset control circuits, rather than building from

scratch every time, for every action, countless ad hoc circuitries each encasing countless neurons. There is some evidence that implicit learning can persist indeed, given the lower requirements for attention (an often impaired function in MS patients) and declarative memory, and – presumably – its diffused brain representation. For sure, implicit learning remains possible in most stroke and cerebellar syndromes [39, 40, 41]. The teaching paradigm proposed here is also tailored to the needs of MS patients commonly encountered in rehabilitation settings, who present with some degree of cognitive impairment preventing attention and memory consolidation. There is evidence that when unconscious performances such as APAs or overall balance during gait have to be trained, avoiding explicit instructions and allowing the patient to fail repeatedly is the optimal procedure to foster implicit learning [41].

The individual training program: the need for a decision tree prescription

Rehabilitation exercise is mainly based on the teaching–training relationship between therapist and patient. This entails relevant differences between the rehabilitative and the conventional biomedical research paradigms [42]. Specificities of the paradigm are summarized in Box 23.2.

The proposal of multiple treatments following a decision tree (often referred to as "triage" in clinical jargon) rather than of single treatments is not common in biomedical research. The randomized double trial to "groups" was overemphasized by the growth of biological and pharmaceutical research, which is mostly looking for effectiveness on "mean" individuals, independently from the therapist. What follows is a summary of the decision tree applied in the author's unit of rehabilitation in the case of patients with balance deficits, which include the majority of MS patients. A paper is in preparation providing operational details.

Main branches of a decision tree for exercise prescription in MS ataxia: the case for balance

Before any prescription of a balance exercise program can be made, there has to be a four-step functional diagnosis (see below), corresponding to four classes of impairment of motor control. This is only a basic proposal. Other programs may be suitable as well.

(1) The capacity to overcome visual preference in selecting motor strategies is tested. This can be performed on an EquiTest™ platform or by means

---

Box 23.2 Research in rehabilitation: a paradigm spanning from biology to behavior

The identification of "whole-person" variables, the quasi-experimental designs, and the selection of proper statistics are the three pillars of the specificity of rehabilitation research. These are summarized under the following points (1), (2), and (3), respectively.

(1) The goals of the therapeutic effort are behavioral in essence, such as independence, fatigue, risk of falling, and the like. Such "latent" personal traits cannot be extrapolated from conventional physical–chemical measurements (e.g., latencies in somatosensory evoked potentials, muscle strength, etc.): outcome measurement must rely on questionnaires, which are often far from able to provide true linear measures, unless dedicated statistical modeling is applied [43]. Only recently has the neurological community acknowledged the need for research specifically addressing the construction of questionnaires based on modern "item–response" theory [44].

(2) The trial designs must take into account that randomization and blindness are often impossible and, whenever this gold standard can be approximated, it may not correspond to real treatment conditions. In a learning–teaching paradigm the "subjective" patient–therapist interactions cannot be taken as a source of bias: rather, they are an intended component of the prescription (the right therapist for the right patient) and one of the determinants of success or failure. Also, the treatment necessarily includes many "ingredients" some of them explicit and known (e.g., cooling a spastic muscle before exercise) and some others implicit and unknown (e.g., the patient's motivation and mental fatigue, the therapist's skills in any given procedure, etc.). This entails the need to validate treatment programs as a whole, according to the logic of decision trees [45]: each patient may receive a distinct program, yet according to reproducible rules.

(3) Statistics should be adapted to this context. First, the struggle for "significance" is not always justified. The "$p < 0.05$" (or less) dogma was developed to minimize the risk of false-positive results. Unavoidably, this weakens the capacity for accepting true-positive results (the statistical "power"). Yet a high power is advisable when pilot studies on small samples aim at testing original hypotheses, and the risk of side effects is minimal, as for most exercise treatments. Also, the prescription of sets of treatments implies following decision "nodes" which, in statistical language, represent interactions (if/then conditions) across critical levels of two or more variables. If the various ingredients are managed as independent variables through conventional regression models, the "main effects" (the impact of an independent variable, "all other staying the same") can be detected or denied (on the basis of statistical significance) much more easily than their many potential interactions, which are difficult to be even foreseen. Dedicated statistics such as the CART (Classification and Regression Tree model) or similar techniques may help in identifying the interactions (the "combinations" of outcome measures and/or of treatments) allowing functional grouping of the patients, with respect to their susceptibility to a given rehabilitation program [46].

of a less expensive technique, like the "visual dome." First proposed by A. Shumway-Cook [47], this is a simple "Chinese lantern" which encases the patient's head to provide a stable visual field despite the patient's movements. Visual preference should be counteracted by "weaning the patient off" vision, by imposing movements under unreliable visual cues (e.g., walking whilst wearing the "lantern").

(2) The overall responsiveness of the vestibular reactions should be tested. Here the term "vestibular" is used to mean not only the transduction of head accelerations at the inner ear but, also, the functioning of vestibular–spinal circuits. Perhaps the simplest test is to ask patients to stand on a tilting platform, to observe the speed, strength, and symmetry of their ankle muscles (the so-called "tendon dance" of olden-day neurology). Exercises will aim at stimulating brisk vestibular responses, e.g., by making subjects stand and move on a tilting table.

(3) Motor strategies should be observed with care. In general, the more subjects tend to use their upper limbs to retain balance (parachute reactions) the more ineffective their reactions will be: arm waving is of little help in displacing the CM. Also, ankle and hip strategies should be selected properly: in close vicinity to fall limits, and well within the fall limits, respectively. Exercises will be focused on asking for various performances while the unwanted strategies are prevented or hindered (the simplest example being binding the upper limbs to the trunk).

(4) Last, the capacity of the postural muscles is linked into the proper sequence and timing should be tested. This can be easily done with the biofeedback device shown in Fig. 23.4 but, also, by careful palpation of a pair of muscles, e.g., a "focal" and a remote "postural" one. Exercises will aim at improving postural chaining, according to the description given above.

Of course, other impairments may well contribute to balance deficits, e.g., deficits in joint mobility, weakness of key muscles due to diseases other than MS, central fatigue, apraxia, and so forth.

From a more general standpoint, within each class the exercises can be grouped into three families:

(a) Exercises aiming to stimulate a weakened mechanism of motor control by increasing the functional demands (e.g., tilting exercises for deficits in vestibular response, walking on soft surfaces and the like, asking for better timing across focal and postural muscles in complex tasks, etc.).

(b) Exercises aiming to develop adaptation through protective mechanisms (e.g., walking with a cane or under careful visual guidance).

(c) Exercises aiming at the first goal, whilst preventing an excessive shift towards adaptation mechanisms (e.g., walking whilst wearing a "conflict dome," thus counteracting the patient's visual preference). This approach is by far the most promising.

A wide variety of exercises may be invented and proposed, provided they are consistent with the foregoing diagnostic frame. The key point here remains that each of the four classes of impairments should be linked to a family of exercises, each including a potentially infinite series of tasks. Thus, the therapist is left a lot of leeway in the selection of individual exercise procedures, their sequence, and their dosage.

Outcome measurement

Balance and coordination are whole-person performances, i.e., what it is now called "activity" in the WHO model of disability [48]. Activities can only be tested by measuring task-level variables and/or behaviors and/or subjective perceptions. The current most common scales for outcome measurement in ataxia are deemed to be unsatisfactory [15]. What follows is the measurement approach in the author's rehabilitation unit. The various tests described below share the focus on balance, and therefore correlate moderately (Spearman ρ around 0.6, unpublished results): in fact, they investigate the "balance" phenomenon from distinct standpoints, so that they are not redundant and make up an integrated battery.

Task level

The capacity to control balance while relying on kinesthetic, vestibular or visual information is investigated through the EquiTest™ battery of "dynamic" (i.e., on a moving platform) posturography, which is called the Sensory Organization Test (SOT) (see Fig. 23.3) and the related tests based on fast slipping and rotations of the platform (known as the Motor Control and the Adaptation test, respectively) [27].

The battery implemented in the Balance Master™ force platform [49] test is adopted for posturography

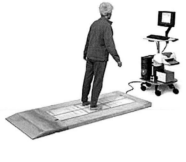

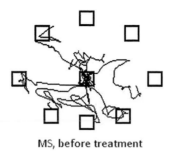

MS, before treatment

Fig. 23.6. The "limits of stability" test on the BalanceMaster™ platform. The subject is requested to "reach" visual targets on a PC screen, by leaning on a force plate recording the approximate displacement of the body's CM. The graphic display is given in the three "spidernet" drawings referring to a normal adult (bottom left), an MS patient suffering from imbalance before and after a series of exercise sessions (top right and bottom right, respectively). (The picture is reproduced with permission from http://www.onbalance.com. The graphs give personal results.)

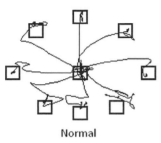

Normal

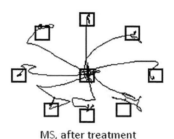

MS, after treatment

on a static force platform. Conventional static posturography explores the stability of the center of pressure (CP), taken as a proxy of the CM, on a force platform. Tests on a firm surface both with eyes open and closed are of limited sensitivity so that tests based on voluntary oscillations are preferred. Figure 23.6 provides a sample of the "limits of stability" test within the BalanceMaster™ battery. The displacements of the CP are filtered in order to approximate the actual displacements of the CM. The subject stands on a firm force platform. At a "go" signal he/she is requested to lean as far as possible in various directions. The subject's CM and the targets are represented on a PC screen. Actually, reaching the target requires that the body CM be moved rather close to the limits of falling. The path of the CM is analyzed quantitatively (length, precision of targeting, etc.). Although qualitative, the graphs given in Fig. 23.6 give perhaps the most impressive idea of the potential effectiveness of the treatment approach.

Behavioral level

The EquiScale questionnaire is adopted [50]. Scores are assigned to eight simple tasks (e.g., leaning forward, resisting nudges on the sternum, pivoting around either lower limb, etc.). The EquiScale is an adaptation for MS patients of the popular Berg balance scale, which was originally conceived for geriatric patients. The new questionnaire was refined in order to match the MS impairments, and it was validated through Rasch analysis, perhaps the most valid statistical model complying with the contemporary item–response theory [43].

Subjective perception level

The Dizziness Handicap Inventory–short form (DHIsf) is adopted [51]. The subject assigns scores to 13 items investigating the impact of balance deficits in daily life. Sample questions include: "Do quick movements of your head increase your problem?" and "Because of your problem do you avoid heights?" The questionnaire derives from a longer form proposed for patients with dizziness, and it too was refined and validated through Rasch analysis. This test is useful in stratifing chronic patients with respect to their disability. This kind of outcome can only be appreciated from a long-term perspective.

Ataxia: also a cognitive and metabolic impairment

There is growing evidence that motor incoordination, the hallmark of ataxia, may contribute to other impairments up to now considered as entirely distinct. A demonstration is available for cognitive impairments. In patients suffering from remitting–relapsing MS, a significant association was found between cognitive deficits and cerebellar lesions [52]. Fatigue, also, may be ataxia-related. Its organic substrate in MS remains unknown [53]. Ataxia entails "inefficiency" of the neural program that translates the motor intention into the proper pattern of muscle contractions (see Fig. 23.1). A sense of fatigue might reflect the increased attentive "cost" required whenever a muscle is recruited in conflict with postural needs [22, 54], which is often the case for ataxia [55]. Recently a metabolic not just an attentive cost was demonstrated for "postural effort" [56]. Healthy subjects standing on a force platform were asked to perform voluntary rhythmic adduction/abduction movements of the upper limbs held horizontal. This action entailed a more than twofold metabolic cost when performed isodirectionally (i.e., both arms rotating clockwise or anticlockwise) rather than antidirectionally (i.e., in mirror pattern toward the midline of the trunk). Unlike mirror movements, isodirectional movements generate a rotator torque along the vertical axis of the body, needing a postural chain spreading caudally down to the ground. The energetic cost of ataxia may be difficult to demonstrate in daily activities, mostly relying upon short-lasting anaerobic actions, yet it may well be a determinant of the fatigue symptom. This may make rehabilitation of ataxia indirectly effective on fatigue, too.

The need for specific clinical trials

The poor evidence of the effectiveness of any specific exercise approach has been already mentioned [3]. The approach proposed here is evidence-based in its diagnostic components (see the SOT and Balance Master measures, the questionnaire scores, etc.). The same holds for most of the old-established exercise procedures. Yet, there is a paucity of specific trials on decision trees as a whole. Methodological difficulties are relevant in the whole field of rehabilitation, as described in Box 23.2 above. Research in MS patients is complicated by the interaction between disability and an unstable disease. Therefore, clinical trials in the field of rehabilitation should be considered a priority.

Conclusions

Whole-body balance and precision in intended actions can now be investigated from a unified sensory–motor perspective, based on evidence from a growing body of physiological research. Rational hypotheses of exercise treatments may now be generated. Outcome studies, however challenging they can be, should be fostered in order to validate and refine the already available, rational exercise protocols.

Acknowledgments

This work was supported by:

F.I.S.M. Italian Foundation for Multiple Sclerosis, Grant cod. 2005/R/20

F.I.R.S.T project 2007, Università degli Studi di Milano

Italian Ministry of Health, ricerca finalizzata 2006

Italian Ministry of Health, ricerca finalizzata 2008

References

1. Kesselring J. Long-term management and rehabilitation in multiple sclerosis. In: Siva A, ed. *Frontiers in Multiple Sclerosis*. London: Martin Dunitz, 1999:243–252

2. Bastian A J. Mechanisms of ataxia. *Phys Ther* 1997;**77**:672–5

3. Deuschl G, Bain P, Brin M. Consensus statement of the Movement Disorder Society on Tremor Ad Hoc Scientific Committee. *Mov Disord* 1998;**13**(Suppl 3):2–23

4. Cordo P J, Nashner L M. Properties of postural adjustments associated with rapid arm movements. *J Neurophysiol* 1982;**47**:287–302

5. Babinski J. De l'asynergie cérébelleuse. *Rév Neurol* 1899;**7**:806–16

6. Bastian A J. Learning to predict the future: the cerebellum adapts feedforward movement control. *Curr Opin Neurobiol* 2006;**16**:645–9

7. Oie K S, Kiemel T, Jeka J J. Multisensory fusion: simultaneous re-weighting of vision and touch for the control of human posture. *Brain Res Cogn Brain Res* 2002;**14**:164–76

8. Baccini M, Rinaldi L A, Federighi G, *et al*. Effectiveness of fingertip light contact in reducing postural sway in older people. *Age Ageing* 2007;**36**:30–5

9. Bakker M, Allum J H, Visser J E, *et al*. Postural responses to multidirectional stance perturbations in cerebellar ataxia. *Exp Neurol* 2006;**202**:21–35

10. Parsons L M, Bower J M, Gao J H, *et al*. Lateral cerebellar hemispheres actively support sensory

acquisition and discrimination rather than motor control. *Learn Mem* 1997;**4**:49–62

11. Katz D B, Steinmetz J E. Psychological functions of the cerebellum. *Behav Cogn Neurosci Rev* 2002;**1**:229–41

12. Michaelis J. Mechanical methods of controlling ataxia. *Baillière's Clin Neurol* 1993;**2**:121–39

13. Casadio M, Sanguineti V, Morasso P, Solaro C. Abnormal sensorimotor control, but intact forcefield adaptation, in multiple sclerosis subjects with no clinical disability. *Mult Scler* 2008;**14**:330–42

14. Mills R J, Yap L, Young C A Treatment for ataxia in multiple sclerosis. *Cochrane Database Syst Rev* 2007; CD005029

15. Riazi A, Cano S J, Cooper J M, *et al.* Coordinating outcomes measurement in ataxia research: do some widely used generic rating scales tick the boxes? *Mov Disord* 2006;**21**,9:1396–1403

16. Tesio L. The wobbly hip: a sign of proximal ataxia and risk of falling. *Eur Medicophys* 2001;**37**:197

17. Gielen S. Review of models for the generation of multi-joint movements in 3-D. *Adv Exp Med Biol* 2009;**629**:523–50

18. Hallett M. Volitional control of movement: the physiology of free will. *Clin Neurophysiol* 2007;**118**:1179–92

19. Baldissera F, Rota V, Esposti R. Anticipatory postural adjustments in arm muscles associated with movements of the contralateral limb and their possible role in interlimb coordination. *Exp Brain Res* 2008;**185**:63–74

20. Hogan N, Bizzi E, Mussa-Ivaldi F A, Flash T. Controlling multijoint motor behaviour. *Exerc Sports Sci Rev* 1987;**15**:153–90

21. King L A, Horak F B. Lateral stepping for postural correction in Parkinson's disease. *Arch Phys Med Rehab* 2008;**89**:492–9

22. Baldissera F, Borroni P, Cavallari P, Cerri G. Excitability changes in human corticospinal projections to forearm muscles during voluntary movement of ipsilateral foot. *J Physiol* 2002; **539**:903–11

23. Cerri G, Borroni P, Baldissera F. Cyclic H-reflex modulation in resting forearm related to contractions of foot movers, not to foot movement. *J Neurophysiol* 2003;**90**:81–8

24. Tesio L. Biomechanics of the muscular–skeletal system. In: Baldissera F, Porro C A eds. Fisiologia e biofisica medica. 4th ed. Milan: Poletto Editore, 2009:281–308 (In Italian.)

25. Tesio L, Colombo B. "Luxury" recruitment of remote fixator muscles: a sign of organic weakness. (Abstract.) *Mov Disord* 1992:7(Suppl):156

26. Lochart D B, Ting L H. Optimal sensorimotor transformations for balance. *Nat Neurosci* 2007;**10**:1329–36

27. Nashner L M, Peters J F. Dynamic posturography in the diagnosis and management of dizziness and balance disorders. *Neurol Clin* 1990;**8**:331–49

28. Ioffe M E, Chernikova L A, Ustinova K I. Role of cerebellum in learning postural tasks. *Cerebellum* 2007;**6**:87–94

29. Boyd L, Winstein C. Explicit information interferes with implicit motor learning of both continuous and discrete movement tasks after stroke. *J Neurol Phys Ther* 2006;**30**:46–57

30. Schmidt R A. Motor control and learning: a behavioral emphasis. 2nd ed. Champaign, IL: Human Kinetics Publishers, 1988

31. Orrell A J, Eves F F, Masters R S, Macmahon K M. Implicit sequence learning processes after unilateral stroke. *Neuropsychol Rehab* 2007;**17**:335–54

32. Tesio L, Gatti R, Monzani M, Franchignoni FP. EMG-feedback from two muscles in postural reactions: a new pocket device for the patient-therapist pair. *J EMG Kinesiol* 1996;**6**:277–9

33. Green D M. Temporal auditory acuity. *Psychol Rev* 1971;**78**:540–51

34. Krakauer J W, Shadmehr R. Consolidation of motor memory. *Trends Neurosci* 2006;**29**:58–64

35. Huang V S, Shadmehr R. Evolution of motor memory during the seconds after observation of motor error. *J Neurophysiol* 2007;**97**:3976–85

36. Sale DG. Neural adaptation to resistance training. *Med Sci Sports Exerc* 1988;**20**(5 Suppl):S135–45

37. Perez M A, Wise S P, Willingham D T, Cohen L G. Neurophysiological mechanisms involved in transfer of procedural knowledge. *J Neurosci* 2007;**31**:1045–53

38. Deliagina T G, Beloozerova I N, Zelenin P V, Orlovsky G N. Spinal and supraspinal postural networks. *Brain Res Rev* 2008;**57**:212–21

39. Morton S M, Bastian A J. Cerebellar contributions to locomotor adaptations during splitbelt treadmill walking. *J Neurosci* 2006;**26**:9107–16

40. Ioffe M E. Brain mechanisms for the formation of new movements during learning: the evolution of classical concepts. *Neurosci Behav Physiol* 2004;**34**:5–18

41. Orrell A J, Eves F F, Masters R S, Macmahon K M. Implicit sequence learning processes after unilateral stroke. *Neuropsychol Rehab* 2007;**17**:335–54

42. Tesio L. Outcome research in rehabilitation: variable construction, trial design and statistical inference. In: Soroker H, Ring H, eds. *Advances in Physical and Rehabilitation Medicine*. Bologna: Monduzzi Editore, 2003:499–505

43. Tesio L. Measuring persons' behaviours and perceptions: Rasch analysis as a tool for rehabilitation research. *J Rehab Med* 2003;35:1–11

44. Hobart J C, Cano S J, Zajicek J P, Thompson A J. Rating scales as outcome measures for clinical trials in neurology: problems, solutions, and recommendations. *Lancet Neurol* 2007;6:1094–105

45. Tesio L. Case-mix classification systems: the specific case for rehabilitation medicine. *Eur Medicophys* 2003;39:201–4

46. D'Alisa S, Miscio G, Baudo S, *et al.* Depression is the main determinants of quality of life in multiple sclerosis: a classification–regression (CART) study. *Disabil Rehab* 2006;28:307–14

47. Shumway-Cook A, Horak FB. Assessing the influence of sensory interaction of balance: suggestion from the field. *Phys Ther* 1986;66:1548–50

48. WHO. International classification of functioning, disability and health (ICF). Geneva: WHO, 2001

49. Jbabdi M, Boissy P, Hamel M. Assessing control of postural stability in community-living older adults using performance-based limits of stability. *BMC Geriatr* 2008;8:1–8

50. Tesio L, Franchignoni F P, Battaglia M A, Perucca L. A short measure of balance in multiple sclerosis:

validation through Rasch analysis. *Funct Neurol* 1997;12:255–65

51. Tesio L, Alpini D, Perucca L, Cesarani A. The short-form of the Dizziness Handicap Inventory: construction and validation through Rasch analysis. *Am J Phys Med Rehab* 1999;78:1–10

52. Valentino P, Cerasa A, Chiriaco C, *et al.* Cognitive deficits in multiple sclerosis patients with cerebellar symptoms. *Mult Scler* 2009;15:854–9

53. Leocani L, Colombo B, Comi G. Physiopathology of fatigue in multiple sclerosis. *Neurol Sci* 2008; 29(Suppl 2):S241–3

54. Baldissera F, Rota V, Esposti R. Postural adjustments in arm and leg muscles associated with isodirectional and antidirectional coupling of upper limb movements in the horizontal plane. *Exp Brain Res* 2008; 190:289–305

55. Tesio L, Perucca L, Bellafà A. A model for fatigue generation and exercise prescription in multiple sclerosis patients. *Neurol Sci* 2006;27(suppl 4):S300–3

56. Esposti R, Esposito F, Cè E, Baldissera F. Difference in the metabolic cost of postural actions during iso- and antidirectional coupled oscillations of the upper limbs in the horizontal plane. *Eur J Appl Physiol* 2009;108:93–104

Chapter 24

Sexual problems in multiple sclerosis

Per Olov Lundberg

Sexual dysfunction is a common but underestimated symptom of multiple sclerosis (MS). Sexual problems may occur in the absence of severe disability [1]. In a questionnaire study of 98 MS patients 30 of them reported that they had had sexual difficulties, but only six had revealed this to their physicians [2].

Women

Thus, sexual dysfunction may occur even in early and mild cases of MS. Half of the women in a controlled study of 25 females with MS aged 20–42 and with a low handicap score reported sexual problems. None of them had had any sexual problems before the start of the disease [3]. In this study 25 women with migraine matched for age and parity served as controls. Here sexual problems were few and mild.

Changes in sexual function become very common during the evolution of the disease. In a study of 47 women with advanced MS (median expanded disability status scale [EDSS] 6.5) 60% reported decreased sexual desire, 36% decreased lubrication, and 40% diminished orgasmic capacity during the course of the disease [4, 5]. These figures are all highly significantly ($p < 0.0001$) different from the figures from the 1996 national survey on sexuality and health in the same country (Sweden). In a review [6] of a series of studies from other countries reduced interest was reported by 29–86% of female MS patients, reduced sensation by 43–62%, reduced orgasmic capacity by 24–58%, vaginal dryness by 12–40%, and dyspareunia by 6–40%. For MS typical sensory dysfunction in the genital area was experienced by 62% of the women in the study of Hulter and Lundberg [4]; 77% had weakness of the pelvic floor.

Although most MS patients report a continued diminished sexual desire during the course of the disease, a few patients may experience a temporary increase in desire just during an episode. Thus, what has been called hypersexuality has been described. In one, a case of MS with onset at the age of 12 years, hypersexuality and pansexuality were observed [7].

Sensory disturbances seem to be a very important mechanism behind sexual problems in MS women. Because of severe external dysesthesiae some patients reported that during a certain period they could not bear direct genital or even non-genital skin contact from their partner. The dysesthesiae were of maximum intensity from the beginning of an episode of neurological symptoms, but resolved fairly rapidly as is usual in multiple sclerosis.

Other important symptoms of sexual dysfunction in women with MS are deterioration of orgasmic capacity, intensity, and quality. In most cases the orgasmic sensations are reduced. They become shorter-lasting, less intense, and/or less agreeable. These changes may be temporary. Brainstem lesions seen on magnetic resonance imaging (MRI) seem to be of particular importance for anorgasmia [8]. However, better orgasms have also been noticed. The orgasms may be more easily triggered, longer-lasting, stronger, and more pleasant. Paroxysmal attacks of different types are common in MS. Attacks of pelvic pain is one type of such attacks [9]. In such cases carbamazepine could be tried. Sometimes the patients seek help for chronic deep genital pain, the mechanism of which is unknown.

Men

Most male patients (37–86%) report diminished sexual desire during the course of the disease, according to Ghezzi [6]. Some patients may experience a temporary decrease just during an episode,

---

Multiple Sclerosis: Recovery of Function and Neurorehabilitation, eds. J. Kesselring, G. Comi, and A. J. Thompson. Published by Cambridge University Press. © Cambridge University Press 2010.

in others the problem is continuous. When this phenomenon is transitory and concurrent with an episode of new symptoms the decrease in desire should be considered to be caused by a cerebral MS lesion; however, the localization of such a lesion is not known.

Erectile dysfunction is of course the most notable sexual dysfunction in men with MS [10–15]. Figures given in the literature vary between 34% and 80% (see review by Ghezzi [6]). There are no indications of insufficient arterial inflow to the penis or venous outflow. In men dysesthesiae as described above do not seem to create such severe problems as in women, probably because of the sexual intercourse technique used.

Problems with ejaculation are also frequent; 34–61% have been reported. Since positron emission tomography (PET) studies during sexual activity have shown distinct increased regional blood flow foremost in the ventral tegmental area but not in the hypothalamus or limbic cortex during orgasm/ejaculation in normal men this particular brain area might be a candidate area for ejaculatory control [16]. Another candidate area is the amygdala [17].

Common symptoms in both sexes

The majority of patients with multiple sclerosis at some stage of the disease suffer from the combination of lower urinary tract symptoms with sexual dysfunction. This has of course a negative impact on the quality of life of patients as well as causing concern to caregivers and family [18]. The use of aids such as catheters to manage incontinence also creates problems. Sexual dysfunction in MS male patients correlates strongly with bladder and bowel sphincter dysfunction, but more mildly with motor and sensory dysfunction in the legs [6, 19–22]. Correlation with disability scale, clinical course, or disease duration is poor. Sexual dysfunction in MS women correlates with bladder and bowel dysfunction [3, 4, 6, 23, 24], but more mildly with motor and sensory dysfunction in the legs [4]. Correlation is poor with disability scale, clinical course, and disease duration.

The most common autonomic symptoms in MS are, besides disorders of micturation and impotence, sudomotor and gastrointestinal disturbances and orthostatic intolerance [25]. Sexual dysfunction is also correlated with lesions in the pons as detected

by MRI [22]. All these autonomic dysfunctional symptoms can result in sexual dysfunction during particular types of sexual intercourse.

Other problems related to MS, such as muscle contractions in the lower limbs, and paroxysmal motor and sensory disturbances triggered by sexual intercourse, can indirectly exert a negative effect on the patient's sex life as well as causing social and physical changes. Spasticity is especially problematic during intercourse for MS patients. On the other hand, many have reported a temporary relief of spasticity after an orgasm. Some women even use vibrators regularly to induce orgasms and in such a way treat their spasticity.

Fatigue is a very typical and troublesome symptom for many MS patients. In addition, depression and cognitive impairment cause important problems for a normal sexual life [8].

It may be difficult to decode what kind of sexual dysfunction is caused by the central nervous system lesions and what is caused by other factors. Sexual dysfunction, not particularly well defined, has been correlated with MRI findings of the brainstem and pyramidal abnormalities as well as with total area of lesions on MRI and lesions in the pons [8, 22].

Neurophysiology

Changes in sexual functions in MS patients usually start rather abruptly and correlate in time both with neurological symptoms from the sacral segments and as mentioned with bladder and bowel dysfunction. Neurophysiological studies may give further indications of involvement of those parts of the nervous system controlling pelvic structures. Genital sensory evoked potential (SEP) abnormalities are common in men with MS and sexual dysfunction [26]. One of the causes of sexual dysfunction in men with MS may be genital somatosensory pathway disruption, with sparing of the efferent tracts in some men. Gruenwald *et al.* [27] found a significant correlation between decreased clitoral vibration sensation and orgasmic dysfunction. There was also a correlation between cerebellar deficit and orgasmic dysfunction. Neurophysiological data such as cortical evoked potentials of the dorsal nerve of the clitoris or pudendal nerve [22, 28] as well as measurement of vibratory thresholds in the clitoris [29] imply that pudendal somatosensory innervation is necessary for one type of female sexual stimulation, stimulation through the clitoris.

Treatment

Sildenafil is an effective treatment for erectile dysfunction in men with multiple sclerosis. Among men with MS and erectile dysfunction 89% of the patients receiving sildenafil compared with 24% of patients receiving placebo reported improved erectile function [30]. Since there are only insignificant amounts of phosphodiesterases in the female genitalia [31], one can not expect much effect from phosphodiesterase inhibitors like sildenafil in women with MS [32]. Women and men with MS usually are not hypogonadal needing substitution but estrogen substitution is recommended in postmenopausal women with MS. Hyperprolactinemia and even galactorrhea have been found in one-third of 27 MS patients [33]. In such cases treatment with bromocriptine could be tried. The use of water-soluble lotions or even baby oil can be used in cases with insufficient lubrication.

To compensate for a sensory loss in the clitoris the use of external vibration and/or more direct stimulation of the anterior vaginal wall (G-spot area) are recommended, possibly with the aid of a dildo. For treatment of dysesthesia drugs such as carbamazepine and selective serotonin reuptake inhibitors (SSRIs) could be tried.

Rehabilitation

Sexual symptoms in MS patients can be divided into three groups [34]. Primary sexual dysfunction includes those directly caused by MS lesion in certain areas of the brain and spinal cord essential for sexual functioning. Secondary sexual dysfunction relates to other physical neurological symptoms caused by the MS pathology, and tertiary refers to psychological, social, and cultural issues that interfere with sexual functioning. These distinctions are important in the rehabilitation process. In this process one must also remember that the coping mechanism is different in a disorder that is or may be progressive than in a disorder that is stationary. There is always a fear of recurrence and/or progression. A regression into the role of a handicapped person may be overwhelming. The ways to help the patient may be very different dependent upon the pre-morbid personality including the degree of sexual function before the start of the disease. Even if many MS patients are relatively young, their previous sexual experiences also play a role.

References

1. Demirkiran M, Sarica Y, Uguz S, Yerdelen D, Asian K. Multiple sclerosis patients with and without sexual dysfunction: are there any differences? *Mult Scler* 2006;**12**:209–14

2. O'Sullivan S S, Hardiman O. Detection rates of sexuál dysfunction among patients with multiple sclerosis in an out-patient setting: can this be diagnosed? *Ir Med J* 2006;**100**:304–6

3. Lundberg P O. Sexual dysfunction in female patients with multiple sclerosis. *Int Rehab Med* 1981;**3**:32–4

4. Hulter B, Lundberg P O. Sexual function in women with advanced multiple sclerosis. *J Neurol Neurosurg Psychiatry* 1995:**59**:83–6

5. Hulter B. Sexual function in women with neurological disoders. Acta Universitatis Upsaliensis: Thesis 873. Uppsala: 1999

6. Ghezzi A. Sexuality and multiple sclerosis. *Scand J Sexol* 1999;**2**:125–40

7. Lopez-Meza E, Corona-Vazquez T, Ruano-Calderon L A, Ramirez-Bermudez J. Severe impulsiveness as the primary manifestation of multiple sclerosis in a young female. *Psychiat Clin Neurosci* 2005;**59**:739–42

8. Barak Y, Achiron A, Elizur A, *et al.* Sexual dysfunction in relapsing–remitting multiple sclerosis: magnetic resonance imaging, clinical, and psychological correlates. *J Psychiatr Neurosci* 1996;**21**:255–8

9. Miró J, García-Moncó C, Leno C, Berciano J. Pelvic pain: an undescribed paroxysmal manifestation of multiple sclerosis. *Pain* 1988;**32**:73–5

10. Valleroy M, Kraft G. Sexual dysfunction in multiple sclerosis. *Arch Phys Med Rehab* 1984;**65**:125–8

11. Minderhoud J M, Leemhuis J G, Kremer K, Labon E, Smits P M L. Sexual disturbances arising from multiple sclerosis. *Acta Neurol Scand* 1984;**70**:299–306

12. Kirkeby H J, Poulsen E U, Petersen T, Dørup J. Erectile dysfunction in multiple sclerosis. *Neurology* 1988;**38**:1366–71

13. Betts C D, Jones S J, Fowler C G, Fowler C J. Erectile dysfunction in multiple sclerosis. *Brain* 1994;**117**:1303–10

14. Mattson D, Petrie M, Srivastava K, McDermott M. Multiple sclerosis: sexual dysfunction and its response to medications. *Arch Neurol* 1995;**52**:862–8

15. Ghezzi A, Malvestiti G M, Baldini S, Zaffaroni M, Zibetti A. Erectile impotence in multiple sclerosis patients. *J Neurol* 1995;**242**:123–6

16. Holstege G, Georgiadis J R, Paans A M J, *et al.* Brain activation during human male ejaculation. *J Neurosci* 2003;**23**:9185–93

17. Redoute J, Stoleru S, Gregoire M C. Brain processing of visual stimuli in human males. *Hum Brain Mapp* 2000;**11**:162–77

18. Fernández O. Mechanisms and current treatment of urogenital dysfunction in multiple sclerosis. *J Neurol* 2002;**249**:1–8

19. Ghezzi A, Zaffaroni M, Baldini S, Zibetti A. Sexual dysfunction in multiple sclerosis male patients in relation to clinical findings. *Eur J Neurol* 1996;**53**:462–6

20. Zivadinov R, Zorzon M, Bosco A, *et al.* Sexual dysfunction in multiple sclerosis. II: Correlation analysis. *Mult Scler* 1999;**5**:428–31

21. Zorzon M, Zivadinov R, Bosco A, *et al.* Sexual dysfunction in multiple sclerosis: a case-control study. I: Frequency and comparison of groups. *Mult Scler* 1999;**5**:418–27

22. Zivadinov R, Zorzon M, Locatelli L, *et al.* Sexual dysfunction in multiple sclerosis: a MRI, neurophysiological and urodynamic study. *J Neurol Sci* 2003;**210**:73–6

23. Beck K P, Warren K G, Whitman P. Urodynamic studies in female patients with multiple sclerosis. *Am J Obst Gyn* 1981;**139**:273–6

24. Hennessey A, Robertson N P, Swingler R, Compston D A. Urinary, faecal and sexual dysfunction in patients with multiple sclerosis. *J Neurol* 1999;**246**:1027–32

25. Haensch C A, Jürg J. Autonomic dysfunction in multiple sclerosis. *J Neurol* 2006;**253**(Suppl 1):1/3–1/9

26. Yang C C, Bowen J D, Kraft G H, Uchio E M, Kromm B G. Physiologic studies of male sexual dysfunction in multiple sclerosis. *Mult Scler* 2001;**7**:249–54

27. Gruenwald I, Vardi Y, Gartman I, *et al.* Sexual dysfunction in females with multiple sclerosis: quantitative sensory testing. *Mult Scler* 2007;**13**:95–105

28. Yang C C, Bowen J R, Kraft G H, Uchio E M, Kromm B G. Cortical evoked potentions of the dorsal nerve of the clitoris and female sexual dysfunction in multiple sclerosis. *J Urol* 2000;**164**:2010–13

29. Hulter B, Lundberg P O. Genital vibratory perception threshold (VPT) measurements in women with sexual dysfunction and/or sexual pain disorders. *Sexologies* 2006;**15**:S33

30. Fowler C, Miller J, Sharief M for the **Sildenafil Study Group**. Viagra (sildenafil citrate) for the treatment of erectile dysfunction in men with multiple sclerosis. *Ann Neurol* 1999;**46**:497

31. Uckert S, Ellinghaus P, Albrecht K, Jonas U, Oelke M. Expression of messenger ribonucleic acid encoding phosphodiesterase isoenzymes in human female genital tissues. *J Sex Med* 2007;**4**:1604–9

32. DasGupta R, Wiseman O J, Kanabar G, Fowler C J. Efficacy of sildenafil in the treatment of female sexual dysfunction due to multiple sclerosis. *J Urol* 2004;**171**:1189–93

33. Kira J, Harada M, Yamaguchi Y, Shida N, Goto I. Hyperprolactinemia in multiple sclerosis. *J Neurol Sci* 1991;**102**:61–6

34. Foley F W, Sanders A. Sexuality, multiple sclerosis and women. International MS Support Foundation, 2004. www.imssf.org/sex3.shtml

Bulbar problems in multiple sclerosis

Susan L. McGowan, Lucy Rodriguez, and Clare Laing

Introduction

Speech and swallowing disturbances in multiple sclerosis (MS) may be related to involvement of multiple neural systems, of which demyelination in the brainstem is one. Others include lesions in the cerebellum and demyelination in the extrapyramidal system. There is no one pattern of swallowing or speech disturbance associated with MS and the range of dysfunction is described in this chapter. Respiratory impairment in MS is also described. Although the three systems of swallowing, speech, and respiration are described separately, there is interdependence in function – they are to a large extent dependent on each other for optimum performance. The reciprocity between breathing and swallowing implies that a breakdown in one system may affect the other. The primary concern in dysphagia is airway protection; thus a comprehensive dysphagia management program will involve assessment of breath support, coordination, and airway protection when swallowing. In speech, poor breath support impacts sentence length, voice volume, and speech intelligibility.

Dysphagia

Normal swallowing function is thought to occur in four stages: oral preparatory (moving the food up to the mouth), oral (voluntarily preparing, controlling, and manipulating the bolus in the mouth), pharyngeal (the involuntary transfer of the bolus through the pharynx subsequent to a swallow trigger), and esophageal (peristalsis through the esophagus). Thus swallowing is a complex task requiring the precise orchestration of 31 pairs of smooth and skeletal muscles supplied by five cranial nerves.

Multiple sclerosis is not characterized by a single disorder of swallowing; swallow dysfunction may occur in any of the four stages. This is pertinent to individuals with MS where difficulties with oral preparation often impact on bolus volume and oral priming which in turn may overload and compound a weak pharyngeal stage. Thus managing brainstem symptoms of dysphagia in MS may involve correcting or adapting the voluntary "oral" component of swallowing which has more to do with cortical control.

Incidence of dysphagia

Dysphagia has been recognized as a clinical finding in MS since as early as 1877. Prevalence rates can be as high as 43% [1, 2] and swallowing abnormalities seem to be more frequent in individuals with MS than generally believed [3].

Pathophysiology of dysphagia

The central neural swallowing pathway is located in the medullary brainstem region. The ventromedial reticular formation (near the nucleus ambiguus – NA) and the nucleus tractus solitarii (NTS) appear to have a central role in the control of swallowing and its coordination with respiration. The NTS is the primary sensory nucleus or "architect" for the swallowing reflex. It receives afferent information directly from the facial, glossopharyngeal, and vagus cranial nerves and indirectly from the trigeminal nerve (via the trigeminal sensory nucleus in the pons). The NTS also receives input from the "swallowing cortex" (a discrete area located in the frontal lobe, anterior to the sensorimotor cortex) and instructs the NA (through the corticobulbar pathway through the internal capsule) to execute the motor swallowing

Multiple Sclerosis: Recovery of Function and Neurorehabilitation, eds. J. Kesselring, G. Comi, and A. J. Thompson.
Published by Cambridge University Press. © Cambridge University Press 2010.

Table 25.1 Swallow physiology [3, 4, 7, 8, 9, 10]

Poor oral bolus formation and transportation
Residue in valleculae
Delayed trigger
Reduced hyolaryngeal elevation, affecting upper esophageal sphincter opening
Reduced airway closure

Sources: Based on De Pauw et al. 2002 [3], Abraham and Yun 2002 [4], Herrera et al. 1990 [7], Wiesner et al. 2002 [8], Logemann 1998 [9], and Merson and Rolnick 1998 [10].

Table 25.2 Reported symptoms of dysphagia in MS [1, 3, 12, 13]

Coughing and choking during the meal
Altered feeding habit
Nasal regurgitation and excessive salivation
Sticking of the bolus
Anxiety and/or fear about swallowing

Sources: Based on Abraham et al. 1997 [1], De Pauw et al. 2002 [3], Hughes et al. 1994 [12], and Daly et al. 1962 [13].

response. The NA is the primary motor nucleus of the glossopharyngeal, vagus, and spinal accessory nerves, and it also has neural connections with the trigeminal, facial, and hypoglossal motor nuclei.

The brainstem is the "central pattern generator," in that it retains the fundamental control of coordination of sequential muscle activity of the pharynx, larynx, cricopharyngeus and of the esophageal stage of swallowing. Innervation is bilateral, thus either side of the brainstem can coordinate pharyngeal and oesophageal stages.

If demyelinization occurs in the brainstem sensori-motor pathways such as cranial nerves VII, IX, X, or XII, then oropharyngeal dysphagia may occur [4, 5]. However, cerebellar dysfunction in symptomatic patients has also been implicated which may give rise to oral stage dysphagia [1, 2]. Dysphagia has also been reported in one case due to the opercular syndrome in MS [6].

There is a growing appreciation that there are inconsistencies in the clinical characteristics of dysphagia in MS. The pattern of dysphagia in MS has only been described from one-off assessments. No data are available that track the development and change in dysphagia through the MS disease process. Table 25.1 charts swallowing physiology using instrumental swallowing assessments.

Dysphagia may develop early or late in the disease process. It is widely recognized that the frequency of dysphagia rises with increasing disability. However, there is some controversy as to whether expanded disability status scale (EDSS) scores alone facilitate identification of dysphagia on the basis of severity. Several authors have found EDSS scores did not identify dysphagic patients [4, 5] while other studies report higher EDSS scores for symptomatic patients

[1, 11]. Calcagno et al. [5] reported that patients with ≥3 score on the brainstem functional system of EDSS showed a risk of developing dysphagia nearly three times greater as compared with other MS patients. Dysphagia is also reported in patients with minimal disability [1, 3]. Therefore, there is a need for caution in the use of EDSS scores alone to alert physicians to the possibility of dysphagia. The data, rather, show that dysphagia is not only associated with end-stage disease in MS, but may also occur in patients with minimal disability.

Symptoms of dysphagia in MS

The symptoms of dysphagia reported by individuals with MS are shown in Table 25.2, listed in order of frequency of occurrence.

The presenting symptoms of dysphagia may be one or more of the following:
- weight loss
- dehydration
- chest infections
- halitosis
- drooling of saliva.

Therefore case history taking should involve consideration of all these specific symptoms.

This is important for three main reasons.

(1) An individual who chronically aspirates is at risk of developing pneumonia, although the link between aspiration and the potential development of pneumonia is not fully understood.

(2) It is easy to miss other dysphagia symptoms if the individual does not show any symptoms of aspiration.

(3) Individuals may often not divulge dysphagia symptoms independently. Whether this is due to a perceptual problem with an underlying cognitive

or sensory base, or a reflection of weak questionnaires which lack sensitivity and specificity is as yet unknown. In addition, Abraham et al. [1] and Herrera et al. [7] described an inconsistency between self-reports and clinical instrumental findings of dysphagia. Thus individuals may deny any dysphagia symptoms, yet show patterns of dysphagia through instrumental tests.

Over the last ten years, the problems inherent in self-report by individuals with MS have become more apparent and inconsistencies in individual's self-reports are increasingly appreciated amongst dysphagia clinicians. Detection of dysphagia through physician inquiry alone is likely to lack sensitivity, and may lead to dysphagia not being recognized. This has led some authors to recommend instrumental tools as part of comprehensive evaluation.

Assessment of dysphagia

The *Multiple Sclerosis: National Clinical Guidelines for Diagnosis and Management* [14] makes the following recommendation:

> R160: Any person with MS who has difficulty swallowing for more than a few days should be assessed by a neurological rehabilitation team to review the need for:
> - Adjustments to or provision of seating that will increase ease and safety of swallowing and feeding
> - Chest physiotherapy
> - Short term use of NG tube, especially if recovery is anticipated.

Diagnostic tools

Diagnostic tools that are available through multidisciplinary collaboration comprise:
- swallowing questionnaires (SWAL-QOL [15] and M.D. Anderson Dysphagia Inventory [16])
- bedside screening assessment
- instrumental tests of videofluoroscopy (VFS) and fiberoptic endoscopic evaluation of swallowing (FEES).

Swallowing questionnaires

These may have limited value given the inconsistencies in self-reporting, but when used with caregivers, their sensitivity in highlighting dysphagia symptoms may be maximized. Indeed caregivers have an important role in assisting with identification of symptoms of dysphagia.

Bedside screening assessment

This can lack sensitivity and specificity, yet this may be improved with the additional use of the timed water swallow test [2] and with the input of interdisciplinary team members (Table 25.3). In addition, an assessment of swallowing function and feeding approach in the individual's natural environment will help to identify any impact of cognitive difficulties on feeding behavior which in turn impacts on management advice.

Instrumental tests

Videofluoroscopy (VFS) is a modified barium swallow, conducted with the individual seated and using small quantities of food and fluid consistencies. It is usually performed by a radiologist and a speech and language therapist. Results of VFS should be interpreted in the light of the clinical history as it is recognized that VFS is just a snapshot in time. It is unknown whether there are specific clinical features in MS that correlate with dysphagia identified through VFS.

Fiberoptic endoscopic evaluation of swallowing (FEES) involves the insertion of a nasendoscope which overhangs the pharynx, allowing direct visualization of the pharynx and larynx before and after the swallow. It is normally performed by an otolaryngologist and a speech and language therapist.

Both VFS and FEES provide invaluable instrumental tools, guiding not only the assessment but also the management of swallowing. During each procedure, swallow strategies and techniques can be trialed to maximize the efficiency and safety of swallowing.

Management of dysphagia
The role of the interdisciplinary team

An individual with MS requires timely access to specialist neurology and neurological rehabilitation services where the patient is located and which provide interdisciplinary assessment and management when needed [14, 17]. New dysphagia symptoms may occur as a result of relapse, further brainstem/cerebellar deterioration, or swallow decompensation due to infection, cognitive, or physical decline.

In addition to the medical professional, the interdisciplinary team (IDT) involved in dysphagia management will ideally comprise a speech and language therapist, dietitian, physiotherapist, occupational therapist, psychologist, and clinical nurse specialist

Table 25.3 Interdisciplinary team roles in dysphagia management

Speech and language therapist	Comprehensive assessment of swallow function including the impact of dysphagia upon the individual's quality of life
	Provision of information to patient and carers on general signs and symptoms of dysphagia and individually tailored information in order to support self-management
	Introduction of strategies that increase the likelihood of successful eating and drinking
	Training of carers in feeding skills when physical and/or cognitive impairments limit safe or efficient self-feeding
	Informing decisions regarding need for non-oral route feeding
	Advice on oral hygiene and saliva management
Dietitian	Assessment of nutritional status
	Provision of individualized dietary advice to prevent deterioration of nutritional status
	Advice on need for prescribable nutritional supplementation
	Involved in decision regarding timing of non-oral route feeding and provides education regarding appropriate options
Physiotherapist	Postural advice and activation of the trunk to improve head alignment for swallow and to optimize respiratory function
	Specialist seating advice to support postural alignment
	Chest physiotherapy
Occupational therapist	Posture management within feeding tasks
	Devising strategies to integrate available movement and control in the most effective and efficient manner possible during self-feeding
	Introduction of adaptive cutlery/feeding equipment
	Advice on fatigue management
Neuropsychologist	Assessment of cognition
	Information to patients, carers, and the wider interdisciplinary team (IDT) regarding cognitive difficulties such as impaired attention, judgment, or memory, that may contribute to the risk factors for aspiration and choking
	Advice on strategies to manage cognitive impairments
	Provision of advice in the context of the IDT regarding capacity issues, e.g., acceptance of non-oral route feeding
	Assessment of mood and advice on management
Clinical nurse specialist	Detection of swallowing difficulties on assessment of any person who presents with signs or symptoms of cerebellar or bulbar dysfunction such as abnormality of eye movements, ataxia or slurring of speech or ataxia, asking patients if they have difficulties with chewing, swallowing food or fluids
	Asking patients who have poor sitting posture of difficulty with transfers if they experience difficulties chewing or swallowing
	Asking any person who has experienced a chest infection if they have experienced problems swallowing
	Asking patients if they have altered diet due to swallowing problems
	Assess nutritional intake and weight
	Training of patient and family re percutaneous endoscopic gastrostomy (PEG) feeding regimes and use of equipment
	Maintenance of tissue viability and monitoring for presence of infection at PEG insertion site
	Supervision of nutritional and medication regimes acting as a link worker to expert IDT colleagues

in MS. Each professional has a specific yet complementary role within the IDT (Table 25.3). The speech and language therapist usually leads the IDT in dysphagia management and provides a comprehensive assessment of the presenting dysphagia, formulating an individually tailored management plan which takes into account the wishes of the patient and the findings and advice of the full IDT.

Rehabilitation of dysphagia

There are two aims of dysphagia intervention:

(1) Prevention of morbidity and disability through:
- reducing the risk of aspiration-related illnesses and choking
- maintaining adequate nutrition and hydration.

(2) Addressing and managing quality-of-life issues pertaining to the psycho-social effects of dysphagia including:
- anxiety/fear associated with oral intake
- embarrassment leading to avoidance of eating in public
- social isolation and low self-esteem [18, 19].

Few studies have reported upon the efficacy of swallowing rehabilitation specifically for the MS population. However, there is supporting evidence in the literature for the introduction of a variety of compensatory strategies to maximize safety of oral intake in individuals with MS [5]. These may be highly effective in reducing distressful coughing or choking and associated high levels of anxiety regarding oral intake.

Swallowing rehabilitation may include one or more of the following options.

(1) *Use of specific swallow postures* An example is the chin tuck, effective in the management of a delay in swallow reflex trigger which is a relatively common feature of dysphagia in MS. The chin tuck position aims to keep food/liquid residue in the valleculae long enough to facilitate triggering of the swallow reflex [9].

(2) *Modification of food and fluid consistencies to compensate for reduced oral-stage abilities* Foods can be modified to soft/moist or puree consistencies where there are difficulties in chewing and bolus control. Liquids can be thickened artificially to syrup or custard consistency where there are oral-stage difficulties

in liquid bolus control. However the pharyngeal stage of swallowing must be adequate to clear residue post swallow. Many people find thickened fluids unpalatable and more acceptable natural alternatives include thick milkshake drinks, smoothies, and liquidized soups.

(3) *Modification of food and fluid consistencies to compensate for fatigue* Many individuals with MS experience variable fatigue levels during the day with some reporting increasing fatigue levels during a meal time associated with the effort of eating. Eating the main meal earlier in the day when less fatigued and eating foods which require less effort to chew such as soft moist foods/uniform food consistencies can be helpful.

(4) *Specific advice from the IDT* This includes optimum posture of head and neck for swallowing, use of adaptive equipment, non-distractible environment, essential prompts, and specialist seating.

(5) *Providing medication in alternative forms* Swallowing medications in tablet form can be particularly difficult for some individuals with MS. If required and where possible, medications should be taken in suspension form. If pharmacologically appropriate, tablets can be crushed and mixed with foods/fluids.

(6) *Advice to carers* When an individual with MS is no longer able to feed themselves safely and efficiently as a result of physical or cognitive disability, and oral intake is still viable, carers will require instruction on feeding techniques including: optimum rate of feeding; bolus size; presentation of food/liquids; use of verbal prompts for safety; oral hygiene care, and management of choking.

(7) *Use of specific swallow maneuvers* Either VFS or FEES can be used to identify abnormalities in swallowing physiology and trial maneuvers [9]. One example of a maneuver is the supraglottic swallow for reduced hyolaryngeal elevation and/or reduced airway closure. The supraglottic swallow aims to recoordinate breathing and swallowing and increase tidal volume at the time of the swallow. The usefulness of any swallow maneuver is dictated by cognitive ability, in particular self-monitoring regarding the initiation and sequencing of events, and fatigue. Ongoing supervision with standby prompting is frequently

required for individuals who have a significant cognitive disability.

(8) *Resistance/strength training exercises* Although there have been no studies yet that evaluate the use of tongue muscle strengthening exercises in MS, change in swallowing efficiency in stroke patients with tongue exercises has been found [20]. The timing of introducing these exercises is important to consider – a greater effect may be expected in the remitting stage of MS. Other strength training exercises such as the Shaker exercise [21], shown to improve the strength of the suprahyoid muscles and increase upper esophageal sphincter opening in healthy older adults, have been advocated for use in MS [22]. The Shaker exercise requires intensive repetition of a head flexion movement. This may trigger Lhermitte's sign in some individuals with MS. The prevalence of clinical fatigue as a common and disabling symptom in MS may mitigate against the use of specific strengthening exercises at required levels of intensity in some individuals. This would be a valuable area for future clinical research.

(9) *Use of instrumental tools for treatment* The tools of surface electromyographic (sEMG) biofeedback and transcutaneous electrical stimulation are under investigation in general patient groups. To date, there are no studies evaluating their use in the MS population.

Non-oral route feeding

The introduction of tube feeding should take full account of the perspective of the individual with MS and their family [14]. Temporary nasogastric (NG) tube feeding is recommended in the management of acute-onset dysphagia associated with a relapse or infection. A percutaneous endoscopic gastrostomy (PEG) tube should be considered if any of the following occur: recurrent chest infections; inadequate food and/or liquid intake; prolonged or distressing feeding; NG tube *in situ* for over 1 month [14]. In individuals with MS with increased risk of complications during PEG insertion due to a reduced respiratory reserve, a radiologically inserted gastrostomy that does not require sedation should be considered [22].

Hydration and/or nutrition via NG (in the acute management) or PEG tube can be used to supplement suboptimal oral intake. Quality of life can also be enhanced by enabling enjoyment of small amounts of recommended consistencies orally, whilst ensuring optimum nutrition and hydration is maintained via the non-oral route. Tube feeding can improve nutritional status, reduce risk of aspiration pneumonia associated with oral intake, and minimize the risk of skin breakdown and fatigue associated with malnutrition [23]. Specific attention should be paid to maintaining optimal oral hygiene if individuals are nil by mouth.

Dysarthria

Incidence of dysarthria

The incidence of dysarthria in MS is reported to be between 41% [24] and 51% [25]. Figures from different studies vary widely. This may be due to the severity and stage of the illness in the study group or the sensitivity of the assessments used.

Hartelius *et al.* [25] found that neurological examination significantly underestimated the incidence of dysarthria, identifying only 20% of the 51% affected.

Dysarthria in MS is generally associated with widespread neurological involvement. Moderate or severe speech disorders do not occur in isolation, but tend to coexist with physical and cognitive symptoms [26]. There is a positive correlation between the degree of speech deviation and severity of neurological impairment. Hartelius and Lillvik [27] found that 75% of individuals with moderate or severe dysarthria have progressive MS and the severity of speech disturbance is related to the number of years of progression of the disease. However, no significant correlation has been shown between the degree of speech deficit and the individual's age or time since diagnosis [26].

Presence of severe disease is not always associated with speech changes.
Conversely, when speech problems are moderate or severe, the disease is likely to be disabling. [26]

Features of dysarthria

Charcot included speech disorder in his description of MS in 1877 [28]. He described prolonged phonation of words produced in a measured, slow, and slurred manner as if the individual was suffering from "incipient intoxication." These collective speech features, referred to as scanning speech, were attributed to cerebellar disturbance.

Table 25.4 The most consistent deviant speech features of MS

Harshness

Imprecise articulation/consonant production

Impaired emphasis/stress patterns

Impaired respiratory support

Impaired pitch variation/control

The original belief that dysarthria in MS is exclusively a manifestation of cerebellar involvement has since been shown to be inaccurate. Speech disturbance in MS may be related to involvement of multiple neural systems, namely lesions in the cerebellum, or demyelination in the extrapyramidal system and the brainstem. In the largest scale study of dysarthria in MS, featuring 168 individuals, Darley *et al.* described perceptual speech features consistent with both ataxic and spastic dysarthria [24]. The study described deviations in all components of speech production: respiration, phonation, resonance, and prosody (stress patterning, intonation, and rate).

Two further studies of speech in MS demonstrated the predominance of mixed ataxic–spastic dysarthria in this population [24, 25, 29]. Table 25.4 lists the five deviant speech features common to all three cohorts.

Hartelius *et al.* [25] and Darley *et al.* [24] suggest that distorted consonant articulation is the perceptual quality most influential in producing impressions of speech deviation and decreased intelligibility. Tongue function has also been found to be more severely affected than lip function in individuals with MS. A correlation between tongue function and disease progression has also been demonstrated [27].

Yorkston *et al.* [30, 31] suggested the following classification of the stages of speech disturbance in MS.

Mild dysarthria

Individuals typically show changes in vocal quality that do not interfere with normal speaking rate or intelligibility. The vocal symptoms often relate to harsh voice quality or phonatory instability. These vocal changes rarely limit the ability to function in speaking situations. Individuals with mild dysarthria may complain that symptoms worsen with fatigue.

Moderate dysarthria

This is typically associated with the signs of the vocal changes seen with mild dysarthria, together with prosodic changes such as slow speaking rate and impaired stress. Articulatory imprecision may become evident at this stage.

Severe dysarthria

Individuals at this stage commonly experience involvement of multiple neural systems. Speech symptoms often include impaired respiratory support due to respiratory muscle weakness and hyperfunctional laryngeal behavior due to spasticity. Prosodic disturbance due to ataxia may be reflected in impaired stress, emphasis, and pitch variation. Articulatory disturbance is usually characterized by weakness, poor coordination, and reduced rate.

Assessment of dysarthria

As with all neurological examinations of motor speech disorders, the assessment of speech in MS should include the history of the problem together with a physical and motor speech examination. A cranial nerve examination must be carried out to establish the presence of sensory or motor impairment involving oral musculature. Other assessments include the following.

A standardized clinical dysarthria assessment

One example is the Frenchay Dysarthria Assessment [32]. The administration of a standardized clinical dysarthria assessment is a key feature of the initial evaluation. These assessments are composed of subtests that measure performance of respiration, phonation, oral motor function, articulation, prosody, and intelligibility. The assessment data add to the information available from the neurological examination. The results may also be used to monitor clinical and subclinical disease progression. Clinical dysarthria assessment is highly sensitive to capturing subtle signs of neuromuscular dysfunction. Using formal assessment, Hartelius *et al.* [25] found evidence of pathological speech signs in 11% of a sample of individuals with MS who showed no clinical signs of dysarthria. Formal dysarthria assessment also provides a useful method of differential diagnosis and helps the clinician to classify the type of dysarthria.

Perceptual assessment

In the perceptual assessment of motor speech disturbance many clinicians adopt the terminology and classification system of perceptual rating dimensions produced by Darley *et al.* in 1975 [33]. These rating scales provide descriptors of specific deviant speech features and classic descriptions of what a particular speech disorder sounds like.

Perceptual analysis is usually based on evaluation of taped continuous speech samples. Reductions in overall intelligibility and prosodic disturbance imprecision of articulation are more evident in continuous speech than in repeated or read single words or sentences. Therefore, clinical dysarthria tests and perceptual assessments should be used complementarily.

Quantifiable tests of speech intelligibility

These tests form an important part of the assessment procedure. The Assessment of Intelligibility of Dysarthric Speech defines single word and sentence intelligibility, rate, and the communication efficiency of speech [34]. These quantitative data may be used to monitor the progression of speech impairment and the effectiveness of treatment.

Acoustic analysis

This involves the use of a range of specialized physiological instruments to assess the functioning of the major components of speech production. It may be used to describe articulatory timing and vocal characteristics of MS. Acoustic analysis of speech features in MS may be used to assess the timing of syllables and other speech events and the distribution of energy across different speech sounds. These assessments provide very specific information about articulation and the coordination of respiration and phonation in speech.

Management of dysarthria: therapy/intervention

Early intervention

The presence of preclinical signs of tongue dysfunction, characterized as decreased rate and endurance, has been shown in a significant proportion of people with MS [27, 35, 36]. This feature may be a precursor to the development of clinical dysarthria. What is less clear, however, is the number of individuals with preclinical signs who will later progress to clinical motor speech disturbance. Hartelius argues that tongue dysfunction should be a target for early intervention in an attempt to maintain motor speech function [27].

Early intervention may provide essential time to meet the challenges of dysarthria before the progression of concomitant physical, sensory, and cognitive difficulties. Input at an early stage may prove more successful in maintaining function than intervention provided later when impairment and functional limitations are more severe: "Early intervention may circumvent barriers such as cognitive decline and fatigue that hinder new learning" [26].

Early involvement in the management of speech disorders in MS is also supported by studies which suggest that mild communication problems in MS may result in important changes in communicative participation [30, 37].

Intervention aimed at the remediation of prosodic disturbance has also been shown to be more effective in individuals with early stage MS compared with those who have later stage disease [38].

The over-rehabilitation of individuals with MS – i.e., therapy at the earliest sign of speech disorder – has been suggested by teaching strategies that can be used during periods of relapse [39].

The challenges and aims of the treatment of dysarthria in MS are well recognized. In planning treatment the impact of fatigue on the individual's ability to participate in therapy needs to be considered. Intensive input is not always appropriate for this group of patients. Intervention is determined by the general characteristics and severity of the dysarthria.

Treatment of articulatory disturbance

Articulation is frequently a focus of therapy because of the impact that imprecise consonant production has on overall intelligibility. The aim of therapy is to establish more precise and effective articulation. Individuals may be provided with guidance on the control, coordination, and direction of articulators in the production of specific sounds in order to normalize articulatory targets. Speech tasks are usually carried out in a graded manner and are made more difficult by altering the complexity of the sound structure of words and the length of utterance. Individuals may be encouraged to compensate by adopting alternative articulatory postures or by exaggerating articulatory movements.

Treatment of prosodic disturbance

Impaired stress may be addressed using contrastive stress drills where the individual is taught how to alter stress position in words. A key aim is to develop the ability to self-monitor intonation. Where increased rate is an issue, individuals may be taught rate reduction strategies such as developing improved phrasing and breath grouping. The use of alphabet boards may be implemented where the speaker points to the first letter of each word as it is spoken thus slowing rate. This is also helpful in cueing the listener to what is being said.

Treatment of respiratory impairment

Impaired expiration can impact on the ability to generate adequate pressure for speech production. In these circumstances it is helpful to establish an adequate and consistent subglottal air pressure in order to achieve adequate loudness and controlled exhalation during speech. Establishing respiratory support may be achieved by using tasks to generate consistent air pressure, which may include breathing and sustained phonation exercises. An individual's ability to self-monitor respiration during speech is key to the success of these approaches, and they may be taught to recognize when the respiratory supply is diminishing.

Treatment of phonatory disorders

Disorders of vocal fold adduction may occur in MS resulting in phonatory instability or incoordination. Hyperadduction results in a strained–strangled voice quality and harshness. Hypoadduction produces a reduced volume with a breathy, hoarse quality. These disorders may be addressed through the implementation of different voice exercises. Improved vocal fold adduction may also be achieved using a program known as the Lee Silverman Voice Treatment (LSVT®)[40]. This has been successfully employed on a large scale with patients with Parkinson's disease. The program uses high-effort vocal exercises to maximize phonatory and respiratory function. This technique has been shown to be of particular value to individuals with MS whose main symptom is reduced volume, and may also improve their phonatory stability [41]. An enhancement in the coordination of phonation and respiration can be attained by carrying out respiratory and voice onset exercises.

Functional communication techniques

Individuals may be encouraged to make efficient verbal repairs by being provided with feedback to alter particular speech dimensions. Linguistic modifications such as reducing sentence complexity or length may help. The speaker may be advised to identify explicitly the topic of conversation using key words to help cue in the listener. The role of the communication partner is valuable. They may be instructed to notify the speaker of their level of comprehension by repeating each word or sentence as it is said or to seek clarification as soon as they have failed to understand. Suggestions to modify particular environments by reducing noise levels and altering poorly lit surroundings may also be appropriate.

Augmentative and alternative communication systems

As MS progresses, augmentative and alternative communication (AAC) systems can be introduced to compensate for communication loss. Early assessment and implementation of AAC systems is important in order that the individual may be involved in identifying their communication needs [42]. Such AAC systems range from low-technology strategies such as communication charts or books to high-technology communication devices such as voice-output communication aids. These can be adjusted to meet the motor abilities of the individual. The effective use and acceptance of AAC systems is reliant upon support from communication partners. These individuals, just as for those using AAC, require instruction and support.

Respiratory function

Respiratory muscle weakness is common in individuals with MS, although the incidence is uncertain. It can occur at any stage of the disease process [43]. Respiratory complications are recognized as the major cause of morbidity and mortality in individuals with advanced MS.

The central pattern generator for respiration is located in the brainstem (ventral and lateral medulla) and produces rhythmic synaptic drive for motoneurons controlling the phrenic, intercostal, and abdominal muscles of respiration.

Pulmonary impairments may be due to a number of factors: bulbar involvement affecting laryngeal and pharyngeal function [44], cerebellar involvement [45], and/or tonal and strength changes in muscles involved in respiration [46]. In a series of 19 patients, Howard et al. reported that bulbar dysfunction increased the risk of aspiration and lower respiratory tract infection [44].

Acute respiratory failure reflecting extensive bulbar disease manifests in altered ventilatory patterns, acute loss of voluntary control of respiration, and apnea. Ventilatory support may be required. In advanced stages of the disease, atelectasis, aspiration, and pneumonia may be seen.

Individuals may describe difficulty coughing or removing airway secretions or dyspnea but there is a low overall rate of symptom reporting. Cognitive impairment may contribute to this low rate.

Specific tests of respiratory muscle strength are rarely performed in the MS population. Pulmonary function testing is an insensitive indicator of respiratory muscle weakness. Thus clinical assessment is a better predictor of respiratory muscle weakness than spirometry [46]. The effect of respiratory muscle training remains to be determined [47, 48].

Conclusion

The MS population is a varied group which requires individually tailored treatment approaches for bulbar problems. Further research is needed in specific treatment techniques applied to individuals with MS. An example is LSVT® – its use and efficacy in treatment of voice, speech intelligibility, and dysphagia in idiopathic Parkinson's disease is documented, although its effects in MS remain unknown [49]. There remains a wide variety of treatment interventions available, which, applied carefully to the individual within an interdisciplinary context and recognizing the reciprocity between the speech, respiratory, and swallowing systems, should result in functional gains and impact on quality of life.

References

1. Abraham S, Scheinberg L C, Smith C R, LaRocca N G. Neurologic impairment and disability status in outpatients with multiple sclerosis reporting dysphagia symptomatology. *J Neuro Rehab* 1997;**11**:7–13

2. Thomas F J, Wiles C M. Dysphagia and nutritional status in multiple sclerosis. *J Neurol* 1999;**246**:677–82

3. De Pauw A, Dejaeger E, D'hooghe B, Carton H. Dysphagia in multiple sclerosis. *Clin Neurol Neurosurg* 2002;**104**:345–51

4. Abraham S S, Yun P T. Laryngopharyngeal dysmotility in multiple sclerosis. *Dysphagia* 2002;**16**:69–73

5. Calcagno P, Ruoppolo G, Grasso M G, De Vincentiis M, Paolucci S. Dysphagia in multiple sclerosis: prevalence and prognostic factors. *Acta Neurol Scand* 2002;**105**:40–3

6. Pender M P, Ferguson S M. Dysarthria and dysphagia due to the opercular syndrome in multiple sclerosis. *Mult Scler* 2007;**13**:817–19

7. Herrera W, Zeligman B E, Gruber J, *et al.* Dysphagia in multiple sclerosis: clinical and videofluoroscopic correlations. *J Neuro Rehab* 1990;**4**:1–8

8. Wiesner W, Wetzel S G, Kappos L, *et al.* Swallowing abnormalities in multiple sclerosis: correlation between videofluoroscopy and subjective symptoms. *Eur Radiol* 2002;**12**:789–92

9. Logemann J A. Evaluation and treatment of swallowing disorders. 2nd ed. Austin, TX: Pro-ed, 1998

10. Merson R A, Rolnick M I. Speech-language pathology and dysphagia in multiple sclerosis. *Phys Med Rehab Clin N Am* 1998;**9**:631–41

11. Thomas F J, Hughes T A T, Wiles C M. Swallowing problems and nutritional status in multiple sclerosis. *Eur J Neurol* 1996;**3**(Suppl 2):2

12. Hughes J C, Enderby P M, Langton Hewer R. Dysphagia and multiple sclerois: a study and discussion of its nature and impact. *Clin Rehab* 1994;**8**:18–26

13. Daly D D, Code C F, Andersen H A. Disturbances of swallowing and esophageal motility in patients with multiple sclerosis. *Neurology* 1962;**12**:250–6

14. National Collaborating Centre for Chronic Conditions. Multiple sclerosis: national clinical guideline for diagnosis and management in primary and secondary care. London: National Institute for Clinical Excellence, 2004

15. McHorney C, Robbins J, Lomax K, *et al.* The SWAL-QOL and SWAL_CARE outcomes tool for oropharyngeal dysphagia in adults. III: Documentation of reliability and validity. *Dysphagia* 2002;**17**:97–114

16. Chen A Y, Frankowski R, Bishop-Leone J. The development and validation of a dysphagia specific quality-of-life questionnaire for patients with head and neck cancer: the M. D. Anderson dysphagia inventory. *Arch Otoloaryngol Head Neck Surg* 2001;**127**:870–6

17. Department of Health. National service framework for long-term conditions. London: The Stationery Office, 2005

18. Ekberg O, Hamdy S, Woisard V, Wuttge-Hannig A, Primitivo O. Social and psychological burden of dysphagia: its impact on diagnosis and treatment. *Dysphagia* 2002;**17**:139–46

19. Threats T T. Use of the ICF in dysphagia management. *Sem Speech Lang* 2007;**28**:323–33

20. Robbins J A. Tongue strengthening: dysphagia intervention and prevention. *Proc 13th Annual Dysphagia Research Society Mtg*, Montreal, Canada, 2004

21. Shaker R, Kern M, Bardan E, *et al.* Augmentation of deglutitive upper esophageal sphincter opening in the elderly by exercise. *Am J Physiol* 1997;**272**(35): G1518–22

22. Prosiegel M, Schelling A, Wagner-Sonntag E. Dysphagia and multiple sclerosis. *Int MS J* 2004;**11**:22–31

23. Payne A. Nutrition and diet in the clinical management of multiple sclerosis. *J Hum Nutr Dietet* 2001;**14**:349–57

24. Darley F L, Brown J R, Goldstein N P. Dysarthria in multiple sclerosis. *J Speech Hear Res* 1972;**15**:229–45

25. Hartelius L, Runmarker B, Andersen O, Nord L. Prevalence and characteristics of dysarthria in a multiple sclerosis incidence cohort: relation to neurological data. *Folia Phoniatr Logop* 2000;**52**:160–77

26. Yorkston K M, Klasner E R, Bowen J, *et al.* Characteristics of multiple sclerosis as a function of the severity of speech disorders. *J Med Speech-Lang Pathol* 2003;**11**:73–84

27. Hartelius L, Lillvik M. Lip and tongue function differently affected in individuals with multiple sclerosis. *Folia Phoniatr Logop* 2003;**55**:1–9

28. Charcot J M. Lectures on the diseases of the nervous system. London: New Sydenham Society, 1877

29. Fitzgerald F J, Murdoch B E, Chenery H J. Multiple sclerosis: associated speech and language disorders. *Austr J Hum Commun Disord* 1987;**15**:15–33

30. Yorkston K M, Miller R M, Strand E A. Management of speech and swallowing in degenerative disease. Austin, TX: Pro-ed, 1995

31. Yorkston K M, Beukelman D R, Strand E A, Bell K R. Management of motor speech disorders in children and adults. Austin, TX: Pro-ed, 1999

32. Enderby P M. Frenchay dysarthria assessment. San Diego, CA: College Hill Press, 1983

33. Darley F L, Aronson A E, Brown J R. Motor speech disorders. Philadelphia, PA: WB Saunders, 1975

34. Yorkston K M, Beukelman D R. Assessment of intelligibility of dysarthric speech. Austin, TX: Pro-ed, 1981

35. Murdoch B E, Spencer T J, Theodoros D G, Thompson E C. Lip and tongue function in multiple sclerosis. *Motor Control* 1998;**2**:148–60

36. Murdoch B E, Theodoros D G. Speech and language disorders in multiple sclerosis. London: Whurr Publishers, 2000

37. Yorkston K M, Klasner E R, Swanson K M. Communication in context: a qualitative study of the experiences of individuals with multiple sclerosis. *Am J Speech Lang Pathol* 2001;**10**:126–37

38. Hartelius L, Wising C, Nord L. Speech modification in dysarthria associated with multiple sclerosis: an intervention based on vocal efficiency, contrastive stress and verbal repair strategies. *J Med Speech Lang Pathol* 1997;**5**:113–39

39. Kraft G H. Rehabilitation principles for patients with multiple sclerosis. *J Spinal Cord Med* 1998;**21**:117–20

40. Ramig L, Pawlas A, Countryman S. The Lee Silverman Voice Treatment (LSVT): a practical guide to treating the voice and speech disorders in Parkinson's disease. Iowa City, IA: National Center for Voice and Speech, and LSVT Foundation, 1995

41. Sapir S, Pawlas A A, Ramig L O, *et al.* Effects of intensive phonatory-respiratory treatment (LSVT) on voice in two individuals with multiple sclerosis. *J Med Speech Lang Pathol* 2001;**9**:141–51

42. Porter P B. Intervention in end-stage of multiple sclerosis: a case study. *Augment Altern Commun* 1989;**5**:125–7

43. Gosselink R, Kovacs L, Decramer M. Respiratory muscle involvement in multiple sclerosis. *Eur Respir J* 1999;**13**:449–54

44. Howard R S, Wiles C M, Hirsch N P, *et al.* Respiratory involvement in multiple sclerosis. *Brain* 1992;**115**:479–94

45. Grasso M G, Lubich S, Guidi L, Rinnenburger D, Paolucci S. Cerebellar deficit and respiratory impairment: a strong association in multiple sclerosis? *Acta Neurol Scand* 2000;**101**:98–103

46. Smeltzer S C, Skurnick J H, Troiano R. Respiratory function in multiple sclerosis: utility of clinical assessment of respiratory muscle function. *Chest* 1992;**101**:470–84

47. Koseoglu B F, Gokkaya N K O, Ergun U, Inan L, Yesiltepe E. Cardiopulmonary and metabolic functions, aerobic capacity, fatigue and quality of life in patients with multiple sclerosis. *Acta Neurol Scand* 2006;**114**:261–7

48. Fry D K, Pfalzer L A, Chokshi A R, Wagner M T, Jackson E S. Randomized control trial of effects of a 10-week inspiratory muscle training program on measures of pulmonary function in persons with multiple sclerosis. *J Neurol Phys Ther* 2007;**31**:162–72

49. El Sharkawi A, Ramig L, Logemann J A, *et al.* Swallowing and voice effects of Lee Silverman Voice Treatment (LSVT®): a pilot study. *J Neurol Neurosurg Psychiatry* 2002;**72**:31–6

Chapter 26

Back home

Carlo Pozzilli and Emanuela Onesti

Background

Multiple sclerosis (MS) is associated with various symptoms and functional deficits resulting in a range of progressive impairments and handicap. Symptoms that contribute to loss of independence and restrictions in social activities produce continuing decline in quality of life. Management of MS requires a multidisciplinary approach including drug therapy, psychological counseling, and physiotherapy.

Neurorehabilitation has been shown to alleviate the burden of MS symptoms by improving self-performance and independence. Even though rehabilitation has no direct influence on disease progression, this kind of intervention recovers personal ability to participate in social activities, thereby improving quality of life. These findings suggest that quality of life is determined by disability and handicap more than by functional deficits and disease progression. Treatment should be adapted depending on: the individual patient's needs, the demands of their immediate environment, the type and degree of disability, and treatment goals. Improvement persists frequently for several months beyond the treatment period, mostly as a result of reconditioning, adaptation, and use of medical and social support at home.

Even though in recent years much progress has been made in MS therapeutic research, a concomitant advance in supporting of patients in their daily routine and in improving their assistance is not so apparent [1]. In fact, if the primary aim of pharmacological treatment of MS is the prevention of clinical relapses and the reduction of progression of the disease, emphasis on the improvement of the patient's quality of life in terms of maintaining his/her job and social activities is required. New and more specific guidelines about the different treatments in relation to the different phases of the disease and about the clinical follow-up of MS patients are also needed.

Patients in some countries (especially the UK) are not managed only in hospitals [2]. There is evidence that the majority of patients with progressive MS need major long-term support in their home or in the community rather than hospital care. Specialized care at home has had variable success as an alternative way of providing organized multidisciplinary care for various diseases [3, 4]. Multiple sclerosis represents a high economic burden, with indirect costs greatly exceeding direct costs [5], and for this reason if for no other, better understanding of the clinical effectiveness and costs of supplementary home assistance and home exercise rehabilitative programs is needed.

Overview of rehabilitation in multiple sclerosis

Physical rehabilitation is commonly administered to MS patients, but little attention has been given to the development of effective and different rehabilitation strategies for these patients [6].

Some publications have described the role of neurorehabilitation in MS [7–11]. More recently controlled studies have demonstrated the efficacy of rehabilitation in disability and quality of life [12, 13]. Other studies have shown that rehabilitation can also improve the fitness of MS patients [14] and reduce their fatiguability [14, 15]. Some studies were made with an inpatient rehabilitation program [12, 13, 16, 17], others were carried out with an outpatient rehabilitation program [15, 18].

Evidence on the advantage of one method of organization of care over others is inconclusive, and direct comparisons of different methods of organized

Multiple Sclerosis: Recovery of Function and Neurorehabilitation, eds. J. Kesselring, G. Comi, and A.J. Thompson.
Published by Cambridge University Press. © Cambridge University Press 2010.

MS care to identify the best strategy for managing MS patients are still lacking. The multiplicity of MS symptoms and the way in which they interact creates a complex model of disability that requires support from a whole medical team with a high level of experience in this specific medical area, and collaboration with social services. In patients with a chronic illness, suffering may result not only from their physical limitations, but also from the psycho-social consequences of having a chronic condition. Moreover, for the management of MS patients, the design of specific rehabilitative projects for the different phases of the disease is needed: in the first phase of disease, counseling and educational programs about the symptoms management and the prevention of possible secondary damage (retraction, postural habit); in the intermediate phases, specifying personal programs according to the clinical and functional circumstances; in the advanced phases, planning the prevention and reduction of secondary damage, maintaining of vertical and sitting positions, improving the nursing and management of the patient by the caregiver.

The choice of setting for the rehabilitative project can vary: it might be in a day hospital, in a department of intensive rehabilitation, in an outpatients' department, or in the patient's home. Among the advantages of home rehabilitation are the involvement of family, the opportunity to treat the most serious patients, compatibility with work commitments of caregivers, and access to patients who are unable to come out of their home. On the other hand, the disadvantages are the difficulty of organizing treatment especially in uncomfortable locations, the difficulty of bringing the multidisciplinary team to the home, the impossibility of using specific instrumental equipment, and the lack of socialization for the patient.

Moreover, apart from the personal suffering, the financial consequences for the patients with MS and their family are enormous, as is the economic burden for society. Cost areas consist of expensive medical treatments, lost earnings for both patients and caregivers, and the provision of social services [19, 20]. Patients with MS have often complex needs that require an input from a wide range of community services. Despite a shift of emphasis in recent years from hospital to community care, many people with moderate or severe disease still fail to receive adequate assistance. It is still common that the burden of care falls on the family and unpaid carers [21]. Medical and therapeutic measures capable of promoting health and independence, and preventing medical complications, are often not put into practice [12, 13, 18], and the urgent need for a review of community services in MS has been highlighted [1, 22].

The organization of MS centers

During the last 20 years several hospitals and universities have given particular attention to MS, and specific MS centers have been created; they became structures of reference for patients both for diagnosis and for treatment. The welfare model for MS replaces the idea of "occasional" assistance such as that offered by a normal outpatient department, offering instead a model of a complete *taking care of* the patient. Patients with MS and their caregivers have the opportunity to access and enjoy information, facilities, health services, and provision of contacts with the relevant professional figures. The addition of a home care package in this welfare program, and a multidisciplinary approach with integration of the various medical disciplines and health competences (such as a specialized nurse, psychologist, urologist, ophthalmologist, etc.) could be very useful. The MS patient is at the center of this welfare intervention. Adequate information permits patients to evaluate carefully their own choices, to plan the future, and to adhere better to treatments; all this is intended to give the patients a measure of control of their life as a whole.

Initial and intermediate phases

The neurologist, the nurse, the physiotherapist, the psychologist, and the other expert figures in the MS center have to establish a relation of trust with the patient so as to discuss his/her needs frankly and realistically. The patient has to be sustained in his/her relationships with their partner and with relatives, above all when difficult interpersonal situations arise, which are often correlated with a superficial or poor knowledge of the disease. The cooperation of patients is also important when they start a preventive treatment, as such treatments are often associated with some adverse events that could compromise their continuation. A study has established that about 44% of MS outpatients have poor compliance, stopping preventive therapy during the first 3 years of treatment [23]. A similar percentage was also found in a more recent study on a cohort of relapsing–remitting MS [24], but in several multicenter studies of a similar duration, the percentage of non-compliant patients was usually about 10%. The reason for this discrepancy is that often patients in a protocol study receive the best attention. The nurse has the specific task of guiding the patient in the management of therapies, assisting the neurologist in the control of adverse events, and thus improving the compliance with the treatment. Moreover, other strategies aimed at improving the quality of life of MS patients are a better level of physical activity, a good diet, and psychological support [25]. Promotion of fitness in MS patients can avoid muscle atrophy, fatigue, depression, and circulatory problems. A study has shown that aerobic training improves physical and psychic well-being in patients with MS [18], and more recently yoga has been found useful for the same purpose [26]. It is important to achieve a low-fat diet and with plenty of water, so as to avoid the risk of obesity and to prevent urinary infections. A program aimed at promoting a good state of health does not leave out the psycho-social aspect in relation to adaptation at the disease. For the patient to have contact with "healthy" subjects and constant support from family and friends leads to better adjustment to the disease [27]. Despite the possible worsening of the disease, if patient learns to face it in a positive way, quality of life can be maintained.

Advanced phase

The approach to the patient in the advanced phase of disease is necessarily multidisciplinary, and rehabilitation can lead to a reduction of the disability and an improvement in the quality of life.

Services are usually in short supply, and the patient often has to wait many months to access the rehabilitation service or to obtain a wheelchair. In this phase of the disease, for patients with more severe disability, the role of national social associations (for example, the Associazione Italiana Sclerosi Multipla [AISM] in Italy provides several centers throughout the country) is very important.

Home-based care for MS

Home-based care is a model of care for severely disabled patients who are still living at home but usually spend long periods in hospital. It is a service that provides active treatment by healthcare professionals in the patient's home for conditions that

otherwise would require acute hospital inpatient care. The establishment of alternative models of care other than hospitalization for patients with chronic disease represents an important challenge for today's healthcare systems, and home care is now recommended for various diseases such as cancer, diabetes, and neurological conditions.

Specialized care at home has achieved some success as an alternative mode of multidisciplinary care, and several observational studies have suggested that the outcome in terms of physical independence is equally good in patients treated at home compared to those receiving conventional hospital services [28]. This is supported by evidence from a large randomized controlled trial, which showed that intensive specialist home care for defined conditions attained outcomes similar to, if not better, than those realized in hospitals [3]. Another controlled trial on managing acute stroke patients at home showed that there were no differences in the hospital admission rates, functional recovery, social outcome, or carer stress between the intervention and control groups [29].

"Hospital at home" schemes have grown in importance in health services in both Europe and North America. This is partly because of rising inpatient costs, which increase the pressure on hospitals to reduce the length of stay. Several randomized controlled trials comparing "hospital at home" care with hospital inpatient care have been undertaken in elderly medical patients [30, 31], in people with terminal illness [32, 33], and in those who need follow-up care after a stroke or myocardial infarct [34, 35].

Another study compared the safety, effectiveness, tolerability, and costs of a hospital-at-home program with conventional acute hospital inpatient care [36]. Costs included hospital care, home care, community services, and personal healthcare expenses. Significantly more patients receiving care at home reported high levels of satisfaction, as did more of their relatives. Relatives of the care-at-home group reported significantly lower scores on the Carer Strain Index. However, the mean cost per patient was almost twice as much for patients treated at home ($6524) as for standard hospital care ($3525).

Tsai et al. compared the outcomes of a hospital-based home care model with those of a conventional outpatient follow-up for mentally ill patients [37]. The outcome measures used were disease maintenance behavior, psychotic symptoms, social function, service satisfaction, and costs. The cost for each patient was the sum of costs for all direct mental health services. The cost-effectiveness ratio showed that the costs of the hospital-based home care model (4.3) were lower than those of conventional outpatient follow-up (13.5) and that over a 1-year period, the hospital-based home care model was associated with improvement in mental conditions, social functional outcomes, and service satisfaction. The improved outcomes and the lower costs in the hospital-based home care program support the view that it is the most cost-effective of the two.

Costs caused by MS have been well studied in Europe in recent years [38–40]. A large study performed in France found that the mean cost per patient is estimated at €44 400 [41]. Disease-modifying therapies represented 11.5% of total costs. Costs increased from €16 000 for patients with an expanded disability status scale (EDSS) score of 1 to €76 000 for patients with an EDSS score of 8–9. The average cost of a relapse was assumed to be represented by the difference of €3500 in total costs between patients with and without a relapse during the previous 3 months. These results are strikingly similar in all aspects to those found in the other European countries.

For MS patients, home-based care should be considered as a complement to hospital care and community support. Patients suffering from chronic conditions such as MS are likely to require long-term provision of care, with fewer occurrences of "emergencies" and more requests for social support and help for caregivers.

Recently, a group of experts have outlined the principal features of a home care program, with suggestions for its realization [40, 42]. More specifically, a randomized controlled study has shown an improvement of quality of life in patients treated with a home-based care model compared to a control group treated according to a traditional scheme in the MS center of reference, without involving an increase in the healthcare costs [41, 43]. Specifically, it was a randomized controlled trial in which 201 patients participated. The patients were randomized to home (intervention) or hospital care (control) in a ratio of 2 : 1. Randomization was stratified by age and EDSS score. Patients randomized to home-based care ($n = 133$) were monitored through home visits and telephone follow-up. The home-based care multidisciplinary team included two neurologists, an urologist, a rehabilitation physician, a psychologist, a physical therapist, a nurse, a social worker, and a coordinator. This team collaborated with the patient, physician, and caregiver in designing individualized clinical care and in coordinating home services as appropriate for the individual patient, intervening directly at the patient's home when required. Instead, patients randomized to routine hospital care ($n = 68$) were followed as usual in their MS referral centers; for them, no more than a week or two were required to obtain an outpatient appointment, and hospital admission was rapid in cases of need. A brief monitoring phone call once a month was used to obtain information about the patient's medical visits and hospital admissions in the previous month.

All patients were assessed at baseline and 1 year after randomization with validated measures of physical and psychological impairment and quality of life, including EDSS, functional independence measure (FIM), mini-mental state examination (MMSE), clinical depression questionnaire (CDQ), fatigue severity scale (FSS), state trait anxiety inventory (STAI), state trait anger expression inventory (STAXI), and 36-item short form health survey questionnaire (SF-36). The economic analysis was conducted only on direct healthcare costs (cost of inpatient, outpatient, and home care services); indirect costs (lack of productivity of patients and of caregivers) and non-medical costs were not included.

Data on the follow-up assessment at 12 months were available in 188 patients (123 in the intervention group and 65 in the control group). The two groups were similar in all baseline measured variables, including functional and cognitive abilities. Many of the patients were unemployed or retired people and were in the progressive phase of the disease. No significant differences between intervention and control groups were detected for outcome measures, including EDSS, FIM, MMSE, CDQ, FSS, STAI, and STAXI. There was a trend in favor of the intervention group for changes in depression as measured by the CDQ score. A decrease in CDQ score was seen in the intervention group (-7.8%) while it was slightly increased ($+0.7\%$) in the control group ($p = 0.11$).

In respect of the SF-36 scale, an improvement in eight SF-36 subscales was observed in the intervention group, while a less consistent increase of the score was detected just in four SF-36 scales in the control group. In particular the intervention group had a significant improvement in bodily pain ($p = 0.0001$), emotional role ($p = 0.0001$), general health ($p = 0.0001$), and

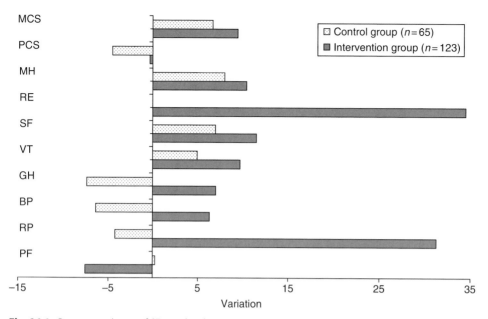

Fig. 26.1. Percentage change of SF-36 subscales in intervention (home care) and control (hospital care) groups after 1 year of follow-up. In the intervention group an improvement was observed in eight SF-36 subscales, in particular bodily pain ($p = 0.0001$), emotional role ($p = 0.0001$), general health ($p = 0.0001$), and social functioning ($p = 0.001$). In contrast, in the control group a less consistent increase in the score was detected just in four SF-36 scales. MCS, mental component score; PCS, physical component score; MH, mental health; RE, emotional role; SF, social functioning; VT, vitality; GH, general health; BP, bodily pain; RP, physical role; PF, physical functioning.

social functioning ($p = 0.001$) when compared with the control group (Fig. 26.1). In addition, scores of SF-36 dimensions were reduced to two summary scores: a physical component (PCS) and a mental component (MCS). There was a significant difference between the two groups in favor of the intervention group for both PCS ($p = 0.0001$) and MCS ($p = 0.0001$).

Moreover, at 12 months home-based care presented a saving of €822 per patient compared with the controls, mainly as result of a reduction in hospital admissions. Instead, the needs of patients receiving home-based care increased for problems requiring both medical care and nursing, social, and psychological support. This study showed that a comprehensive home-based follow-up intervention implemented by an interdisciplinary team and designed specifically for patients with MS improves some aspects of their quality of life without increasing the cost of care. The study indicated also that home-based management does not influence the most common measures of neurological disability (EDSS, FIM); anyway, physicians are usually more concerned than patients about the physical manifestations of disease, while the patients identified role limitations caused by

emotional problems as the most important determinant of their overall quality of life.

Another randomized, controlled cross-over trial was carried out involving 40 patients with MS [42]. Patients received physiotherapy either at home or in hospital. Benefit was seen in the primary outcome measure, the Rivermead Mobility Index, in those patients receiving physiotherapy, irrespective of location.

Solari et al. in an further study showed the effect of an inpatient rehabilitation program for 3 consecutive weeks consisting of twice-daily exercise periods, each 45 minutes long [13]. At the end of the period, the patients were instructed in a self-administered exercise program to perform at home. Fifty ambulatory MS patients were assigned to 3 weeks of inpatient physical rehabilitation (study treatment) or exercises performed at home (control treatment). The control treatment consisted of the home exercise program which included passive (stretching, mobilization) and active interventions. For patients with an EDSS score ≤4.5, the main goals were normalization of postural control, facilitation of a normal gait pattern, increasing the range of movement, and maximizing muscle power and endurance. For patients with an

EDSS score >4.5, instruction on the appropriate use of mobility aids and orthoses as well as refinement of compensatory strategies were also part of the program. Impairment, as assessed by the EDSS, was not influenced by the rehabilitation program in either group. At the end of the intervention the study group improved significantly in disability as assessed by the FIM motor domain, compared with controls ($p = 0.004$), and the improvement persisted at 9 weeks ($p = 0.001$). The study group also improved in overall health-related quality of life profile compared with controls; however, the difference was significant only for the mental composite score at 3 ($p = 0.008$) and 9 weeks ($p = 0.001$).

Furthermore, Patti et al. carried out a study in order to evaluate the effectiveness of a short period (6 weeks, 6 days per week) of a individualized outpatient rehabilitation program in people with progressive MS [43, 44]. One hundred and eleven patients were randomly assigned to the treatment group and 53 to the control group. Each patient in the treatment group was treated with a individualized, goal-oriented rehabilitation program following a multidisciplinary team assessment (neurologist, physiatrist, physiotherapist, speech therapist, nurse, psychologist, urologist, family members, volunteers). The treatment group was also trained in the home exercise program for a further 6 weeks. The control group was instructed in a home exercise program to be carried out for 12 weeks [45, 46]. Thirty two patients (55.1%) of the treatment group and four of the control group improved on the FIM particularly in locomotion, self-care, and transfers ($p < 0.001$). By contrast the control group showed no change. Instead, impairment, as assessed by the EDSS and functional systems, was not influenced by a short outpatient rehabilitation program.

However, Shapiro et al. [44, 47] developed a "maintenance" rehabilitation program which could be considered as "extended" home outpatient rehabilitation. This extended exposure to rehabilitation (5 hours, 1 day per week for 1 year) generated significant benefit in patients with chronic progressive MS. Patients who participated in this treatment program experienced fewer symptoms, less fatigue, and had a lower rate of decline in physical function compared with a control group [15]. A more recent study by Wiles et al. showed that a course of physiotherapy improved the mobility of MS patients who walk 5 meters with or without a mechanical aid; the authors concluded that physiotherapy improves

subjective well-being and mood without difference in efficacy between home- and hospital-based therapy [42, 45]. But they also found that home therapy was more costly.

The management of relapses could also be run at home. Robson et al. showed in 1998 that the cost of a 4-day relapse treatment regimen for an inpatient was close to US$1180 (approximately €810) [48]. The cost was lower if the treatment was administered in the MS outpatient clinic or if treatment was initiated in the clinic but completed at home. In Chataway et al.'s study, patients who had a clinically significant MS relapse within 4 weeks of onset were randomly assigned administration of a 3-day regimen of intravenous methylprednisolone either in an outpatient clinic ($n = 69$) or at home ($n = 69$) [46, 49]. The MS relapse management scale (MSRMS) was developed to measure patients' experiences of relapse management as the primary outcome. Economic costs were also evaluated. Coordination of care was significantly better in the home treatment group (median score 4.5) than in the hospital treatment group (12.1; $p = 0.024$). Administration of steroids was equally safe and effective in either location. No direct medical costs in addition to the charge for healthcare at home were reported; by comparison, direct medical costs incurred by hospital patients were significantly higher than those incurred by patients treated at home.

A more recent multi-center study investigated 807 MS patients who received intravenous methylprednisolone at home [50]. Home treatment was well tolerated, 93.8% of patients were satisfied with the cure approach, and 98% requested to receive future treatment courses at home as well. The overall cost savings of home-based treatment versus hospital-based treatment were evaluated at €1 091 482 over a period of 3 years. This kind of management could be also very useful for office-based neurologists who do not have a hospital in their immediate surrounding area.

Patients with MS represent an appropriate population for the application of home care based on social support, nursing care, rehabilitation, and the administration of drugs, as a complementary element of a hospital care program. In fact, a comprehensive home-based follow-up intervention implemented by an interdisciplinary team and designed specifically for patients with MS can improve some aspects of their quality of life with little or no increase in the cost of care. Coordinated multidisciplinary care is of greater benefit than medical care alone and may result in a reduction of number of acute hospital admissions [47, 51]. A survey of community-based services for people with MS advocates a professional healthcare service in every district and the development of a directory detailing services with appropriate expertise for all the various problems associated with the disease [48, 52]. The authors restate the need for a multidisciplinary, specialist, expert, and coordinated service, and advocate an ongoing educational program for all professional staff who come into contact with people with MS. The ideal model is extremely difficult to achieve and more studies are necessary [1].

It is safe to say that there are two basic assumptions implicit in establishing home-based healthcare: that it is preferred by patients, and that it is economically advantageous [49] [53].

Recently, a Cochrane Review was conducted comparing the effects of a hospital-at-home program with inpatient hospital care [50, 54]. Twenty-two trials were included in this update. Allocation to hospital at home resulted in a small reduction in hospital length of stay, but hospital at home increased the overall length of care. Patients assigned to hospital at home expressed greater satisfaction with care than those in hospital, while the view of their carers was varied. Although increasing interest in the potential of hospital at home services as an alternative form of patient care, this review provided insufficient objective evidence of economic benefit.

The caregiver

One of the most important features in a home-based care project is the family member who most supports the patient, the so-called *caregiver*, who receives instructions and help from the formal multidisciplinary team. The MS patient is at the center of a support net established on the one hand by the medical MS center team, and on the other by his or her own family. The concept of the burden of care is defined as the physical, psychological, financial, and social discomfort and disruption experienced by the principal caregiver of a family member.

The caregiver can experience the effects of the disease, both in terms of the emotional repercussions, and of the social (isolation) and financial problems (loss of work days) [5]. Commonly, caregivers of people with MS also exhibit less satisfaction with their quality of life in comparison to the general population.

In one study the relationship between depression in caregivers and the health status profiles of MS patients was examined [51, 55]. One-hundred and thirty-three patients were evaluated at baseline and 1 year later with measures of physical and psychological impairment and health status (SF-36). Caregivers' psychological morbidity was assessed by the profile of mood state (POMS) at the same time points. Depression in caregivers was related to physical, emotional, and health status of the patients at baseline and at 12-months follow-up. Changes in the degree of depression of caregivers were also associated with modifications in disability and health status of the patients. It suggests that the caregiver could be a legitimate and independent target for more focused welfare strategies.

Consequently, the inclusion of caregivers in the medical team must become a milestone point in the organization of a welfare service. At the same time, it is important to sustain the same caregivers with respite support because too much intensive activity could be the cause of stress and emotional tension that might have repercussions on the patient.

Development of home-care services

Another important question is whether these kinds of assistance and the possible correlated benefit can be replicated in the real world. Practice development, staff training, and the social services budget need to be developed specifically for this aim. The resulting process will not only be realistic, but it will also result in prevention of delays and better care for patients at home.

So, the objectives to be achieved in the near future can be summarized as follows.

To identify prognostic variables that will help to identify patients suitable for management at home and those requiring hospital-based care

Criteria to definite hospital admission could be: swallowing problems, double incontinence, difficulty in organizing travel outside the home, patients who live alone.

To describe the organizational aspects of different strategies of MS care

For patients with disabling disease (e.g., persistent neurological deficit affecting continence, mobility, or self-care abilities) a multidisciplinary steering group must set up a supervisory structure of the operational aspects. The team should consist of a medical director, a social services director, a head nurse, a physiotherapist, a physiatrist, an occupational therapist, some consultants (neuropsychologist, psychiatrist, continence advisor, neuro-urologist, neuro-ophthalomologist, dietician), a speech and language therapist, and a nurse. The skills of the various healthcare professionals could be called upon depending on the specific needs of the individual patient. Rehabilitation should be goal-oriented and highly focused. The individual's expectations should be appropriately managed and re-evaluated at regular intervals. Investigations and medical treatment for patients being managed at home is the responsibility of the specialist MS medical team. Appointments for all tests, including specialized blood tests and neuroimaging, should be arranged on the same day so that the patient does not have to keep returning repeatedly to the hospital. Moreover, neuro-rehabilitation for MS often requires attention to highly individualized disparate symptoms that range from fatigue and spasticity to cognitive impairments and reduced bladder and bowel control [52, 56]. In any case, the assessment from the multidisciplinary MS team should use the social services and beneficial association budget to buy personal care to maintain the patient at home.

To evaluate the acceptability of various strategies to patients and to professionals involved in care provision

The major advantage of treatment at home is its flexibility in adapting treatment, especially rehabilitation, to the patients' needs in their own environment. Some advantages in terms of a higher level of quality of life in patients managed at home can be reflected in significantly greater patient satisfaction compared with other strategies. The major areas contributing to this satisfaction are the opportunity to talk about MS and related problems with visiting professionals, a better organization of services at home, and a high level of personal contact with the specialist team. Perhaps, although carers share these views, they might tend to be less satisfied than patients with the amount of therapeutic input and contact with the specialist team. Professional acceptance of domiciliary care is more difficult to assess because of the relatively small numbers of professionals involved and their relatively slight involvement in the day-to-day care of the patient.

Conclusion and recommendations for future research

The patients' and carers' perceptions of services, their satisfaction with the care provided, and the acceptability of different forms of care need to be examined carefully. Devising a real measurement of the care process is complex, presenting the specific problem of quantifying its quality. In addition, specialist management consists of several elements working together and it may be difficult to discriminate the individual processes. Exploring the relationships between patient satisfaction, individual variables (such as the patient's characteristics), the level of residual independence, and the development of focused management strategies will be very useful.

A great expansion of future studies will be possible if health and social services are well funded. It is well known that the real-world effectiveness of proven interventions may be different from their efficacy in a study, depending on the structure of the population and the proportion of patients eligible for the chosen intervention. Hence, it is important to evaluate interventions in different clinical settings.

It is also argued that such maintenance rehabilitation does not require the intensive and expensive care of an acute inpatient hospital, but rather, specialized rehabilitation can be provided on an outpatient basis [53, 54, 57, 58]. The effectiveness of this care, especially compared with inpatient treatment, remains a central question for further research.

In conclusion, a home care system has the potential to improve the quality of discharges and to facilitate the functioning of the hospital/community interface. Essential components of this kind of management include: involving people in their own care, coordination of care, multidisciplinary teamwork, and integration of specialist expertise. Active and conscious participation of patients, a tight collaboration between families, healthcare professionals, political and social authorities, and charity associations can really contribute to the creation of a modern and qualified welfare system able to satisfy the multiple needs of patients and their families.

References

1. Freeman JA, Thompson AJ. Community services in multiple sclerosis: still a matter of chance. *J Neurol Neurosurg Psychiatry* 2000;**69**:728–32

2. Shah E, Harwood R. Acute management: admission to hospital in stroke: epidemiology, evidence and clinical practice. 2nd ed. Oxford: Oxford University Press, 1999

3. Sheppard S, Harwood D, Gray A, Vessey M, Morgan P. Randomized controlled trial comparing hospital at home with in-patient hospital care. I: Three months follow-up of health outcomes. *BMJ* 1998;**316**:1786–91

4. Sheppard S, Iliffe S. Effectiveness of hospital at home compared to inpatient care. Oxford: Cochrane Library, 1999.

5. Amato MP, Battaglia MA, Caputo D, *et al.* The costs of multiple sclerosis: a cross-sectional, multicenter cost-of-illness study in Italy. *J Neurol* 2002;**249**:152–63

6. Thompson A. Multiple sclerosis: symptomatic treatment. *J Neurol* 1996;**243**:559–65

7. DeLisa JA, Hammond MC, Mikulic M, Miller RM. Multiple sclerosis. II: Common physical disabilities and rehabilitation. *Am Fam Physician* 1985;**32**:157–63

8. DeLisa JA, Hammond MC, Mikulic M, Miller RM. Multiple sclerosis. I: Common functional problems and rehabilitation. *Am Fam Physician* 1985;**32**:127–32

9. Scheinberg L, Smith CR. Rehabilitation of patients with multiple sclerosis. *Neuro Clin* 1987;**5**:585–600

10. Erikson RP, Lie MR, Wineinger MA. Rehabilitation in multiple sclerosis. *Mayo Clin Proc* 1989;**64**:818–28

11. Svensson B, Gerdle B, Elate J. Endurance training in patients with multiple sclerosis: five case studies. *Phys Ther* 1994;**74**:1017–26

12. Freeman JA, Langdon DW, Hobart JC, Thompson AJ. The impact of inpatient rehabilitation on progressive multiple sclerosis. *Ann Neurol* 1997;**42**:136–44

13. Solari A, Filippini G, Salmaggi A, La Mantia L, Farinotti M. Physical rehabilitation has a positive effect on disability in multiple sclerosis patients. *Neurology* 1999;**52**:57–62

14. Spencer MK, Mino L, Hicks RW. Impact of aerobic training on fitness and quality of life in multiple sclerosis. *Ann Neurol* 1996;**39**:432–44

15. Di Fabio R, Soderberg J, Choi T, Hansen C, Shapiro RT. Extended outpatient rehabilitation: its influence on symptom frequency, fatigue and functional status for persons with progressive multiple sclerosis. *Arch Phys Med Rehab* 1998;**79**:141–6

16. Aisen ML, Sevilla D, Fox N. Inpatient rehabilitation for multiple sclerosis. *J Neurol Rehab* 1996;**10**:43–6

17. Kidd D, Howard RS, Losseff NA, Thompson AJ. The benefit of inpatient neurorehabilitation in multiple sclerosis. *Clin Rehab* 1995;**9**:198–203

18. Petajan JH, Gappmaier E, White AT, *et al.* Impact of aerobic training on fitness and quality of life in multiple sclerosis. *Ann Neurol* 1996;**39**:432–41

19. Whetten-Goldstein FS, Goldstein LB, Kulas ED. A comprehensive assessment of the cost of multiple sclerosis in the United States. *Mult Scler* 1998;**4**:419–25

20. Parkin D, Jacoby A, McNamee P, *et al.* Treatment of multiple sclerosis with interferon beta: an appraisal of cost-effectiveness and quality of life. *J Neurol Neurosurg Psychiatry* 2000;**68**:144–9

21. Carton H, Loos R, Pacolet J, Versieck K, Vlietinck R. Utilization and cost of professional care and assistance according to disability of patients with multiple sclerosis in Flanders (Belgium). *J Neurol Neurosurg Psychiatry* 1998;**64**:444–50

22. Stolp-Smith KA, Atkinson EJ, Campion ME, O'Brien PC, Rodriguez M. Health care utilisation in multiple sclerosis: a population based study in Olmsted Country, MN. *Neurology* 1998;**50**:1594–600

23. Onesti E, Bagnato F, Tomassini V, *et al.* Interferon beta treatment of MS in the daily clinical setting: a 3-year post-marketing study. *Neurol Sci* 2003;**24**:340–5

24. Tremlett HL, Oger J. Interrupted therapy: stopping and switching of the beta-interferons prescribed for MS. *Neurology* 2003;**61**:551–4

25. Stuifbergen AK, Roberts GJ. Health promotion practices of women with multiple sclerosis. *Arch Phys Med Rehab* 1997;**78**:(Suppl 5):3–9

26. Oken BS, Kishiyama S, Zajdel D, *et al.* Randomized controlled trial of yoga and exercise in multiple sclerosis. *Neurology* 2004;**62**:2058–64

27. Maybury CP, Brewin CR. Social relationship, knowledge and adjustment to multiple sclerosis. *J Neurol Neurosurg Psychiatry* 1984;**47**:372–3

28. Wade DT. Epidemiologically based needs assessment: stroke. London: National Health Service Management Executive, 1992.

29. Wade DT, Langton Hewer R, Skilbeck CE, Bainton D, Burns-Cox C. Controlled trial of home care service for acute stroke patients. *Lancet* 1985;**i**:323–6

30. Stuck AE, Aronow HU, Steiner A, *et al.* A trial of in-home comprehensive discharge assessment for elderly people living in the community. *N Eng J Med* 1995;**333**:1184–9

31. Naylor MD, Brooten D, Campbell R, *et al.* Comprehensive discharge planning and home follow-up of hospitalized elders: a randomized clinical trial. *JAMA* 1999;**281**:613–20

32. Cummings JE, Hughes SL, Weaver F, *et al.* Cost-effectiveness of Veterans Administration hospital-based home care: a randomized clinical trial. *Arch Intern Med* 1990;**150**:1274–80

33. Bredin M, Corner J, Krishnasamy M, *et al.* Multicentre randomized controlled trial of nursing intervention for breathlessness in patients with lung cancer. *BMJ* 1999;**318**:901–7

34. Anderson C, Rubenach S, Mhurchu CN, *et al.* Home or hospital for stroke rehabilitation? Results of a randomized controlled trial I: Health outcomes at 6 months. *Stroke* 2000;**31**:1024–31

35. Jolly K, Bradley F, Sharp S, *et al.* Randomized controlled trial of follow-up care in general practice of patients with myocardial infarction and angina: final results of the Southampton heart integrated care project (SHIP). *BMJ* 1999;**318**:706–11

36. Harris R, Ashton T, Broad J, Connolly G, Richmond D. The effectiveness, acceptability and costs of a hospital-at-home service compared with acute hospital care: a randomized controlled trial. *J Health Serv Res Policy* 2005;**10**:158–66

37. Tsai SL, Chen MB, Yin TJ. A comparison of the cost-effectiveness of hospital-based home care with that of a conventional outpatient follow-up for patients with mental illness. *J Nurs Res* 2005;**13**:165–73

38. Kobelt G, Berg J, Lindgren P, Fredrikson S, Jönsson B. Costs and quality of life of patients with multiple sclerosis in Europe. *J Neurol Neurosurg Psychiatry* 2006;**77**:918–26

39. Orlewska E, Mierzejewski P, Zaborski J, *et al.* A prospective study of the financial costs of multiple sclerosis at different stages of the disease. *Eur J Neurol* 2005;**12**:31–9

40. Sobocki P, Pugliatti M, Lauer K, Kobelt G. Estimation of the cost of MS in Europe: extrapolations from a multinational cost study. *Mult Scler* 2007;**13**:1054–64

41. Kobelt G, Texier-Richard B, Lindgren P. The long-term cost of multiple sclerosis in France and potential changes with disease-modifying interventions. *Mult Scler* 2009;**15**:741–51

42. Palmisano L, Thompson A, Miller D, *et al.* Toward the standardization of a home-based care delivery system in multiple sclerosis: report of a round table held in Bari, Italy, on April 10, 1999. *MS Management* 2000;**7**:26–32

43. Pozzilli C, Brunetti M, Amicosante AM, *et al.* Home based management in multiple sclerosis: results of a randomized controlled trial. *J Neurol Neurosurg Psychiatry* 2002;**73**:250–5

44. Patti F, Ciancio MR, Cacopardo M, *et al.* Effects of a short outpatient rehabilitation treatment on disability of multiple sclerosis patients: a randomized controlled trial. *J Neurol* 2003;**250**:861–6

45. Wiles CM, Newcombe RG, Fuller KJ, *et al.* Controlled randomized crossover trial of the effects of physiotherapy on mobility in chronic multiple sclerosis. *J Neurol Neurosurg Psychiatry* 2001;**70**:174–9

46. Patti F, Sellaroli T, Reggio A. Il trattamento multiintegrato della sclerosi multipla: progetto neuroriabilitativo e terapia farmacologia sintomatica. Naples: Scientifiche Cuzzolin, 1998.

47. Shapiro RT, Soderberg J, Hooley M, *et al.* The multiple sclerosis achievement center: a maintenance approach toward a chronic progressive form of the disease. *J Neuro Rehab* 1998;**2**:21–3

48. Robson LS, Bain C, Beck S, *et al.* Cost analysis of methylprednisolone treatment of multiple sclerosis patients. *Can J Neurol Sci* 1998;**25**:222–9

49. Chataway J, Porter B, Riazi A, *et al.* Home versus outpatient administration of intravenous steroids for multiple-sclerosis relapses: a randomized controlled trial. *Lancet Neurol* 2006;**5**:565–71

50. Créange A, Debouverie M, Jaillon-Rivière V, *et al.* Home administration of intravenous methyl-prednisolone for multiple sclerosis relapses: the experience of French multiple sclerosis networks. *Mult Scler* 2009;**15**:1085–91

51. Pozzilli C, Pisani A, Palmisano L, *et al.* Service location in multiple sclerosis: home or hospital? In: Fredrikson S, Link H, eds. *Advances in Multiple Sclerosis.* London: Martin Dunitz, 1999:173–80

52. Wade DT, Green Q. A study of services for multiple sclerosis: lessons for managing chronic disability. In: Comprehensive review of service provision in one region in the UK. London: Royal College of Physicians, 2001.

53. Gundersen L. There's no place like home: the home care alternative. *Ann Intern Med* 1999;**131**:639–40

54. Shepperd S, Iliffe S. Hospital at home versus in-patient hospital care. *Cochrane Database Syst Rev* 2005; CD000356

55. Pozzilli C, Palmisano L, Mainero C, *et al.* Relationship between emotional distress in caregivers and health status in persons with multiple sclerosis. *Mult Scler* 2004;**10**:442–6

56. Kraft GH. Rehabilitation principles for patients with multiple sclerosis. *J Spinal Cord Med* 1998;**21**:117–20

57. Barnes MP, Radermacher H. Neurological rehabilitation in the community. *J Rehab Med* 2001;**33**:244–8

58. Wade D. Community rehabilitation, or rehabilitation in the community? *Disabil Rehab* 2003;**25**:875

Index